Psychosomatics

Psychosomatics
Box 4010
500 West Putnam Avenue
Greenwich, CT 06830

PSYCHIATRIC ILLNESS IN PHYSICIANS

PSYCHIATRIC ILLNESS IN PHYSICIANS

Edited by

SAMUEL E. D. SHORTT, M.D., Ph.D.

Department of Family Medicine
Queen's University
Kingston, Ontario, Canada

CHARLES C THOMAS • PUBLISHER
Springfield • Illinois • U.S.A.

Published and Distributed Throughout the World by

CHARLES C THOMAS • PUBLISHER
2600 South First Street
Springfield, Illinois, 62717, U.S.A.

ISBN 0-398-04638-7

Library of Congress Catalog Card Number: 81-21320

With THOMAS BOOKS *careful attention is given to all details of manufacturing and design. It is the Publisher's desire to present books that are satisfactory as to their physical qualities and artistic possibilities and appropriate for their particular use.* THOMAS BOOKS *will be true to those laws of quality that assure a good name and good will.*

Printed in the United States of America
CU-RX-1

Library of Congress Cataloging in Publication Data

Main entry under title:

Psychiatric illness in physicians.

Bibliography: p.
Includes index.
1. Physicians--Mental health. I. Shortt, S. E. D. (Samuel Edward Dole), 1947- . [DNLM: 1. Mental disorders. 2. Physician impairment. 3. Physicians--Psychology. WA 305 P974]
RC451.4.P5P78 616.89'008861 81-21320
ISBN 0-398-04638-7 AACR2

CONTRIBUTORS

Bissell, Leclair, M.D., President and Chief Executive Officer, Edgehill Newport Inc., Newport, Rhode Island

Bittker, Thomas, E., M.D., Department of Neuropsychiatry, Arizona Health Plan, Phoenix, Arizona

Brighton, Jane R., A.B.

Buxton, William D., M.D., Virginia State Board of Medicine, Portsmouth, Virginia

Carroll, George J., M.D., Virginia State Board of Medicine, Portsmouth, Virginia

Coburn, David, Ph.D., Assistant Professor, Department of Behavioral Science, Faculty of Medicine, University of Toronto, Toronto, Ontario, Canada

Cramond, W. A., O.B.E.M.D., F.R.A.N.Z.C.P., F.R.C. (Psych) Director, Mental Health Services, Health Commission of New South Wales, Sydney, Australia; Honorary Professor in Clinical Psychiatry, University of Sydney

Duffy, John C., M.D., Professor, Department of Psychiatry, School of Medicine, Uniformed Services University of the Health Sciences, Bethesda, Maryland

Epstein, Lynn Chaikin, M.D., Instructor, Department of Psychiatry and Department of Pediatrics, Assistant Professor, Department of Psychology and Counseling, Johns Hopkins University School of Medicine, Baltimore, Maryland

Evans, James, L., M.D., F.A.P.A., Assistant Clinical Professor of Psychiatry, George Washington University, Washington, D.C.

Green, Robert, C., Jr., M.S., M.D., Assistant Professor of Clinical Medicine, Virginia State Board of Medicine, Portsmouth, Virginia

Hilberman, Elaine, M.D., Associate Professor, Department of Psychiatry, University of North Carolina, Chapel Hill, North Carolina

Hunter, Rosemary, M.D., Special Lecturer, Department of Psychiatry, University of North Carolina School of Medicine, Chapel Hill, North Carolina

Jones, Robert, W., M.A., Adjunct Professor of Sociology, Rutgers Center of Alcohol Studies, New Brunswick, New Jersey

Jovaisas, Al V., University of Toronto, Ontario, Canada

Klein, Henriette, M.D., Special Lecturer, Department of Psychiatry, Columbia University College of Physicians and Surgeons, New York, New York

Konanc, Judy, Ph.D., Assistant Professor, Department of Psychiatry, University of North Carolina School of Medicine, Chapel Hill, North Carolina

Krell, Robert, M.D., F.R.C.P. (C.), Associate Professor, Department of Psychiatry, University of British Columbia, Vancouver, B.C., Canada

Lin, Tsung-Yi, M.D., Professor of Psychiatry, Department of Psychiatry, University of British Columbia, Vancouver, B.C., Canada

Litin, Edward M., M.D., Formerly of the Mayo Clinic, Rochester, Minnesota

Mausner, Judith S., M.D., Professor, Department of Community and Preventive Medicine, The Medical College of Pennsylvania, Philadelphia, Pennsylvania

Mawardi, Betty Hosmer, Ph.D., Associate Professor, Division of Research in Medical Education, Case Western Reserve University School of Medicine, Cleveland, Ohio

McArthur, Charles, Ph.D., Harvard University Health Services, Cambridge, Massachusetts

Miles, James. E., M.D., D.P.M. (Lond.), F.R.C.P.(C.), Associate Professor, Department of Psychiatry, University of British Columbia, Vancouver, B.C., Canada; Head, Department of Psychiatry, Shaughnessy Hospital, Vancouver, B.C., Canada

Modlin, Herbert C., M.D., Menninger Foundation, Topeka, Kansas

Montes, Alberto, M.D.

Mumford, Emily, Ph.D., Professor of Psychiatry and Preventive Medicine, Department of Psychiatry, University of Colorado Medical Center, Denver, Colorado

Murray, Robin, M., M.D., M. Phil., M.R.C.P., M.R.C. Psych., Sub-Dean and Senior Lecturer, Institute of Psychiatry, The Bethlehem Royal Hospital and the Maudsley Hospital, London, England

Parlow, J., Division of Studies in Medical Education, Faculty of Medicine, University of Toronto, Toronto, Ontario, Canada

Perez-Reyes, Maria, M.D., Associate Professor, Department of

Psychiatry, University of North Carolina School of Medicine, Chapel Hill, North Carolina

Perlin, Seymour, M.D., Clinical Professor of Psychiatry, Department of Psychiatry, George Washington University Medical School, Washington, D.C.

Rose, Daniel K., M.D., Family Physician, Healdburg, California

Rosow, Irving, Langley Porter Neuropsychiatric Institute, San Francisco, California

Rothman, A. I., Division of Studies in Medical Education, Faculty of Medicine, University of Toronto, Toronto, Ontario, Canada

Sanders, Shirley, Ph.D., Assistant Professor, Department of Psychiatry, University of North Carolina School of Medicine, Chapel Hill, North Carolina

Scagnelli, Joan, Ph.D., Assistant Professor, Department of Psychiatry, University of North Carolina School of Medicine, Chapel Hill, North Carolina

Shaffer, John, W., Ph.D., Associate Professor, Department of Psychiatry and Behavioral Science, The Johns Hopkins University School of Medicine, Baltimore, Maryland

Shortt, S.E.D., Ph.D., M.D., C.C.F.P., Associate Professor, Department of Family Medicine, Queen's University, Kingston, Ontario, Canada

Sobowale, Nancy Corbin, A.B., Harvard University Health Services, Cambridge, Massachusetts

Steppacher, Robert C., M.D., Associate Professor, Department of Psychiatry, The Medical College of Pennsylvania, Philadelphia, Pennsylvania

Thomas, Caroline Bedell, M.D., Professor Emeritus of Medicine, Department of Medicine, The Johns Hopkins University School of Medicine, Baltimore, Maryland

Vaillant, George E., A.B., M.D., Professor, Department of Psychiatry, Harvard Medical School, Cambridge, Massachusetts

Waring, E. M., M.D., D. Psych., F.R.C.P. (C.), F.A.B.P.N., Director of Psychiatric Education; Associate Professor, Department of Psychiatry; Assistant Dean — Continuing Medical Education, University of Western Ontario, London, Ontario, Canada

Watterson, Donald J., M.D., Clinical Professor, Department of Psychiatry, University of British Columbia, Vancouver, B.C., Canada

PREFACE

DURING medical school and later, as a resident and practitioner, I, like many other physicians, gradually became aware of a considerable degree of psychopathology within the profession. Such an awareness, in turn, raised a host of questions: How does emotional illness present in the physician? What are the etiological factors? How is it treated? and, How may it be prevented? The articles that comprise this volume are an attempt to provide answers from the current literature. I am grateful to the many contributing authors and to the journals in which their work first appeared. For those readers who wish to explore a particular topic in greater depth, suggestions for further reading have been included.

Despite the diversity of perspectives revealed in the various articles, two common themes emerge. First, the ancient medical dictum, Physician heal thyself, if taken literally, leads to anguish and folly. It must now be replaced by a new admonition: Doctor, find professional help. One purpose of this volume is to make those in need – and their families and friends – aware that such assistance is both available and efficacious. A second theme common to most of the selections is that a preventative approach to physician impairment is essential. Doctors, it must be realized, constitute a distinct "high-risk group" and must be observed with the same vigilance that any particularly vulnerable group deserves. To encourage a realistic awareness among medical students and practitioners is the other major objective of this book.

It is a pleasure to acknowledge financial support arranged by the Dean of Medicine at Queen's University. Technical assistance was provided by the Department of Medical Photography. I have benefitted, as well, by discussions of the issues raised in this book with the residents in the Department of Family Medicine, with my colleagues Doctor Tony Johnson, Doctor Simon Ramesar, Doctor John Swift, and Peter Burbidge, and with my wife, Doctor Meri Bukowskyj.

S.E.D. Shortt

CONTENTS

PSYCHIATRIC ILLNESS IN PHYSICIANS

Introduction

Chapter 1

PSYCHIATRIC ILLNESS IN PHYSICIANS

S.E.D. SHORTT

FOR most practitioners medicine is a rewarding career, but for some it becomes a journey through despair. Indeed, psychiatric illness among physicians is serious and not uncommon. Evidence of significant psychiatric disturbance has been found in 10 percent of medical students[1] and of persons graduating in medicine from Johns Hopkins University between 1948 and 1964.[2] A survey of British Columbia physicians from 1970 to 1974 estimated the incidence of psychiatric illness at 1.27 percent per year.[3] Despite these figures, our knowledge of the topic is scant, a deficiency that may inhibit our ability to deal effectively with disturbed physicians. In an attempt to rectify the situation this chapter examines the subject, with reference to classic articles in the field and reports appearing since the publication of two important reviews.[4,5]

DRUG ABUSE

Drug addiction is an illness to which physicians are inordinately susceptible. Studies in the 1960s suggested that drug abuse was the primary diagnosis in approximately one in five cases of physicians receiving inpatient psychiatric treatment.[6-8] Compared with their social peers, physicians are twice as likely to misuse mood-altering drugs.[9]

Typically the physician becomes addicted in his or her late thirties or early forties but avoids therapy for two to three years. Meperidine hydrochloride (Demerol®) is the drug most commonly misused, though morphine and amphetamines are also misused, and alcohol is often abused as well.[10,11] Physical disease is frequently cited by the addicts as a cause of the drug abuse, in some cases justifiably[7] and in others without basis.[12] Other causes given by the addicts include overwork,[11] a family tragedy and addiction of the spouse.[10] Many appear to deny their addiction, and premature cessation of therapy is common.[9] However, perhaps three quarters

Originally published in *Canadian Medical Association Journal.* "PSYCHIATRIC ILLNESS IN PHYSICIANS," Vol. 121, 1979, 283-288 by S.E.D. Shortt.

of addicted physicians can be rehabilitated and returned to active, though supervised, practice.[10]

Traditionally the physician's ready access to drugs has been blamed for the high incidence of addiction in the profession. It is strange that a similar misuse of drugs is not well documented among dentists or pharmicists, who, for example, when they commit suicide, do not do so with drugs as often as physicians do.[13] Further, though it has been suggested that the addicted physician frequently demonstrates aspects of the "oral character," it appears that many "relatively well-adjusted physicians"[8] become dependent on drugs and that "doctors at the healthy as well as the pathological end of the continuum show a relative excess of drug use."[9] Clearly the nature of drug abuse among physicians and the characteristics of individual addicts require further study.

ALCOHOLISM

Alcoholism, like drug abuse, is not infrequent among physicians. A recent Scottish study found that male doctors were 2.5 times more likely than other men of the same social class to enter hospital because of alcoholism.[14] It is doubtful whether these figures can be explained by the medical profession's greater access to psychiatric help or by the particular frequency of alcoholism in Scotland. Physicians in England appear to enter hospital frequently for the treatment of alcoholism, though no more so than a socially matched control group,[15] and the standardized mortality for cirrhosis of the liver of the physicians is 2.5 times that of the general population.[16] Among hospitalized North American physicians alcoholism is a significant problem,[6,8,17] though it does not appear that they are treated for alcoholism[18] or perhaps abuse alcohol[9] more frequently than a comparable group.

A recent study in the United States has shed light on certain aspects of alcoholic physicians.[19] Perhaps contrary to expectation, such individuals are not necessarily the least talented of the profession; 54 percent of those studied were from the upper third of their medical classes. Abuse of other drugs was frequently present, as were the usual physical stigmata of chronic alcoholism and a high rate of suicide. Of the sample 49 percent had been arrested for impaired driving and 38 percent had been jailed. Nevertheless, 54 percent had not experienced any change in job status and many stated that their alcoholism had never resulted in injury to their patients. While few had shared their problems with peers, a surprising 78 percent had requested professional help of their own volition, and 71 percent of these had remained in treatment for two or more years. Unfortunately the tone of the study may be unduly optimistic, for the group examined consisted of "recovered" alcoholics; greater knowledge is required of the untreated and those who have relapses before definitive statements on cause and prognosis are justified.

MARITAL DISCORD

Often linked to drug abuse and alcoholism are marital and family discord, which may precipitate or result from psychiatric illness. Among British doctors hospitalized for phychiatric reasons divorce is 20 times more frequent than among nonphysician patients.[7] Similar discrepancies, though of lesser magnitude, have been noted in an American study.[18] Physician patients have been said to show little interest in their children[11] and, compared with controls, tend to remain aloof from family responsibilities and activities.[18] Such evidence of marital disharmony, moreover, is not confined to the physician who is demonstrably ill. On the contrary, a 30-year follow-up study of college students selected for physical and emotional well-being documented a high frequency of unstable marriage, sexual maladjustment and divorce among those who became physicians.[20]

Not only do physicians suffer from these problems, but also their spouses not infrequently find it necessary to seek phychiatric help. A recent Canadian study of hospitalized wives of physicians suggested that such women were typically in their late 30s, though their illness had been present for half a dozen years.[21] Most had married in their early 20s and had had two or three children. Drug and alcohol abuse were common, as were complaints of unsatisfactory sexual relations, thoughts of suicide and somatic disturbances. Depressive neuroses and personality disorders, especially hysterical or passive-aggressive, were the most common diagnoses. These findings agree with those of an earlier American study that, however, noted a higher proportion of psychotic disorders.[22] In both studies the physician husbands were described by their wives as cold, rigid and distant. Of the 70 husbands only two had received psychiatric care, and conjoint therapy was not actively sought. In both studies a frequent complaint from the patients was the lack of time spent with their husbands and the relative isolation of the physicians from family affairs. This is in marked contrast to the optimism expressed by medical students' wives, who anticipated little difficulty adjusting to this aspect of their future role.[23]

On the basis of these findings it has been suggested that the underlying marital disorder may stem from the personalities of the spouses and the nature of the medical profession. A "dependent, histrionic woman with an inordinate need for affection and nurturing"[21] is attracted to a physician whom she construes as "omnipotent, understanding, and protective."[22] Unfortunately the successful physician may well be detached, aloof and a compulsive worker — precisely the type of husband unable to gratify his wife's demands. Her depressions, addictions and threats may be attempts to assume the role of a patient in order to extract care from her physician husband.

SUICIDE

With a conscience tortured by the problem of addiction or a family life in disarray the physician frequently experiences profound depression. One result of this emotional turmoil is suicide. In Britain physicians commit suicide 1.5 times more often than other individuals of the same social class.[24] This situation in the United States has been, until recently, much less clear. Studies prior to 1970, which were largely based on incomplete records of the American Medical Association, suggested that the rate of suicide among physicians did not exceed that of the general population.[25,26] Investigations using other sources of information and indicating the opposite results were based on too few cases to warrant firm conclusions. A study of causes of death in Oregon between 1950 and 1961, for example, revealed only eight suicides by doctors,[27] and a review of all suicides in Tulsa, Oklahoma, between 1937 and 1956 noted only five such cases.[28] Recent and methodologically rigorous studies have arrived at more accurate estimations. In one study close scrutiny of American Medical Association files, validated when necessary by individual death certificates or physicians' letters, showed that the rate of suicide among physicians was 1.15 times that of the general population for males and three times for females.[29] Another study, based on a computerized review of California death certificates for a 3-year period, found that the rate of suicide among doctors of both sexes was twice that of non-physicians.[18]

Male physicians who commit suicide are usually between 45 and 65 years old, in contrast to female physicians who commit suicide, 40 percent of whom are under 40.[29] Drug ingestion is the most common method,[13] but male physicians frequently use firearms.[29] It has been suggested that certain specialists, particularly psychiatrists,[26,30] are suicide-prone, though this statement has recently been disputed.[13] Drug addiction and the depression associated with financial or practice difficulties may be implicated as causal factors.[30] However, suicide among male doctors correlates most closely with retirement from practice or divorce,[13] while among female physicians suicide appears to occur most frequently during medical training.[29,31] Suicidal ideas are common among physicians hospitalized for psychiatric reasons.[17] It is clear that prevention requires more detailed investigation into the cause of suicide among physicians.

PSYCHIATRIC CARE

Almost half the physicians who commit suicide feel that psychiatric treatment has nothing to offer them.[30] Yet many other emotionally disturbed physicians stop short of self-destruction and seek, or are compelled to seek, psychiatric care. The size of the physician psychiatric patient population is difficult to estimate; the ratio of physicians to other psychiatric patients has been reported to vary from 1:2000 at a general hospital to 1:37 at a private clinic.[32] The most informative recent study was of Scottish physicians, who were demonstrated to have twice the rate of admission to psychiatric facilities as other men of the same social class.[33] The figures proved only that Scottish physicians were more likely to receive psychiatric care; they did not establish that the rate of illness was higher among physicians than among their peers. Given, however, the reluctance with which doctors approach psychiatric treatment, it seems probable that the incidence of emotional illness among them is appreciably greater than in the general population.

Physicians are usually hospitalized in their late 40s or early 50s,[6,8,17] after approximately 16 years of practice.[7] The earliest sign of illness may be a "gradually developing chaotic everyday life."[32] Psychiatric care prior to admission is unusual.[5] Referral is rarely from a general practitioner, but more often from a physician friend of the patient,[18,33] and committal occurs in 5% to 30% of cases.[8,17,18,33] The average stay in hospital varies from less than 2 weeks to more than 5 weeks.[6,17,32] The diagnosis differs according to the type and location of the treatment centre. A Scottish study noted a low incidence of personality and behaviour disorders, while an American group recorded a surprisingly high rate of schizophrenia.[18,33] Nevertheless, it seems reasonable to accept the results of a Pennsylvania study that found over two thirds of the physician patients to be depressed.[17] It is generally agreed that abuse of drugs, including alcohol, is a common secondary diagnosis.[5,8,15,17,33] Typically the patients blame overwork or marital discord for their problems,[17] and they tend to exhibit masochism, hypochondriasis, altruism, reaction formation and suppression as defense mechanisms.[20,34] Although physician patients appear to be discharged more rapidly than nonphysicians,[33] 10 percent to 25 percent of physicians insist on leaving hospital prematurely, compared with 1 percent to 2 percent of nonphysicians,[17,18,21] and many physicians refuse to cooperate in follow-up treatment.[6,7]

Physicians present particular difficulties as psychiatric inpatients. Many have delayed seeking treatment[7,8,32] and have complicated their condition by self-diagnosis and self-medication.[35] Often little pressure is brought to bear by colleagues or family, who believe, as does the physician, that doctors are capable of evaluating their own emotional status. Once hospitalized, physicians frequently attempt to direct their own therapy, while remaining aloof from other patients.[7,15] This refusal to accept the "sick role"[36] may be given unwitting support by the psychiatrist, who may identify with the physician patient and minimize the extent of the illness.[5,18,37] In fact, a recent study suggested that, for the physician, being a "special patient" results in inferior care.[34] When compared with controls, physicians had significantly fewer family interviews and involuntary confinements and significantly more suicide attempts, covert out-of-town admissions and drug abuse. As well, physicians tended to have shorter stays in hospital and fewer readmissions, and were treated with a greater number of drugs. All of these factors may suggest that disturbed physicians receive deficient care.

Despite this pessimistic view of psychiatric treatment of doctors, opinions regarding prognosis are mixed. A recent British study suggested that 2 years after discharge one third of physicians will no longer by listed in the medical register, compared with one fifth of a healthy control group.[15] This confirmed the finding of an earlier study with a 1-year follow-up period.[17] Yet, as emphasized by an American study in which fewer than 60 percent of physician patients continued to practice for 3 years after treatment, the figures are unusually encouraging, given the generally poor prognosis for addiction and schizophrenia (the illnesses of 85 percent of the physicians in the study).[18] A similar positive therapeutic response, especially in addicted physicians, has been noted in other studies.[8] For physicians who avoid self-destruction and instead seek psychiatric help the prognosis, despite the "special patient" handicap, may be equal to or better than that for nonphysician patients.

ETIOLOGIC FACTORS

How is one to account for the seemingly inordinate frequency of psychiatric illness among physicians? Two basic responses to this question are evident in the literature, the first of which may be termed the "role strain" hypothesis. The role of the doctor, the theory states, is socially defined. Society has certain expectations of the physician, who, being a part of society, shares these ideals. The role, to be adequately fulfilled, demands that the doctor "function at a maximum level of competence at all times;"[26] to do less is to negate the role and produce feelings of personal inadequacy and social disapprobation. To correct this inevitable failure the physician may begin to work twice as hard but then will simply find that the failures come with increasing frequency. Overwork here is a symptom rather than a cause of stress[38] and is related to the inherent conflict between the physician's altruistic identity as a healer and the coexistent role as an independent entrepreneur. Moreover, the doctor's ethical credo demands that "he do what he can for everyone who lies within his reach and needs his help."[25] Yet twentieth century developments in medical technology have extended untenably what physicians might do and, therefore, to acquit their role, must do. Physicians ultimately fail to fulfil their own ethical commitments and society's role expectations. Faced with this stressful reality they can make one of two responses: acceptance of their limitations or personally destructive behaviour.

Such an abstruse, essentially sociologic, hypothesis is not readily susceptible to the type of verification required by the medical profession. Nevertheless, a few studies have yielded suggestive observations. An Australian investigation found that clinicians, when compared with both nonclinical physicians and American and Scottish nonphysicians, were "significantly more anxious."[39] The anxiety was directly related to fears of inadequacy in fulfilling the professional role. Similarly, among medical students the perceived sources of greatest stress were those related not to social adaptation but to professional inadequacy.[1,40,41] Such concerns may well be inherent in the health care field, as the high rate of suicide in the allied health professions suggests.[13,28] Certainly both sick physicians[10,11,33] and their emotionally disturbed spouses[21,22] attribute much of the blame for their illness to the strain of the profession. It seems a reasonable conclusion, then, that inherent stresses peculiar to the medical profession may account for the inordinate frequency of psychiatric illness among its members.

A second explanation for physicians' high incidence of psychiatric illness might be termed the "susceptible personality" theory. While less philosophically complex than the role strain hypothesis, it may marshall more objective support. Briefly stated, it takes as its thesis the view that physicians in whom psychiatric illness develops have a vulnerability that antedates their entry to medical school.[4] Individuals of a particular personality type, the obsessive-compulsive, are attracted to medicine or accepted into medical school with disproportionate frequency.[42-44] These individuals are achievement- and endurance-oriented but possess little spontaneous creativity or flexibility.[45,46] Such traits are well rewarded in medical school but ensure frustration in the unstructured world of clinical medicine. The result may be, in some cases, an inability to cope. Complicating this professional inadequacy is the fact that such an individual may find married life difficult[21] and is more predisposed to addiction[11] and depression.[27] At particular risk are medical students[19] and physicians[34] who have a strong family history of mental disturbance. As might be expected, physician patients such as drug abusers have had an unhappy or unstable childhood,[11,20] but a long-term study was unable to show that they differ in this respect from emotionally disturbed, socially matched, non-physician controls.[20] It is clear, however, that the family history, personal development and personality traits of the individual physician are closely related to the presence or absence of psychiatric illness.

These two etiologic explanations for psychiatric illness in physicians represent an old dichotomy — the debate between character and circumstances, environment and heredity. It is, of course, a false duality, for both views must be taken into account. In sum, the stresses peculiar to medicine, in contrast to those of a less demanding profession, precipitate out those who are predisposed to psychiatric illness.

PREVENTION AND TREATMENT

Each form of psychiatric disturbance — whether drug abuse, alcoholism, marital discord, suicide or depression — demands its own form of prevention. The following suggestions are meant to apply to psychiatric illness in a general sense.

The problem must initially be approached at its origin: medical school. Admissions committees must select well-rounded individuals whose academic achievements complement, rather than substitute for, a stable personality. During the undergraduate years psychiatry must, in contrast to what appears to be the case now,[47,48] sustain its credibility both as a specialty and as a potential source of solace should the need arise. Special attention should be focused on the single woman during her training to reduce the high frequency of suicide.

Specific areas that medical school must emphasize are the dangers of drug and alcohol abuse to the profession, the counter-productive nature of overwork, the necessity of continuing self-awareness, the need to develop constructive interests outside medicine and the importance of devoting appropriate time to family life.

These themes may be stressed after medical school by medical societies and continuing education programs. Practitioners must be encouraged to monitor their own emotional status continually and realistically. At the same time they must realize their duty to watch for warning signs among colleagues and, more significantly, must recognize that covering up or remaining tactfully silent does no kindness to an ill physician.[49] Practitioners should be urged to cooperate in and initiate studies on such topics as suicide or sources of stress in clinical practice, for only with greater knowledge does prevention become feasible.

When prevention fails, the physician must be encouraged to seek psychiatric therapy early in the course of the illness. The stigma of such care must be removed and, further, the care must be designed to accommodate the physician's "special status." The doctor, after all, is not a patient like the rest;[50] what is similar is the illness. To ignore the physician's professional identity is to refuse to recognize a host of management problems and, in some cases, the key to diagnosis.

CONCLUSION

Most of the studies quoted in this review, one senses, reveal only the surface of the problem. For example, more than one third of the physicians who committed suicide in one series had had no psychiatric therapy before death.[30] Such people may be the sick who are not seen — individuals who cope with chronic depression or anxiety but for whom life is a continuing agony. To save these doctors from their existential misery, and to minimize psychiatric morbidity in this profession in future, all physicians must be acutely aware of their own vulnerability and that of their colleagues.

REFERENCES

1. Raskin M: Psychiatric crises of medical students and the implications for subsequent adjustment. *J Med Educ* 47: 210, 1972
2. Thomas CB: What becomes of medical students: the dark side. *Johns Hopkins Med J* 138: 185, 1976
3. Watterson DJ: Psychiatric illness in the medical profession: incidence in relation to sex and field of practice. *Can Med Assoc J* 115: 311, 1976
4. Waring EM: Psychiatric illness in physicians: a review. *Compr Psychiatry* 15: 519, 1974
5. Murray RM: Psychiatric illness in doctors. *Lancet* 1: 1211, 1974
6. Duffy JC, Litin EM: Psychiatric morbidity of physicians. *JAMA* 189: 989, 1964
7. a'Brook MF, Hailstone JD, McLauchlan IEJ: Psychiatric illness in the medical profession. *Br J Psychiatry* 113: 1013, 1967
8. Vincent MO, Robinson EA, Latt L: Physicians as patients: private psychiatric hospital experience. *Can Med Assoc J* 100: 403, 1969
9. Vaillant GE, Brighton JR, McArthur C: Physicians' use of mood-altering drugs. A 20-year follow-up report. *N Engl J Med* 282: 365, 1970
10. Green RC Jr., Carroll GJ, Buxton WD: Drug addiction among physicians. The Virginia experience. *JAMA* 236: 1372, 1976
11. Modlin HC, Montes A: Narcotics addiction in physicians. *Am J Psychiatry* 121: 358, 1964
12. Putnam PL, Ellinwood EH Jr.: Narcotic addiction among physicians: a ten-year follow-up. *Am J Psychiatry* 122: 745, 1966
13. Rose KD, Rosow I: Physicians who kill themselves. *Arch Gen Psychiatry* 29: 800, 1973
14. Murray RM: Alcoholism amongst male doctors in Scotland. *Lancet* 2: 729, 1976
15. Franklin RA: One hundred doctors at the Retreat: a contribution to the subject of mental disorder in the medical profession. *Br J Psychiatry* 131: 11, 1977
16. Glatt MM: Alcoholism among doctors (C). *Lancet* 2: 342, 1974
17. Jones RE: A study of 100 physician psychiatric inpatients. *Am J Psychiatry* 134: 1119, 1977
18. Small IF, Small JG, Assue CM, et al: The fate of the mentally ill physician. *Am J Psychiatry* 125: 1333, 1969
19. Bissell L, Jones RW: The alcoholic physician: a survey. *Am J Psychiatry* 133: 1142, 1976
20. Vaillant GE, Sobowale NC, McArthur C: Some psychologic vulnerabilities of physicians. *N Engl J Med* 287: 372, 1972
21. Miles JE, Krell R, Lin TY: The doctor's wife: mental illness and marital pattern. *Int J Psychiatry Med* 6: 481, 1975
22. Evans JL: Psychiatric illness in the physician's wife. *Am J Psychiatry* 122: 159, 1965
23. Eagle JR, Smith BM: Stresses of the medical student wife. *J Med Educ* 43: 840, 1968
24. Suicide among doctors (E). *Br Med J* 1: 789, 1964
25. Craig AG, Pitts FN: Suicide by physicians. *Dis Nerv Syst* 29: 763, 1968

26. DeSole DE, Singer P, Aronson S: Suicide and role strain among physicians. *Int J Soc Psychiatry* 15: 294, 1969
27. Blachly PH, Osterud HT, Josslin R: Suicide in professional groups. *N Engl J Med* 268: 1278, 1963
28. Powell EH: Occupation, status, and suicide: towards a redefinition of anomie. *Am Social Rev* 23: 131, 1958
29. Steppacher RC, Mausner JS: Suicide in male and female physicians. *JAMA* 228: 323, 1974
30. Blachly PH, Disher W, Roduner G: Suicide by physicians. *Bull Suicidol* Dec: 1, 1968
31. Everson RB, Fraumeni JF: Mortality among medical students and young physicians. *J Med Educ* 50: 809, 1975
32. Pearson MM, Strecker EA: Physicians as psychiatric patients: private practice experience. *Am J Psychiatry* 116: 915, 1960
33. Murray RM: Psychiatric illness in male doctors and controls: an analysis of Scottish hospitals in-patient data. *Br J Psychiatry* 131: 1, 1977
34. Waring EM: Medical professionals with emotional illness: a controlled study of the hazards of being a "special patient". *Psychiatry J U Ottawa* 2: 161, 1977
35. Gold N: The doctor, his illness and the patient. *Aust NZ J Psychiatry* 6: 209, 1972
36. Bittker TE: Reaching out to the depressed physician. *JAMA* 236: 1713, 1976
37. Osmond H, Siegler M: Doctors as patients. *Practitioner* 218: 834, 1977
38. Maddison D: Stress on the doctor and his family. *Med J Aust* 2: 315, 1974
39. Cramond WA: Anxiety in medical practice — the doctor's own anxiety. *Aust NZ J Psychiatry* 3: 324, 1969
40. Boyle BP, Coombs RH: Personality profiles related to emotional stress in the initial year of medical training. *J Med Educ* 46: 882, 1971
41. Coburn D, Jovaisas AV: Perceived sources of stress among first-year medical students. *J Med Educ* 50: 589, 1975
42. Ellard J: The disease of being a doctor. *Med J Aust* 2: 318, 1974
43. Myckatyn MM, Miles JE: A profile of today's medical student. *Can Med Assoc J* 109: 1118, 1973
44. Schlageter CW, Rosenthal V: What are "normal" medical students like? *J Med Educ* 37: 19, 1962
45. Baird LL: The characteristics of medical students and their views of the first year. *J Med Educ* 50: 1092, 1975
46. Parlow J, Rothman AI: Personality traits of first year medical students: trends over six-year period 1967-1972. *Br J Med Educ* 8: 8, 1974
47. Light D Jr: The impact of medical school on future psychiatrists. *Am J Psychiatry* 132: 607, 1975
48. Kausch DF: Medical students' attitudes towards the mental health field: a longitudinal study. *J Med Educ* 44: 1051, 1969
49. Edwards G: The alcoholic doctor. A case of neglect. *Lancet* 2: 1297, 1975
50. Sargent DA, Jensen VW, Petty TA, et al: Preventing physician suicide. The role of family, colleagues, and organized medicine. *JAMA* 237: 143, 1977

Incidence

Chapter 2

PSYCHIATRIC ILLNESS IN THE MEDICAL PROFESSION: INCIDENCE IN RELATION TO SEX AND FIELD OF PRACTICE

DONALD J. WATTERSON

THE suicide rates for physicians in England and Wales[1] and in Denmark[2] are significantly higher than those of men of comparable class and age, respectively. In the United States the rate is also high, though there is not yet a consensus that it is significantly higher than that in a comparable socioeconomic population matched for age and sex.[3-8] A rate of 35/100,000 is representative of those reported from the US. Surveys of physician suicides have not been carried out in Canada, but it seems reasonable to assume that the rate would be similar.

Three of the American surveys (carried out in the 1960s) also studied the incidence of physician suicide in relation to field of practice.[6-8] The suicide rate varied with type of professional work, from a low of about 10/100,000 to a high of about 60/100,000, and one of the reports claimed significance for the high rates of suicide among psychiatrists, ophthalmologists and anesthetists, and for the low rates among surgeons, pediatricians, radiologists and pathologists.

During the same decade studies of psychiatric illness in the medical profession were reported.[9-13] They were not epidemiologic in design. Nevertheless, one group of physician-patients had a significant over-representation of psychiatrists[9] and another, of anesthetists,[10] while two of the groups contained a high proportion of physician trainees.[12,13] Psychiatric residents in particular have been found to have a high incidence of neurotic depression[14] and of

Originally published in Canadian Medical Association Journal. "PSYCHIATRIC ILLNESS IN THE MEDICAL PROFESSION: INCIDENTS IN RELATION TO SEX AND FIELD OF PRACTICE," Vol. 115, 1976, 311-317 by D.J. Watterson.

I am much indebted to the psychiatrists of British Columbia and to Doctor W.G. McClure, registrar of the British Columbia College of Physicians and Surgeons, for searching their files to extract the data on which the survey was based; to colleagues in family medicine, ophthalmology and psychiatry for their criticisms and suggestions; to Sara Collinson for reviewing the writing; and to Faith Hunter for preparing the manuscript.

Presented to the annual meeting of the Canadian Psychiatric Association, Sept. 28, 1975.

dropout from training because of emotional disturbance, and an alarmingly high rate of suicide.[15] A rough estimate of the overall psychiatric morbidity of physicians can be calculated from a long-term study carried out by Vaillant, Sobowale and McArthur[16] – namely, 1.13 percent per year.

Physicians suffer from the same types of psychiatric illnesses as comparable nonmedical groups, except for a greater tendency to addiction to drugs.[9–13] Alcoholism is a serious problem, though the incidence seems about the same as in nonmedical groups of similar socioeconomic class.[9–13] Many surveys have demonstrated that abuse of or addiction to drugs is significantly more prevalent among doctors than in the general population.[9,17,18]

The purpose of the study reported in this paper was to clarify the factors in the professional training and working lives of physicians that increase or decrease their tendency to become psychiatrically ill.

AIMS OF THE SURVEY

The aims of the present survey were: (a) to determine variations in the incidence and severity of psychiatric illness among the physicians of British Columbia, related to age, sex, level of training and field of practice; and (b) to test the hypothesis that previously reported suicide rates for various groups of physicians correlate with rates of incidence of psychiatric illness.

The province of British Columbia is a region of Canada particularly suited to such a survey. Largely for geographic reasons few physicians-patients seek treatment outside the province. Most referred for psychiatric consultation and treatment are seen by psychiatrists working largely or part-time in private practice. A small number come to the attention of the College of Physicians and Surgeons under section 55 of the Medical Act.

Naturally some physicians suffering from psychiatric disturbances (particularly when the symptoms are largely physical) are treated by nonpsychiatrist colleagues, but this vaguely defined group was considered outside the scope of this survey.

METHODS

In February 1975 a letter was sent to the 191 psychiatrists in British Columbia explaining the purpose of the survey and requesting their cooperation. They were asked to complete an accompanying form concerning all physician-patients referred for consultation and treatment during the 5 years 1970 through 1974. The required particulars were the year of referral, birth date, sex, field of practice, diagnosis, whether admitted to hospital, outcome and whether an intern, resident or fully qualified practitioner. Hospital records were not searched. Physician-patients who are hospitalized are almost invariable seen by psychiatrists in private practice before, during or after their hospitalization. However, the number of patients admitted to hospital at some point during psychiatric treatment was probably underestimated in this survey.

Responses were received from 134 psychiatrists, 66 being nil responses and 68 listing the requested particulars. The number of physician-patients seen by a given psychiatrist ranged from one to 27. It was judged that the majority of the 57 psychiatrists who did not respond had not had physician-patients between 1970 and 1974 but that a few almost certainly had and presumably did not respond for reasons of confidentiality.

The registrar of the college of Physicians and Surgeons of British Columbia provided comparable anonymous data on the 33 physicians who had been reported to the college over the same 5 years because of impaired functioning due to psychiatric illness or addiction to alcohol or drugs.

In view of the likelihood that some physician-patients were seen by more that one psychiatrist (or by a psychiatrist and the college) it was necessary to have means of differentiating one patient from another. Birth date was chosen as such a means. In most instances the complete birth date was supplied, but in a sizable number only the year of birth was known or the age at the time of referral. It was decided not to exclude the physician-patients whose full birth date was not given, but to scrutinize all particulars supplied (except diagnosis) and make a probable rather than a completely certain differentiation.

Differentiating physician-patients in the small groups of specialties presented no problem; the figures for these groups are certain. However, there was some difficulty in the group of family physicians and the figure of 116 may be in error. Fortunately this is such a large group that the probable error makes no appreciable difference to the statistical findings of the study.

A total of 318 sets of physician data were supplied by psychiatrists and the college. In 34 instances the data were insufficient to allow differentiation and in 37 the same physician-patient was reported from two or more sources; thus, 247 physician-patients constituted the group under study.

The numbers of male and female fully qualified physicians in the various fields of practice, obtained from the medical directories for 1969-70 and 1974-75 published by the college, were averaged. Since the numbers of interns and residents vary from year to year, figures for the 5 years were averaged.

Statistical analysis, when applicable, was carried out by the chi-square method.

FINDINGS

The overall incidence of psychiatric illness among the physicians in British Columbia during 1970-74 as estimated in this survey was 1.27 percent per year.

Differences by level of training in the incidence of psychiatric illness are shown in Table 2-I. Psychiatric residents had an exceptionally high incidence, while there were virtually no differences in psychiatric morbidity among the qualified physicians, the other residents and the interns. There was no significant difference in incidence between the fully qualified male and female physicians. Because breakdown by sex of the resident population between 1970 and 1974 was not obtained, the relative incidence in male and

Table 2-I—Occurrence of psychiatric illness among all physicians in British Columbia, 1970-74, in relation to level of training and sex

Level of training	Average no.* of physicians (and % of total)	No.* of patients (and % of total)	
Qualified physicians			
Male	3291 (84.36) *3278.42*	195 (78.95) *207.58*	
Female	284 (7.28) *284.06*	19 (7.69) *18.04*	
Residents			
Psychiatric	31 (0.80) *42.32*	14 (5.67) *2.68*	$P < 0.005$†
All others	227 (5.82) *227.59*	15 (6.07) *14.41*	
Interns	68 (1.74) *67.71*	4 (1.62) *4.29*	
Total	3901 (100.00)	247 (100.00)	

*Numbers in italics are expected numbers.

†The P values in this and subsequent tables indicate the probability that an observed distribution is due to chance. The probabilities range from 0.05 (1 in 20) to 0.005 (1 in 200), and the significance of difference between actual and expected distributions ranges, correspondingly, from low to high.

female residents is not known.

Undergoing psychotherapy can be a valuable part of psychiatric training. Moreover, residents in psychiatry are facilitated in seeking psychiatric treatment if they show signs of emotional disturbance. The question arises whether the 14 psychiatric-resident patients were referred for treatment because of illness or to gain experience in psychotherapy. Their diagnoses are compared with those of the other resident-patients in Table 2-II. Apart from the fact that three psychiatric residents were being treated for situational conditions, compared with only one of the other residents, the severity of the disorders in the two groups appears similar. This accords with my experience that the primary motive of most psychiatric-resident patients is to seek treatment for manifest psychiatric illness or disorder, though an educational motive usually comes into play during the course of psychotherapy.

Table 2-II—Diagnoses among residents

Diagnosis	No. of resident-patients: Psychiatric	All others	Total
Adult situational reaction	3	1	4
Anxiety reaction	4	5	9
Depressive reaction	3	4	7
Obsessional neurosis	0	2	2
Personality disorders	2	1	3
Borderline psychosis	1	1	2
Schizophrenic reaction	1	0	1
Manic-depressive psychosis	0	1	1
Total	14	15	29

The distribution of resident-patients among the various fields of practice other than psychiatry was unremarkable.

The relation of psychiatric illness to field of practice among fully qualified physicians is shown in Table 2-III. The proportion of patients from a given field of practice was usually remarkably close to the proportion of physicians in the field, the exceptions among the larger fields of practice being internal medicine, ophthalmology, orthopedic surgery, pathology and psychiatry. Statistical analysis of the distribution of patients by field of practice revealed differences, but the probability of their being significant was very low ($P < 0.1$ to 0.05).

However, the findings shown in Table 2-IV are consistent with the hypothesis that the incidence of psychiatric illness is high in the

Table 2-III—Distribution of psychiatric illness by field of practice among fully qualified physicians, 1970-74

Field of practice	Average no. of physicians (and % of total)		No. of patients (and % of total)	
Anesthesiology	161	(4.50)	11	(5.14)
Dermatology	31	(0.87)	0	(0)
Family medicine	1901	(53.17)	116	(54.21)
General surgery	255	(7.13)	15	(7.01)
Medicine	234	(6.55)	7	(3.27)
Neurology	22	(0.62)	0	(0)
Neurosurgery	20	(0.56)	0	(0)
Obstetrics and gynecology	113	(3.16)	6	(2.80)
Ophthalmology	103	(2.88)	13	(6.08)
Orthopedic surgery	69	(1.93)	2	(0.93)
Otolaryngology	53	(1.48)	2	(0.93)
Pediatrics	109	(3.05)	5	(2.34)
Pathology	70	(1.96)	7	(3.27)
Plastic surgery	19	(0.53)	1	(0.47)
Physical medicine and rehabilitation	13	(0.36)	0	(0)
Psychiatry	165	(4.62)	17	(7.94)
Public health	30	(0.84)	2	(0.93)
Radiology	140	(3.92)	5	(2.34)
Thoracic and cardiovascular surgery	15	(0.42)	0	(0)
Urology	52	(1.45)	5	(2.34)
Total	3575	(100.00)	214	(100.00)

fields of practice with high suicide rates. The separate contributions from the psychiatrists and ophthalmologists to the overall high probability of differences were significantly high. The contribution from the group of anesthetists was indeterminable.

Comparable analysis revealed no significant difference in the incidence of psychiatric illness between the fields of practice having low suicide rates (surgery, pediatrics, radiology and pathology) and the other fields of practice collectively, but this finding was not independent and is of low reliance.

The age range among the resident-patients was 22 to 41 years, the median being 30.6 years. The corresponding figures for the fully qualified physicians were 24 to 91 years and 44.5 years. The average age of physician-patients by field of practice ranged from 40 years in psychiatry to 51 years in surgery, but the differences were not significant.

The incidence of psychiatric illness among the family physicians was virtually the same as among the specialists (1.22% and 1.17%

Table 2-IV—Occurrence of psychiatric illness in specialties with high suicide rates, 1970-1974

Field of practice	Average no.* of physicians	No.* of patients		
Anesthesiology	161 *162.29*	11 *9.71*		
Ophthalmology	103 *109.45*	13 *6.55*	$0.005 < P < 0.01$	
				$0.005 < P < 0.01$ (Anesthesiology, Ophthalmology, Psychiatry, All others)
Psychiatry	165 *171.72*	17 *10.28*	$0.025 < P < 0.05$	
All others	3146 *3131.55*	173 *187.45*		
Total	3575	214		

*Numbers in italics are expected numbers.

per year, respectively). However, there were indications that the family practice patients had more severe disorders and less favourable prognoses.

Primary diagnoses are grouped into five categories in Table 2-V. The incidence of psychoneuroses was approximately the same in family physicians and specialists, but the distributions among the remaining four diagnostic categories were significantly different. Specialists were more often referred for situational problems and personality disorders, while the family physician group had a higher incidence of both psychoses and addictions, particularly addiction to drugs (Table 2-VI). Addiction was listed as the primary diagnosis in 23 physicians and as the secondary diagnosis in an additional 35, giving a total of 58 physician-patients (27.1%) who were addicted to alcohol or drugs or both. This included 36 physicians addicted to alcohol (16.8% of all patients) and 32 addicted to various drugs (15.0%). There were no reports of addiction to or abuse of alcohol or drugs among the resident-and-intern-patients. Five of the six patients addicted to narcotics were family physicians. More family physicians than specialists were referred to the College of Physicians and Surgeons of British Columbia because of impaired funtioning and questions of licensure (23 out of a total of 33) and significantly more were hospitalized (35 out of 43; $P < 0.005$).

There were also appreciable differences in outcome between the family physician and specialist patients (Table 2-VII). Relatively more family physicians than specialists were reported as "recovered," but the major contributions to the significant differences in outcome

Table 2-V—Differences in primary diagnosis between family physicians and specialists

Category of primary diagnosis	No.* of patients (n = 214) Family physicians	Specialists	
Adult situational reaction	4 *8.7*	12 *7.3*	0.005 < P < 0.01
Psychoneuroses (anxiety, depressive, obsessional)	60 *58.17*	47 *48.83*	
Personality disorders (including borderline psychosis, sexual deviations)	14 *19.03*	21 *15.97*	
Psychoses (schizophrenic, manic-depressive, organic brain syndrome)	17 *13.59*	8 *11.41*	
Addictions (alcohol, drugs, alcohol + drugs)	17 *12.50*	6 *10.50*	
Subtotal	112	94	
Miscellaneous	4	4	
Total	116	98	

*Numbers in italics are expected numbers.

Table 2-VI—Differences between family physicians and specialists in occurrence of addiction (primary or secondary diagnosis)

Types of addiction	No.* of physicians (n = 3575) Family physicians	Specialists	
Alcohol	13 *13.83*	13 *12.17*	0.025 < P < 0.05
Alcohol + drugs	7 *5.32*	3 *4.68*	
Drugs	18 *11.70*	4 *10.30*	
Not addicted	1863 *1870.16*	1654 *1646.84*	
Total	1901	1674	

*Numbers in italics are expected numbers.

Table 2-VII—Differences in outcome of family physicians and specialists

Category of outcome	No.* of patients (n = 214) Family physicians	Specialists	
Recovered, working satisfactorily	30 *25.28*	20 *24.72*	
Improved, no major recurrences, returned to practice	30 *40.95*	51 *40.05*	
Periodic recurrences, functions marginally	12 *11.12*	10 *10.88*	$0.01 < P < 0.025$
Withdrew from practice, not working	15 *10.62*	6 *10.38*	
Suicide	4 *3.03*	2 *2.97*	
Subtotal	91	89	
Moved from BC	1	0	
Retired	3	0	
Died	1	0	
No follow-up	20	9	
Total	116	98	

*Numbers in italics are expected numbers.

stem from the much smaller proportion of family physicians in the "improved" category and the disproportionately high number who withdrew from practice.

Six of the qualified physicians committed suicide. The two specialists were an ophthalmologist and a psychiatrist. A senior resident in medicine (included among the reported patients) also took his life. The average age of these seven male physicians at the time of psychiatric referral was 39 years, which is unusually low.[6] In two the diagnosis was manic-depressive psychosis; in four, neurotic depression (in three, with associated alcoholism; in one, with drug addiction); and in one, sociopathic personality associated with alcoholism and narcotic addiction.

These seven suicides cannot include all that occurred in the 5-year study period. Any other physicians who took their lives may have been referred for treatment prior to 1970, may never have been referred at all or may simply not have been reported in this survey. For example, a female psychiatric resident who committed suicide in

1970 was not included among the patients reported. The suicide rate of physicians in British Columbia during 1970-74 must therefore have been higher than the rate of 36.5/100,000 calculated on the basis of 7.

DISCUSSION

Adequacies and Limitations of the Survey

There are several indications that the physician-patient group is fairly complete. Data were received from two or more sources for 37 out of 247 patients. The rate of psychiatric referral, 1.27 percent per year, is close to the rate of 1.13 percent per year derived from the study of Vaillant and colleagues.[16] The suicide rate calculated from this survey (> 36.5/100 000) is of the same order as that estimated from the American studies.[6-8]

Statistical analysis of the relations between incidence of psychiatric illness and field of practice did not demonstrate that qualified ophthalmologists and psychiatrists were significantly over-represented but that the data were consistent with the hypothesis that such groups, with high suicide rates, also have a high incidence of psychiatric illness. The significantly high incidence of psychiatric illness among the psychiatric residents was, however, unqualified. Possibilities of statistical analysis regarding relative incidence in other fields of practice were thereupon exhausted. It was not possible from the data of this survey to discover validly which fields were under-represented. The incidence of psychiatric illness appears to have been low in internal medicine and its subspecialities collectively, but a separate survey would be necessary to test that hypothesis.

The study was limited to the physicians of British Columbia; the findings may or may not be true of other provinces or countries.

Etiologic Considerations

In his review of the literature Waring[14] mentioned the common assumption that the stresses that provoke psychiatric illness in the medical profession are the length and arduousness of medical training, the enormous demands of the profession, the responsibility for life-and-death situations and the ready availability of drugs. In his view "these explanations seem somewhat artificial."

The perspective expressed by Pond[13] seems realistic: "It is hard to come by strong evidence that the conditions of work are more than minor precipitating factors in most cases. Mentally ill doctors have had family histories of mental illness, come from unsatisfactory and unhappy homes, and make unsatisfactory adult relationships in marriage, etc., to much the same extent as do their non-medical patients." However, it still seems worth while to attempt to discern some of the "minor precipatating factors."

The following portions of the discussion are confined to the few groups in which the relative incidence or severity of psychiatric illness was determined by statistical analysis of the data. Even so, discussion of the stresses associated with particular professional work can only be speculative.

WOMEN PHYSICIANS: In the general population the suicide rate of females is several times less than that of males at all ages.

Lindhardt and colleagues[2] found that suicide among women physicians contributed excessively to the total number of deaths. Craig and Pitts[7] later showed that the suicide rate of women physicians in the United States was virtually the same as that of male physicians.

Russell, Pasnau and Taintor[15] remarked on the widespread belief that women physicians in training are more liable to psychiatric illness than men and showed by their study of psychiatric residents that this is not so. The present study also showed no appreciable difference in incidence of psychiatric illness between fully qualified male and female physicians.

The evidence, while still slender, suggests that sex per se (at least among physicians) is not a significant determinant of either psychiatric breakdown or suicide.

OPHTHALMOLOGISTS: Blachley, Disher and Roduner[6] speculated that there is a high incidence of suicide in specialties that tend to enhance "the fantasy of omnipotence of the doctor." Ophthalmology is an obvious exception, and the authors fell back on the implausible suggestion that suicide among ophthalmologists is related to their alleged "compulsive perfectionistic traits."

There has been no previous discussion of the incidence of psychiatric illness among ophthalmologists, and the possibility raised by the present study that it is significantly high needs confirmation.

Ophthalmologists quickly dismiss the layman's assumption that operating on the eye is particularly stressful. Some ophthalmologists in British Columbia are aware of their collective proneness to psychiatric illness and to suicide. They are aware of certain stresses in their work and are planning to alleviate these.

The ophthalmologist in private practice typically has a heavy caseload and his appointment book may be filled for months ahead. He runs himself to a tight schedule. After some years of practice in this situation (whether caused by external pressures or self-imposed) he is apt to feel irritably constrained by the straitjacket of his professional life.

Most of his time is spent carrying out refractions. He strives for perfection in this work, and many patients reward him by their cheerful satisfaction from seeing better. He hates the dissatisfied patient if only because he is not paid for having to do the work over again.

The ophthalmologist is naturally confronted by the same mixture of cooperative and uncooperative behaviour in his patients as is any other physician or surgeon, but he needs greater precision of response to questions than doctors in most fields of practice. He runs through a refraction with a patter he has perfected with experience, and becomes frustrated by the patient who cannot tune in and respond helpfully.

Doubtless the majority of ophthalmologists tolerate this frustration, but some are reported to become openly angered by the seemingly stupid or recalcitrant patient or to become explosively irritable in their professional contacts generally. Such reactions to the frustrations of medical practice are obviously not specific to a single specialty, but they are emphasized by ophthalmologists themselves.

Some ophthalmologists point to an additional frustration. The ophthalmologist needs full medical and specialty training for his work as a consultant, but not for uncomplicated refractions. Thus, he may also become frustrated by being professionally underchallenged in a sizable part of his work. This situation was indirectly referred to in the 1975 report of the British Columbia Oto-Ophthalmology Society: "With regard to medical manpower, the Section of Ophthalmology was almost unanimous in its opinion that there are too many ophthalmologists at present practising in this province."[19]

However, after taking these recognized stresses into account, the high incidence of suicide and the possibly high incidence of psychiatric illness among ophthalmologists seem insufficiently explained. It is possible that these high rates may not be upheld by further investigation, that ophthalmologists have unsuspected vulnerability to frustration, or that additional psychological stresses are presently being overlooked.

Perhaps the speculation that working on the eyes of people may be stressful should not be dismissed so abruptly. As well as being the organ of vision, the eye also carries profound symbolic connotations.

PSYCHIATRIC RESIDENTS AND QUALIFIED PSYCHIATRISTS: Psychiatry is the only field of practice with a significantly high incidence of psychiatric illness and of suicide among both residents and qualified specialists. The factor of preselection has often been mentioned in the literature.[1,6,9] It is understandable that some physicians are drawn to the specialty by their personal emotional problems, and it is no overstatement that a degree of neurotic vulnerability is a prerequisite for the would-be psychotherapist. This vulnerability is probably the most important single factor contributing to the high incidence of psychiatric illness and suicide among both psychiatric residents and psychiatrists.

The second contributing factor is the adverse experience of would-be psychiatrists in medical school, a subject recently documented by Light.[20] Duffy[21] wrote that in medical school "a subtle but demeaning attitude toward emotional illness and psychiatric help is all too often inculcated." The main reasons seem to be "the hostile perspective of technical medicine" and the fact that "psychiatry is rated as one of the most poorly taught specialties."[20] The initial high interest in psychiatry wanes and many potentially able clinicians are deterred from entering the specialty.

There are many sources of insecurity for psychiatrists in their varied professional work. The philosophy of psychiatric treatment has always been in transition,[22] and the psychiatrist continues to be in a state of "future shock." The psychiatric clinician is confused by the current "role-diffusion" in his specialty. The psychotherapist is apt to be bewildered by old therapeutic wines being decanted into new bottles with labels that give no clue as to their nature — gestalt therapy, primal therapy, bioenergetics and the like.

The psychotherapist meets his patient in a relatively open confrontation in which his values and integrity are challenged and tested. The practice of psychotherapy can be at times a deeply rewarding personal experience, and at other times a threatening stress. Freeman[23] has suggested that insight can be mistakenly pushed, to the detriment of, or even disaster for, the psychiatrist himself.

The psychiatrist in practice (whether his basic orientation is biological or psychological) must also keep the courage of his convictions in the face of an undeniably high rate among his patients of relapse and readmission to hospital.

All these considerations apply with even greater force to the psychiatrist in training. He may feel professionally disoriented in a specialty still uncertain of its roles. He often has a sense of floundering in the course of interviewing patients, planning treatment or undertaking psychotherapy. He discovers the intense anxiety provoked by seeing his own psychological disorders and psychodynamics mirrored by his patients. These stresses are compounded if his training is insufficiently supportive or educationally inadequate.

Margaret Mead[24] has implied that the psychiatrist (like the ophthalmologist) is underchallenged in part of his work and is professionally frustrated by carrying out psychotherapy with persons whose problems are purely situational and who are not really ill. Possible frustration from this source could be obviated since the majority of patients troubled by essentially situational problems seem willing to accept paraprofessional therapists with adequate training under psychiatric supervision.[25]

FAMILY PHYSICIANS: A curious finding of the present study was the contrast between incidence and severity of psychiatric illness among family physicians, the incidence being no higher than expected but the severity (as judged by several measures) being significantly greater than among specialists. The most likely explanation is that family physicians tend to delay longer than specialists in seeking treatment.

If this were true it might be expected that the suicide rate among family physicians would be the higher. In two of the three American surveys mentioned previously the suicide rates of family physicians and specialists were virtually the same,[6,8] in the third the rate for family physicians was significantly higher ($P < 0.05$ to 0.025).[7]

Diagnostic breakdown between family practitioners and specialists was compared in two previous studies — those carried out by Duffy and Litin[11] at the Mayo Clinic and by Vincent, Robinson and Latt[10] at the Homewood Sanitarium in Guelph, Ont. Both groups found no differences in diagnostic breakdown between family physicians and specialists. However, the patient populations of the two studies were inpatients preselected as the most severely sick from among both the family physicians and the specialists; by contrast, the patient group in this study was representative of physicians referred for psychiatric treatment regardless of kind and degree of disorder.

There may be several reasons why family physicians delay longer than specialists in seeking psychiatric treatment. Many family practitioners in British Columbia are geographically isolated from medical colleagues and may be deterred from arranging a psychiatric consultation by sheer distance.

It has been suggested that family physicians (who make most of the referrals) are more aware than specialists of psychiatric treatment failures and are therefore reluctant to have themselves referred (P.R. Grantham: personal communication, 1975).

The hypothesis of "role-strain" advanced by DeSole, Singer and Aronson[8] applies to some family physicians much more than to specialists. These authors were not referring to strain inherent in a professional role but rather to the strain imposed on physicians by never being able to regress to less demanding roles. The family physician living amidst his patients in a rural area where there is little privacy is particularly subject to such role strain.[13] If he becomes psychiatrically disturbed it is more dislocating to his practice and more embarrassing to him to seek professional help than it is for physicians whose circumstances are less public. He is likely to stay too long on the job until forced to quit or compelled to find psychiatric treatment because of impaired professional functioning. Probably this is the reason for the observation that the family physician more often than the specialist is reported to the College of Physicians and Surgeons by his patients (W.G. McClure: personal communication, 1975).

The family physician may also receive less overall surveillance by his colleagues than the specialist. In a hospital setting the work of family physicians and specialists is equally subject to peer review, but in office practice the quality of work of the specialist is more readily apparent to fellow specialists and referring physicians. This greater professional surveillance may be felt as a pressure, but it may also induce the specialist who needs psychiatric treatment to seek it earlier.

By contrast, it may be relatively late before emotional disturbance in the family physician is noticed by anyone but his patients and family. By the time he has a psychiatric referral he will likely be more severely ill and may have been giving himself medication, occasionally to the point of addiction. The prognosis thereby will have become less favourable. At the end of treatment it is less likely that he will have improved and more likely that he will have withdrawn from medical practice.

RECOMMENDATIONS

Comparable surveys should be carried out in other provinces or countries to explore further the incidence and severity of psychiatric illness among physicians in relation to field of practice. The sections of general practice and of psychiatry of the British Columbia Medical Association should discuss jointly the earlier referral of family physicians for psychiatric treatment. Medical schools should aim at further integration of the teaching and practice of psychiatry with those of the other clinical fields. Finally, university departments of psychiatry should give higher priority to follow-up studies of physicians selected for psychiatric training, with a view to finding a better balance between psychological sensitivity and neurotic vulnerability.

REFERENCES

1. Suicide among doctors (E). *Br Med J* 1: 789, 1964
2. Lindhardt M, Frandsen E, Hamtoft H, et al: Causes of death among the medical profession in Denmark. *Dan Med Bull* 10: 59, 1963
3. Emerson H, Hughes HE: Death rates of male white physicians in the United States, by age and cause. *Am J Public Health* 16: 1088, 1929
4. Dublin LI, Speigelman M: The longevity and mortality of American physicians, 1938-1942; preliminary report. *JAMA* 134: 1211, 1947
5. Dickinson FG, Martin LW: Physician mortality 1949-1951. *JAMA* 162: 1462, 1956
6. Blachley PH, Disher W, Roduner G: Suicide by physicians. *Bull Suicide:* 1, 1968
7. Craig AG, Pitts FN Jr: Suicide by physicians. *Dis Nerv Syst* 29: 763, 1968
8. DeSole DE, Singer P, Aronson S: Suicide and role strain among physicians. *Int J Soc Psychiatry* 15: 294, 1969
9. a'Brook MF, Hailstone JD, McLauchlan IE: Psychiatric illness in the medical profession. *Br J Psychiatry* 113: 1013, 1967
10. Vincent MO, Robinson EA, Latt L: Physicians as patients: private psychiatric hospital experience. *Can Med Assoc J* 100: 403, 1969
11. Duffy JC, Litin EM: *The Emotional Health of Physicians,* Springfield, IL, CC Thomas 1967, p. 52
12. Pearson MM, Strecker EA: Physicians as psychiatric patients: private practice experience. *Am J Psychiatry* 116: 915, 1960
13. Pond DA: Doctor's mental health. *NZ Med J* 69: 131, 1969
14. Waring EM: Psychiatric illness in physicians: a review. *Compr Psychiatry* 15: 519, 1974
15. Russell AT, Pasnau RO, Taintor ZC: Emotional problems of residents in psychiatry. *Am J Psychaitry* 132: 263, 1975
16. Vaillant GE, Sobowale NC, McArthur C: Some psychological vulnerabilities of physicians. *N Engl J Med* 287: 372, 1972
17. Modlin HC, Montes A: Narcotics addiction in physicians. *Am J Psychiatry* 121: 358, 1964
18. Vaillant GE, Brighton JR, McArthur C: Physicians' use of mood-altering drugs. A 20-year follow-up report. *N Engl J Med* 282: 365, 1970
19. Gillanders DA: *General Assembly Reports,* annual report of secretary, BC Oto-Ophthalmology Society, Vancouver, BC Med Assoc, 1975, p 8
20. Light D Jr: The impact of medical school on future psychiatrists. *Am J Psychiatry* 132: 607, 1975

21. Duffy JC: The emotional health of physicians. *Ann Intern Med* 69: 1319, 1968
22. Greenblatt M: Psychaitry: the battered child of medicine. *N Engl J Med* 292: 246, 1975
23. Freeman W: *The Psychiatrist: Personalities and Patterns,* New York, Grune, 1968, p 164
24. Mead M: Quoted from her address to American Psychiatric Association. *Psychiatr News* 10: 27, 1975
25. Watterson DJ, Collinson S: Explorations in co-psychotherapy. *Can Psychiatr Assoc J* 19: 577, 1974

Addenda

Since the prior paper was published it has been confirmed that a significantly higher incidence of suicide among the specialties occurs in psychiatry, but not in ophthalmology.* The speculations about stresses in the practice of ophthalmology may still be of interest, even though there is no evidence of a higher incidence of either suicide or psychiatric illness in the specialty.

*Rich CL, Pitts FN: Suicide by psychiatrists: a study of medical specialists among 18,730 consecutive physician deaths during a five-year period, 1967-72. *J Clin Psychiatry* 41: 261, 1980

Watterson DJ, Alfred B: Deaths among U.S. physicians, January 1, 1969-December 31, 1973. Unpublished.

Chapter 3

WHAT BECOMES OF MEDICAL STUDENTS: THE DARK SIDE

CAROLINE BEDELL THOMAS

WHAT becomes of medical students? In an essay first appearing in the St. Bartholomew's Hospital Reports for 1869, Sir James Paget traced the careers of 1000 of 1226 former pupils (1). Of the thousand he found: 23 achieved distinguished success; 66 achieved considerable success; 507 achieved fair success; 124 achieved very limited success; 56 failed entirely; 96 left the profession; 87 died within twelve years of commencing practice; and 41 died during pupilage.

After defining his categories of success, he described what happened to the "very mixed class" of those who failed entirely, those who left the profession, and those who died. Paget found that nearly 13 percent of his entering medical students were dead within 15 years, "a melancholy list." While he realized that many more facts would be required before the influence of different modes of education on the afterlife of medical students could be deduced, he concluded that "nothing appears more certain than that the personal character, the very nature, the will, of each student had far greater force in determining his career than any helps or hindrances whatever."

What becomes of medical students? More than 100 years later, this question is still of central importance. Medical schools in the United States now admit over 14,000 students a year. These schools vigilantly screen a much larger pool of applicants in an effort to accept only "the best." But who are "the best?" As we better understand the causes of student and physician failure, it becomes essential to take the long view, selecting those who not only will be good medical students but who will become sound physicians as well (2-12). Hallmarks of medical success frequently cited include excellence in

This work was supported by Research Grant 1R01-MH-18819, National Institute of Mental Health.

From Caroline Bedell Thomas, What Becomes of Medical Students: The Dark Side. *The Johns Hopkins Medical Journal, 138:* 185-195, 1976.

postgraduate training, medical specialization and Board certification, academic appointment, research publication, and election to medical and scientific societies. The relationship of such hallmarks of success to characteristics of a cohort of twentieth-century American medical students has already been reported (13-15). In this paper, the same cohort is examined with regard to two fundamental requisites for medical competence: the ability and drive to obtain an M.D. degree and the health necessary to graduate and function as a physician. Our chief concern is with those who failed to fulfill their own expectations of success: (1) the *dropouts*, or those who did not graduate from this medical school, and (2) those who *died prematurely*. We also consider the students with an irregular academic course: (3) those who *dropped back* in medical school and (4) those who *transferred* into medical school.

STUDY POPULATION

The cohort consists of the 1337 medical students whose names appeared in the Johns Hopkins University Circulars from 1947 through 1963 as members of classes to graduate in 1948 through 1964. Every student thus registered received an identification number as a subject in the prospective Study of the Precursors of Hypertension and Coronary Heart Disease. All 13.37 subjects are members of the cohort regardless of whether they (1) dropped out of medical school, (2) fell back into classes graduating later, (3) transferred from another medical school on advanced standing, (4) graduated from some other medical school, or (5) were inactive participants in the Precursors Study. The classes of 1948, 1949, and 1950 were already in medical school when assignment of identification numbers began in March, 1947; 18 students who withdrew from these classes before 1947 are not included.

The population consists of males and females of European ancestry, middle-Eastern males, and far-Eastern males and females. Black students were first admitted to Johns Hopkins in the class of 1965 and, therefore, are not represented in this cohort. For the sake of brevity, the 1301 students of European ancestry are called *white*, and the 36 students of non-European ancestry are called *other*.

ACADEMIC STATUS

Graduation status refers to graduation from the Johns Hopkins University School of Medicine. The *graduate* group received the M.D. degree from this institution. The *nongraduate* group is comprised of all subjects registered in this medical school who left Hopkins without the M.D. degree for any reason, including those who transferred to and graduated from another medical school and those who died as medical students.

Academic standing in medical school is expressed in terms of class standing by thirds. Students in each class were ranked in the top, middle, or bottom third of the class by the Dean's Office at the end of the second and fourth academic year. Those who failed or dropped out for other reasons before the marking period were not included in the ranking.

FINDINGS

Although it would seem simple enough to compare the nongraduates with the graduates in various ways, it turns out to be quite a difficult matter. First, there is clearcut heterogeneity *within* both the graduate and nongraduate groups, not only as to sex and race, but in other important respects. While further subdivision often results in very small numbers, retrospective pooling introduces the possibility of bias. Also, differences in age and secular trends must be borne in mind, even though small numbers make it hard or impossible to measure their influence. Despite these difficulties, the basic facts are presented as a descriptive survey to serve as guideposts for further psychological studies.

The distribution of graduates and nongraduates by sex and race is shown in Table 3-I. Eighty-nine, or 6.7 percent, of all men and women attending the Johns Hopkins University School of Medicine at any time between March, 1947, and June, 1964, left before graduation. Proportionately, compared with white males, twice as many white females and three times as many other males and females did not graduate.

Because the cohort consists of subjects in 17 consecutive medical school classes, their birth years span a wide range (Table 3-II). Birth years of graduates and nongraduates are roughly parallel.

Divergent Academic Pathways

A large majority of students, 1105 men and women, completed the prescribed four-year academic course and graduated at the appropriate time. However, 69 students entered medical school in one class and graduated in a later class. Reasons for dropping back are summarized in Table 3-III. Academic failure accounted for a third of those dropping back. Usually these students failed one

Table 3-I

Distribution of 1337 Precursors Study Subjects in Classes of 1948-1964 by Sex, Race, and Graduation Status

Graduation Status	Total Registered		White Males		White Females		Oriental Males		Oriental Females		Middle Eastern Males	
	No.	%	No.	%	No.	%	No.	%	No.	%	No.	%
Graduates	1248	93.3	1117	94.3	102	87.9	15	78.9	4	80.0	10	83.3
Nongraduates	89	6.7	68	5.7	14	12.1	4	21.1	1	20.0	2	16.7
Total	1337	100.0	1185	100.0	116	100.0	19	100.0	5	100.0	12	100.0

Table 3-II

Distribution of 1337 Precursors Study Subjects in Classes of 1948-1964 by Birth Year and Graduation Status

Graduation Status	Total Registered		Birth Year									
			1900–1909		1910–1919		1920–1929		1930–1939		1940–1949	
	No.	%	No.	%	No.	%	No.	%	No.	%	No.	%
Graduates	1248	100.0	1	0.1	45	3.6	495	39.7	663	53.1	44	3.5
Nongraduates	89	100.0	0	0.0	2	2.2	41	46.1	46	51.7	0	0.0
Total	1337	100.0	1	0.1	47	3.5	536	40.1	709	53.0	44	3.3

course and received D's in one or two others. The degree of their academic failure was less than that of 38 students who were dismissed from the medical school for that reason. The first year was repeated by 19 dropbacks; the second and third years were each repeated by two men.

Another third of the dropbacks incorporated additional academic pursuits in their medical school curricula. Nine students enrolled in M.D.-Ph.D. programs and eight undertook research in basic medical sciences; other pursuits included teaching (four men), tropical medicine (two men), and combined undergraduate and graduate work (one man). Fulfilling the requirements for a Ph.D usually added 4 or 5 extra years between the second and third years of medical school, although some students shortened this time by using elective and vacation quarters. Of the group of 24 men undertaking special academic pursuits, seven graduated in the highest third of their classes; seven graduated in the middle third; and ten graduated in the lowest third.

Seventeen students left school for at least one year because of mental or physical illness; all returned to medical school and graduated. Seven men dropped back for psychological reasons; three of these required hospitalization. Between 1945 and 1949, five students dropped back because of active pulmonary tuberculosis; three of them were born in Germany, China, and Costa Rica, respectively. One of these had x-ray evidence of an inactive apical lesion on admission to medical school which flared up during his third school year. No one entering medical school after 1946 dropped out or died from tuberculosis. Other health problems responsible for the loss of a school year included infectious mononucleosis, infectious hepatitis, and rheumatoid arthritis.

Four men in the group of 69 dropbacks entered the Johns Hopkins School of Medicine on advanced standing. One of them dropped back after his third year because of mental illness. Two men, who had obtained Ph.D.'s in basic science elsewhere, taught part-time on the faculty and took longer than usual to obtain their M.D.'s. One carried out a year of research between the last two years of medical school.

In addition to the four transfer students who dropped back and one who dropped out after transferring, 74 students entered Johns Hopkins on advanced standing from other medical schools and graduated on time. Sixty-four were white males, nine were white females, and one was a middle-Eastern male. Sixty-six students transferred into the third-year class, 39 of whom had attended two-

Table 3-III

Dropbacks: Reasons for Dropping Back in Medical School

Reason	Total* No. = 1301		White Males No. = 1185	White Females No. = 116
	No.	%	No.	No.
Academic failure	24	34.8	24	0
Hospitalized for mental illness	3	4.3	3	0
Emotional disturbance	4	5.8	4	0
Tuberculosis	5	7.2	4	1
Other physical illness or handicap	5	7.2	5	0
Special academic pursuits†	24	34.8	24	0
Personal and family reasons	4	5.8	1	3
Total	69	99.9	65	4

* None of the 36 non-European subjects dropped back.

† See text.

year medical schools. The remaining eight entered in the second year.

A total of 89 students left medical school and did not return. Two-thirds of the dropouts left by the end of the first year and another 21 percent left by the end of the second year. The remaining 12 percent left at various times during the last two years. Academic failure was the principal cause of leaving in the first and, to a lesser extent, in the second year, while overt psychological disorders predominated as reasons for dropping out in the last two years.

Compelling reasons for leaving medical school included dismissal for academic failure or reasons of character, death, and hospitalization for mental illness (Table 3-IV). Other reasons for leaving were less clearcut. Those who left before receiving any grades and those who withdrew after having been warned of low academic standing ostensibly lost interest in becoming physicians or changed their goals. Dislike of anatomy and fear of failure invoked by a given teacher, however, were frequent overtones in the students' decision-making process. These were often more important than the stated reasons, which varied from "decided to go into teaching" to "emotional block" or "painful back." Some left without any explanation. The interplay of academic, family, financial, and emotional stresses for each individual was usually complex.

Nine men included in Table 3-IV dropped back a year or two before dropping out. Seven are included in the first group, "dropped by school for academic failure." Three of these men failed both before and after a repeated year. Three who failed at the end of a year repeated the required work but, of their own volition, did not go on. One dropped back because of mental illness, and his subsequent failure was intertwined with continuing psychological problems which did not appear to require hospitalization. The eighth man, who failed and was repeating his first year, was hospitalized for mental illness in the middle of that year. The ninth man obtained a Ph.D. following two years of medical school; on his return he failed in one course, was warned of low academic standing and withdrew. Although reasons for dropping back and leaving medical school were variably apparent, academic failure was involved sooner or later in each case.

In contrast to the tuberculosis so prevalent among medical students in Paget's day, health problems among Precursors Study dropouts were primarily psychological. Only in the case of one man who died of leukemia was a serious medical disease involved. Including two deaths from suicide, 14 of the 89 dropouts failed to

Table 3-IV

Dropouts: Reasons for Leaving This Medical School

Reason	Total No. = 1337		White Males No. = 1185		White Females No. = 116		Other Males and Females No. = 36	
	No.	%	No.	%	No.	%	No.	%
Dropped by school for academic failure	38	42.7	31	45.6	3	21.4	4	57.1
Dropped by school for reasons of character	4	4.5	3	4.4	1	7.1	0	0.0
Died as a medical student	3	3.4	3	4.4	0	0.0	0	0.0
Hospitalized for mental illness	8	9.0	6	8.8	2	14.3	0	0.0
Left before receiving any grades	14	15.7	13	19.1	1	7.1	0	0.0
Warned of low academic standing and withdrew	8	9.0	5	7.4	2	14.3	1	14.3
Transferred to another medical school*	6	6.7	4†	5.9	2	14.3	0	0.0
Transferred to graduate school*	4	4.5	2	2.9	0	0.0	2	28.6
Personal and family reasons	4	4.5	1	1.5	3	21.4	0	0.0
Total	89	100.0	68	100.0	14	99.9	7	100.0

* Transferred directly; does not include those who obtained an M.D. or other graduate degree after an interval.

† One of these men had transferred *into* Johns Hopkins but shortly dropped out and returned to his original medical school.

graduate because of mental illness or character disturbance.

Proportionately, half as many white females as males left medical school because of academic failure. Also, white females were less than half as likely to leave before receiving any grades. Among the women, personal and family reasons equalled academic failure as a reason for leaving, although only three individuals were involved in each case. In addition, two women who withdrew after being warned of low academic standing were known to have personal or family problems. Four men transferred to other medical schools for personal or family reasons; all graduated. Their moves were associated with the death or illness of a parent, living at home to save money, or moving to be close to wife and children. Two women transferred to other medical schools and graduated on time to be with husband or children, and one woman who left Johns Hopkins for personal and family reasons graduated from another medical school after an interval.

Four students, two of whom were of Oriental ancestry, transferred directly to graduate school. Of the three who received Ph.D.'s in basic science from the Johns Hopkins University, all had failed one subject or been warned of low marks; however all were in good standing when they left medical school at the end of the first or second year. One student lost interest in medicine and left before receiving any grades; he obtained a Ph.D. in liberal arts at another university in preparation for teaching at the college level, a plan he had long considered.

The time of marriage for both graduates and nongraduates is shown in Table 3-V. A greater proportion of nongraduate than graduate men married before medical school, but a smaller proportion married during or after medical school. While it is not surprising that fewer dropouts married during medical school (since their average time in school was shortened), the nongraduates tended to remain single. Although the validity of the comparison is limited by the men in both groups whose marital status is unknown, it appears that three or four times as many nongraduates as graduates did not marry. The pattern for the total group of women is similar to that for men, with the exception that three times as many women remained single. In this cohort, 40.5 percent of all women married before or during medical school and were rarely deterred by marriage from graduating and beginning a career in medicine. As with the men, a greater proportion of female graduates than nongraduates married during medical school. The proportions of female graduates and nongraduates who never married, however, are similar.

The mean age at graduation was 25.9 years for all 1216 men and

Table 3-V

Marital Status of Men and Women by Graduation Status

Marital Status	Men						Women					
	Total		Graduates		Nongraduates		Total		Graduates		Nongraduates	
	No.	%	No.	%	No.	%	No.	%	No.	%	No.	%
Married before medical school	165	13.6	153	13.4	12	16.2	13	10.7	11	10.4	2	13.3
		(14.2)		(13.9)		(21.1)						
Married during medical school	381	31.3	371	32.5	10	13.5	36	29.8	33	31.1	3	20.0
		(32.9)		(33.7)		(17.5)						
Married after medical school	533	43.8	512	44.8	21	28.4	46	38.0	40	37.7	6	40.0
		(46.0)		(46.5)		(36.8)						
Never married*	80	6.6	66	5.8	14	18.9	26	21.5	22	20.8	4	26.7
		(6.9)		(6.0)		(24.6)						
Unknown†	57	4.7	40	3.5	17	23.0	0	0.0	0	0.0	0	0.0
		(—)		(—)		(—)						
Total	1216	100.0	1142	100.0	74	100.0	121	100.0	106	100.0	15	100.0
(Total Known)	(1159)	(100.0)	(1102)	(100.1)	(57)	(100.0)						

Percentages in parentheses are based on the total number of men with *known* marital status.

* As of latest information.

† No recent information.

25.8 years for all 121 women. The "age at graduation" for nongraduates and dropbacks was projected from their ages at the time of entering medical school. Table 3-VI shows the average ages for male and female graduates and nongraduates grouped by marital status. Those married before medical school were slightly older than those in other groups. The male nongraduates were slightly older than the graduates in all groups; this was not true for female nongraduates, however.

Diverse Careers

What kinds of careers have medical school graduates and nongraduates pursued? Although this question encompasses a broader view of the individual lives of Precursors Study subjects than we shall explore here, the primary information is useful. The medical fields of interest for 1263 men and women who graduated from Hopkins or elswhere are shown in Table 3-VII. Specialty interests of deceased physicians are included. The areas of specialization have been sharpened since our early reports, when the later classes were still completing residency training and military service (13,14). Although a few individuals have moved from one specialty to another, the overall distribution of male physicians by specialty has changed little since our most recent report (15). The present study compares specialty choice by sex in this population for the first time. Although internal medicine has been the leading choice for both men and women, it is clear that a greater proportion of men have selected careers in the surgical specialties and a greater proportion of women have entered upon careers in the fields of pediatrics and psychiatry.

Although information about the occupational pursuits of the 89 nongraduates is incomplete, the results of our inquiries are outlined in Table 3-VIII. Fifteen students who did not graduate from Hopkins became physicians; six transferred directly to another medical school and graduated on time, while the rest obtained M.D.'s elsewhere after an interval. Three have gone into pediatrics, three into general practice, two into dermatology, two into thoracic surgery, and one each into anesthesiology, neurosurgery, preventive medicine, psychiatry, and radiology. Ten other nongraduates entered medically related fields on a professional level; the proportion of women doing this is three times that of men.

Twenty-four men and one woman entered other professional fields, including education, law, the ministry, and military service.

Table 3-VI

Age at Graduation* by Marital Status, Sex, and Graduation Status

Marital Status	Men				Women			
	Graduates		Nongraduates		Graduates		Nongraduates	
	No.	Mean Age	No.	Mean Age	No.	Mean Age	No.	Mean Age
Married before medical school	153	28.2	12	30.4	11	27.5	2	31.5
Married during medical school	371	25.5	10	26.5	33	25.8	3	25.7
Married after medical school	512	25.3	21	26.3	40	25.3	6	25.0
Never married†	66	25.9	14	26.0	22	25.8	4	25.2
Unknown ‡	40	25.7	17	26.5	0	0.0	0	0.0
Total	1142	25.8	74	27.0	106	25.7	15	26.1

* See text.
† As of latest information.
‡ No recent information.

Table 3-VII

Distribution of 1263 Physicians* by Primary Medical Specialty Interest and Sex

Specialty†	Total		Males		Females	
	No.	%	No.	%	No.	%
Internal medicine	334	26.4	301	26.1	33	30.3
Pediatrics	117	9.3	96	8.3	21	19.3
Other medical specialties	57	4.5	49	4.2	8	7.3
General surgery	204	16.2	201	17.4	3	2.8
Obstetrics/Gynecology	59	4.7	57	4.9	2	1.8
Ophthalmology	59	4.7	57	4.9	2	1.8
Other surgical specialties	108	8.6	107	9.3	1	0.9
Psychiatry	85	6.7	70	6.1	15	13.8
Pathology	77	6.1	75	6.5	2	1.8
Radiology	29	2.3	26	2.2	3	2.8
Anesthesiology	23	1.8	18	1.6	5	4.6
General practice	53	4.2	47	4.1	6	5.5
Preventive/Administrative/ Legal medicine	29	2.3	25	2.2	4	3.7
Preclinical or biological science	25	2.0	24	2.1	1	0.9
None	4	0.3	1	0.1	3	2.8
Total	1263	100.1	1154	100.0	109	100.1

* Includes 15 who graduated from other medical schools.

† Based primarily on the Directory of Medical Specialists, 16th edition, 1974-1975. If not listed there, then the American Medical Directory, 26th edition, 1973, was used, or earlier editions for those who had died. Those who had not answered the recent A.M.D. questionnaire were classified as in the Directory of Graduates of the School of Medicine of the Johns Hopkins University, 1969.

Table 3-VIII
Occupation of 89 Nongraduates from the Johns Hopkins School of Medicine at Last Information or at Death*

Group	Occupation	Total		Males		Females	
		No.	%	No.	%	No.	%
I.	Physician	14	15.7	11	14.9	3	20.0
	Teaching/research/administration:						
II.	Medically related	10	11.2	6	8.1	4	26.7
III.	College or postgraduate level	15	16.9	14	18.9	1	6.7
IV.	School or indeterminate level	4	4.5	4	5.4	0	0.0
V.	Other professional: law, ministry, military	6	6.7	6	8.1	0	0.0
VI.	Business administration and sales	11	12.4	11	14.9	0	0.0
VII.	Housewife	3	3.4	0	0.0	3	20.0
VIII.	Student	6	6.7	4	5.4	2	13.3
IX.	Clerical/manual skills	3	3.4	2	2.7	1	6.7
X.	None	5†	5.6	4	5.4	1	6.7
XI.	Unknown	12	13.5	12	16.2	0	0.0
Total		89	100.0	74	100.0	15	100.1

* This table includes the 15 physicians who graduated elsewhere who are also included in Table VII.
† Includes one man who transferred directly to another medical school and became a physician.

The eleven men in the business category have reported jobs of varying degrees of responsibility, including laundry superintendent, food and drug coordinator, senior specialist in pharmaceutical sales, and partner in an investment counseling firm. Some are self-employed; others have changed jobs or had apparent gaps in their employment records. Three women reported "housewife" as their occupation. Group VIII includes two married women who are studying for advanced degrees in law and genetics, one man who is studying for a Ph.D. in music, and three men who died in medical school. The two men and one woman in Group IX have been employed as carpenter, orderly, and clerk-typist. All five subjects in Group X listed as having no occupation were hospitalized for mental illness; four of them have died. Of the twelve nongraduates whose occupations are unknown, one man has returned to the Middle East and cannot be traced. Another forged his academic records to enter Hopkins and other medical schools; when last heard about, he was under arrest in Canada for forgery. The others posed a variety of serious problems in communication.

It is important to emphasize that many non-graduates have earned advanced degrees. Of the 25 subjects in Groups II and III, 16 obtained Ph.D. degrees after leaving medical school, and one had a Ph.D. before starting medical school. All four women in medically related fields obtained Ph.D.'s and are currently active in academic teaching, research, or both. None of the four subjects in Group IV, however, have reported any postgraduate study. Those in Group V have all completed the graduate work necessary for their chosen professions. Five members of Group VI have taken graduate work, two in chemistry and three in business administration. Two women in Group VII have obtained Master's degrees in English and Education. The three living subjects in Group VIII are pursuing advanced degrees, as stated above. One man in Group III has a Master of Science and one man in Group IX obtained a Master's degree in Physics. In all, of the 89 dropouts, 15 have obtained M.D.'s, 16 have Ph.D.'s, two are working for Ph.D.'s, six have earned the appropriate degrees to become lawyers, ministers or military experts, one is attending law school, nine have Master's degrees (not counting those who also have Ph.D.'s), and several others have done some graduate work. Thus over half have pursued additional education at the postgraduate level.

Untoward Outcomes

In adults, premature death usually refers to death before age 65 (16). In this report, however, it is defined as death occurring before the age of 60, since none of the very few subjects over that age have died. Causes of death have been ascertained from death certificates and autopsy reports supplemented by physicians' statements and hospital records. Death certificates were obtained for all deceased subjects except two who died in accidents at sea. Autopsies were performed in over two-thirds of the cases; where not performed, the cause of death was usually self-evident, as in certain instances of suicide and in subjects with maligant tumors who had biopsies or operations.

As of November 1, 1975, 49 subjects, or 3.7 percent of the cohort of 1337 subjects, have died prematurely. Forty-three were white males and six were white females. Almost half of the deceased subjects died before reaching the age of 40:

Age	*No.*	*%*
20-29	9	18.4
30-39	15	30.6
40-49	22	44.9
50-59	3	6.1
Total	49	100.0

Causes of death are shown in Table 3-IX. Suicide was the most frequent cause, accounting for at least 34.7 percent of deaths. These 17 subjects killed themselves by the following means:

Barbiturate poisoning	7
Other poisonous substances	2
Firearms	3
Hanging	3
Cutting instrument	1
Jumping from high place	1

The importance of psychological factors in other deaths is sometimes clear and sometimes uncertain. Alcoholism is often viewed as another form of self-destruction. Alcohol-related deaths include two men who died of cirrhosis of the liver and one who died of acute hemorrhagic pancreatitis. Because the cause of death stated on the death certificate may be inaccurate or deliberately misleading, particularly in the case of suicide, it is probable that several deaths included under "accidents" or "other deaths" may, in fact, have been additional suicides. Nine men died in accidents, six involving airplanes and two involving automobiles; one was a boating accident. While some, such as the two tragic crashes of commercial airliners, were clearly accidental, others, such as the single-car automobile accident or the disappearance of a rented Beechcraft piloted by the subject in a flight over the ocean, were ambiguous, and may not have been accidental. Causes of six "other deaths" range from fulminating ulcerative colitis immediately following several stressful events to subacute bacterial endocarditis on a congenitally bicuspid valve in which psychological factors were not obvious. The remaining four include two in which suicide was a possible terminal event.

In two groups the final cause of death was clearly organic, whatever the psychological precursors might have been. Eight men and one woman died from malignant tumors: three from carcinoma of the pancreas, and one each from acute lymphoblastic leukemia, astrocytoma, reticulum cell sarcoma, rhabdomyosarcoma, carcinoma of the tongue, and adenocarcinoma of the lung. Five men died during acute episodes of myocardial infarction. In four, death occurred within a few hours of onset and the diagnosis was confirmed at autopsy.

Psychological disorders which affected Precursors Study subjects took many forms, varying not only from subject to subject but in the same subject from time to time. Because our knowledge of the circumstances surrounding the onset and course of the disorder is often inadequate, we have used an operational definition of mental illness, which embraces psychological disturbances sufficiently profound to lead to a period of hospitalization. A few subjects without known hospitalization are included in this category because their clinical patterns more closely resembled mental illness than emotional disturbance. The term emotional disturbance is used to classify subjects with evidence of psychological problems which appear to have been less pervasive that those of the mental illness group. If mental illness is thought of as comparable to psychosis, then emotional disturbance falls in the area of psychoneurosis. Included in this latter category are subjects with anxiety-tension states, mild depression, psychopathic personality, alcoholism, drug abuse, and those who have received psychotherapy for unspecified reasons.

Of the 54 subjects who have suffered from mental illness, 14 have

Table 3-IX

Causes of Premature Death Among Total Precursors Study Subjects by Sex

Cause of Death	Deaths						Age at Death		
	Total No. = 1337		Males No. = 1216		Females No. = 121		Range	Median	Mean
	No.	%	No.	%	No.	%			
Suicide	17	34.7	13	30.2	4	66.7	22–48	32	34.6
Accident	9	18.4	9	20.9	0	0.0	27–47	34	38.0
Malignant tumor	9	18.4	8	18.6	1	16.7	24–57	45	44.3
Myocardial infarction	5	10.2	5	11.6	0	0.0	42–49	45	45.2
Alcohol-related	3	6.1	3	7.0	0	0.0	33–46	39	39.3
Other cause	6	12.2	5	11.6	1	16.7	21–47	39.5	36.5
Total Deaths	49	100.0	43	99.9	6	100.1	21–57	40	38.6

died; this includes 11 of the 17 suicides. Of the remaining three, all spent considerable time in mental hospitals and two died there; one of these two deaths was alcohol-related. Forty subjects with known episodes of mental illness are living; most of them have regained their equilibrium.

At least 86 subjects have been emotionally disturbed at some time. Emotional disturbance preceded five instances of malignant tumor, two of myocardial infarction, and one of hypertension. In one subject it followed hypertension and malignant tumor, and in another subject it followed autoimmune disease and benign tumor.

Some 84 living subjects have been affected by one of the medical disorders under current investigation to an extent warranting definitive therapeutic intervention. Forty-two subjects have been treated for malignant tumor by some combination of surgery, radiation, and chemotherapy. Twenty-eight subjects have received treatment for essential hypertension. One man with renal hypertension underwent dialysis followed by kidney transplantation. Ten subjects have recovered from myocardial infarctions. One man was hospitalized for coronary insufficiency, and two men had coronary bypass operations for angina pectoris. Peptic ulcer, bronchial asthma and diabetes mellitus, affecting nearly 100 subjects all told, are among the most prevalent disorders we have not yet studied.

Interrelationship of Academic Status and Premature Death

In all, 39 graduates and 10 nongraduates have died (Table 3-X). The percentage of deceased nongraduates is 3.6 times as high as that of graduates, and the proportion of deaths is greater for the nongraduates in each causal group. Three of the 10 nongraduates died in medical school: one committed suicide a few weeks after entering school; the second, who stood in the upper third of his class after his second year, committed suicide in his third year; the third received a warning at the end of his first year and developed acute leukemia in the fall of his second year.

Seven nongraduates died five to 20 years after leaving medical school. Five had left because of academic failure, one because of mental illness and one because of emotional disturbance; the three who first dropped back and then dropped out because of academic failure are included in this group. Three of the seven were in mental hospitals at the time of deaths from suicide, alcohol-related cause, and uncertain cause. The other four died of suicide, malignant tumor, acute myocardial infarction and accident.

Table 3-X

Causes of Premature Death by Graduation Status

Cause of Death	Total Cohort No. = 1337		Graduates No. = 1248		Nongraduates No. = 89	
	No.	%	No.	%	No.	%
Suicide	17	1.3	13	1.0	4	4.5
Accident	9	0.7	8	0.6	1	1.1
Malignant tumor	9	0.7	7	0.6	2	2.2
Myocardial infarction	5	0.4	4	0.3	1	1.1
Alcohol-related	3	0.2	2	0.2	1	1.1
Other cause	6	0.4	5	0.4	1	1.1
Total Deaths	49	3.7	39	3.1	10	11.2

Premature death has also occurred with differing frequency when subgroups of the graduates are compared. Among the 1105 regular graduates, 32 (2.9%) have died, compared with six (4.2%) of the 143 dropbacks and transfer students combined. While this difference is smaller than that in the graduate-nongraduate comparison, the trend is in the same direction. There were two deaths in the dropback group, both from cancer, occurring in two of the 24 subjects who dropped back because of academic failure. Two of the four deaths in the transfer group were from suicide. Thus suicide and cancer predominate as causes of death among former medical students whose academic course was irregular.

The relationship of premature death to academic performance is shown in Table 3-XI. There the 49 deceased subjects are grouped according to overall rank in class at the end of the fourth year, or at the end of the last complete academic year for those who dropped out. Premature death is underrepresented in the middle third, where its prevalence was less than in the upper or lower thirds. This was especially true for the suicide group, which is bimodal in distribution, as is the tiny number of alcohol-related deaths. Those who died in accidents, on the other hand, are evenly distributed by rank in class. Death from myocardial infarction and from other causes was more common among subjects who ranked in the lowest third of their classes. Combining those who failed with those ranking in the lowest third, almost half of those dying prematurely were marked by poor academic performance in medical school.

DISCUSSION

The evidence presented in this survey strongly suggests that

Table 3-XI

Causes of Premature Death by Academic Standing

Rank in Class	Premature Deaths						
	Total	Suicide	Accident	Malignant Tumor	Myocardial Infarction	Alcohol-Related	Other Cause
	No.	No.	No.	No.	No.	No.	No.
First third	15	6	3	4	1	1	0
Second third	9	3	3	2	0	0	1
Third third	18	6	2	2	3	1	4
Failed	5	1	1	0	1	1	1
Died or left without marks	2	1	0	1	0	0	0
Total	49	17	9	9	5	3	6

failure in medical school and failure in life are frequently interrelated. The findings clearly indicate that psychological stamina is of vital importance to the entering medical student if he or she is to reach the goal of becoming a sound physician. Superior intelligence alone is not enough. As Sir James Paget said, "the personal character, the very nature, the will" must be strong if the student is to survive the rigors of medical school, residency training, and the practice and teaching of medicine. The inroads made by premature death and early psychological disorders in this carefully selected cohort represent a substantial loss to medicine and to society, as well as personal tragedies for the victims and their families. As of this time, no more than 90 percent of the 1337 former Johns Hopkins medical students in the classes of 1948 through 1964 are living and active in the medical profession. (The actual proportion is some what smaller, as an uncertain few have left the profession because of illness or change of interest.) While this is a much better record than the 72 percent of successful students reported by Paget, it is a sobering fact that more than 10 percent of the medical students in the Johns Hopkins cohort failed to reach their full potential as physicians.

It is our long-held view that psychological factors contribute in yet undetermined ways to many forms of premature death. In support of this hypothesis, we have already identified several psychological precursors of suicide, mental illness, malignant tumor, hypertension, and coronary occlusion which were present in medical school but went unrecognized (17-23). The present study suggests that poor self-image, damaged self-esteem and covert depression, anger, and fear take their toll when certain students undergo the pressures of medical school. How these sensitive and vulnerable individuals are to be recognized and how they can be fostered and strengthened remains one of the most compelling problems in preventive medicine.

REFERENCES

1. Paget J: What becomes of medical students? *In Selected Essays and Addresses* by Sir James Paget. Paget S, Ed. London: Longmans, Green and Co., pp. 27-32, 1902
2. Johnson DG and Hutchins EB: Doctor or dropout? A study of medical student attrition. *J Med Educ 41* (special issue): 1097-1274, 1966
3. AMA council on Mental Health: The sick physician, impairment by psychiatric disorders, including alcoholism and drug dependence. *JAMA 223*: 684-687,

1973

4. Small IF et al.: The fate of the mentally ill physician. *Amer J Psych 125:* 1333-1342, 1969
5. a'Brook MF, Hailstone JD, and McLaughlan IEJ: Psychiatric illness in the medical profession. *Br J Psych 113:* 1013-1023, 1967
6. Duffy JC and Litin EM: Psychiatric morbidity of physicians. *JAMA 189:* 989-992, 1964
7. Pearson MM and Strecker EA: Physicians as psychiatric patients: Private practice experience. *Amer J Psych 116:* 915-919, 1960
8. Freeman W: Psychiatrists who kill themselves: A study in suicide. *Amer J Psych 126:* 846-867, 1967
9. Modlin HC and Montes A: Narcotics addiction in physicians. *Amer J Psych 121:* 358-365, 1964
10. Blachly PH, Disher W, and Roduner G: Suicide by physicians. *Bull Suicide,* pp. 1-18, Dec 1968
11. Rose KD and Rosow I: Physicians who kill themselves. *Arch Gen Psych 29:* 800-805, 1973
12. Shapiro ET, Pinsker H, and Shale JH: The mentally ill physician as practitioner. *JAMA 232*: 725-727, 1975
13. Thomas CB and Monk MA: Characteristics of male medical students related to their subsequent careers. *Johns Hopkins Med J 127:* 254-272, 1970
14. Westling-Wikstrand H, Monk MA, and Thomas CB: Some characteristics related to the career status of women physicians. *Johns Hopkins Med J 127:* 273-286, 1970
15. Monk MA and Thomas CB: Personal and social factors related to medical specialty practice. *Johns Hopkins Med J 133:* 19-29, 1973
16. Cooper T and Mitchell SC: Arteriosclerosis – A problem in diagnosis, treatment and prevention. *J Chron Dis 22:* 377-380, 1969
17. Thomas CB: Suicide among us: II. Habits of nervous tension as potential predictors. *Johns Hopkins Med J 129:* 190-201, 1971
18. Thomas CB and Greenstreet RL: Psychobiological characteristics in youth as predictors of five disease states: Suicide, mental illness, hypertension, coronary heart disease and tumor. *Johns Hopkins Med J 132:* 16-43, 1973
19. Epstein LC et al.: Clinical prediction of physician suicide based on medical student data. *J Nerv Ment Dis 156:* 19-29, 1973
20. Thomas CB et al.: A prospective study of the Rorschachs of suicides: The predictive potential of pathological content. *Johns Hopkins Med J 132:* 334-360, 1973
21. Thomas CB and Duszynski KR: Closeness to parents and the family constellation in a prospective study of five disease states: Suicide, mental illness, malignant tumor, hypertension and coronary heart disease. *Johns Hopkins Med J 134:* 251-270, 1974
22. Thomas CB, Ross DC, and Duszynski KR: Youthful hypercholesteremia: Its associated characteristics and role in premature myocardial infarction. *Johns Hopkins Med J 136:* 193-208, 1975
23. Harrower M, Thomas CB, and Altman A: Human figure drawings in a pro-

spective study of six disorders: Hypertension, coronary heart disease, malignant tumor, suicide, mental illness, and emotional disturbance, *J Nerv Ment Dis 161:* 191-199, 1975

Alcoholism

Chapter 4

ALCOHOLISM AMONGST MALE DOCTORS IN SCOTLAND

ROBIN M. MURRAY

INTRODUCTION

THERE is a widespread assumption that doctors are especially prone to alcoholism,[1,2] and the "alcoholic doctor" has been the subject of recent discussion,[3-5] but convincing evidence that doctors are a high-risk group has not been forthcoming. In the published series of mentally ill doctors the proportion diagnosed as alcoholic has ranged from 12% to 68%.[6] These studies are, however, open to criticism on the grounds that (a) they were carried out in prestigious hospitals or clinics to which sick doctors would be preferentially attracted, and (b) where controls were used neither they nor the doctor-patients were drawn from populations of known size. Scotland has provided the opportunity for a more definitive study; the Scottish Hospitals Research and Intelligence Unit (S.H.R.I.U.) collects information including diagnosis and occupation regarding all patients in mental hospitals and psychiatric units in general and teaching hospitals,[7,8] and regular censuses are carried out on the Scottish population, thus providing an estimate of the population served by the Scottish psychiatric impatient beds.

METHODS

Information was requested from the S.H.R.I.U. regarding the first admissions to (for the years 1963, 1965, 1968, 1972), and total discharges from (for the years 1963-72) Scottish psychiatric inpatient beds of male medical practitioners who had received a primary diagnosis of alcoholism or alcoholic psychosis (numbers 307 and 322 in the 7th revision and 291 and 303 in the 8th revision of the International Classification of Diseases). A minimum age of 25 years was

From Robin M. Murray, Alcoholism Amongst Male Doctors in Scotland. *The Lancet, 2:* 729-731, 1976. Courtesy of *The Lancet* and the author.

The author is grateful to the S.H.R.I.U. for their unfailing cooperation.

chosen because of the relatively small numbers of qualified doctors below that age. Female doctors were excluded because of potential inaccuracies introduced by the practice of recording the occupation of a married woman as that of her husband. Non-medical social class I males aged 25 years and over were taken as a control group, and similar information was requested regarding their admissions and discharges. The data were provided by the S.H.R.I.U. in the form of computer print-outs, and no attempt was made to obtain the names of, or identify in any way, either the doctors or controls.

The numbers and age-distribution of all male medical practitioners and non-medical social class I males aged 25 years and over residing in Scotland at the time of the 1961 and 1971 censuses were provided by the Registrar General for Scotland (personal communications, 1974 and 1976). Their numbers and age-distribution were then estimated for each of the years 1963-72, assuming population change to be distributed equally over the years 1961-71 and the same trends projected to 1972. These methods have been described fully elsewhere[6] and further details may be obtained from the author.

RESULTS

First Admissions

During the four years studied a total of 48 male doctors and 121 non-medical social class I males aged 25 years and over were admitted for the first time to Scottish psychiatric inpatient beds with a primary diagnosis of alcoholism. (The term alcoholism is henceforth used to refer both to alcoholism and alcoholic psychosis.) These figures represented mean annual first-admission rates for alcoholism of 165 per 100,000 for doctors and 60 per 100,000 for controls; this difference was statistically significant ($P < 0.001$).

All Discharges

Over the ten years 1963-72 there were 272 discharges of male doctors and 651 discharges of non-medical social class I males with a primary diagnosis of alcoholism. These figures accounted for 39.8% and 32.5% respectively of the total discharges (for all diagnoses) of male doctors and other social class I males from Scottish psychiatric inpatient beds. Figure 4-I, which shows the age-specific discharge rates for alcoholism, shows that the rates for both groups were highest between 45 and 54 years but the peak was very much higher for doctors. Of the total 218 discharges of male doctors (for all diagnoses) aged between 45 and 54 years, 127 (58%) were attributable to alcoholism. There were no significant trends in rates for either doctors or controls over the decade.

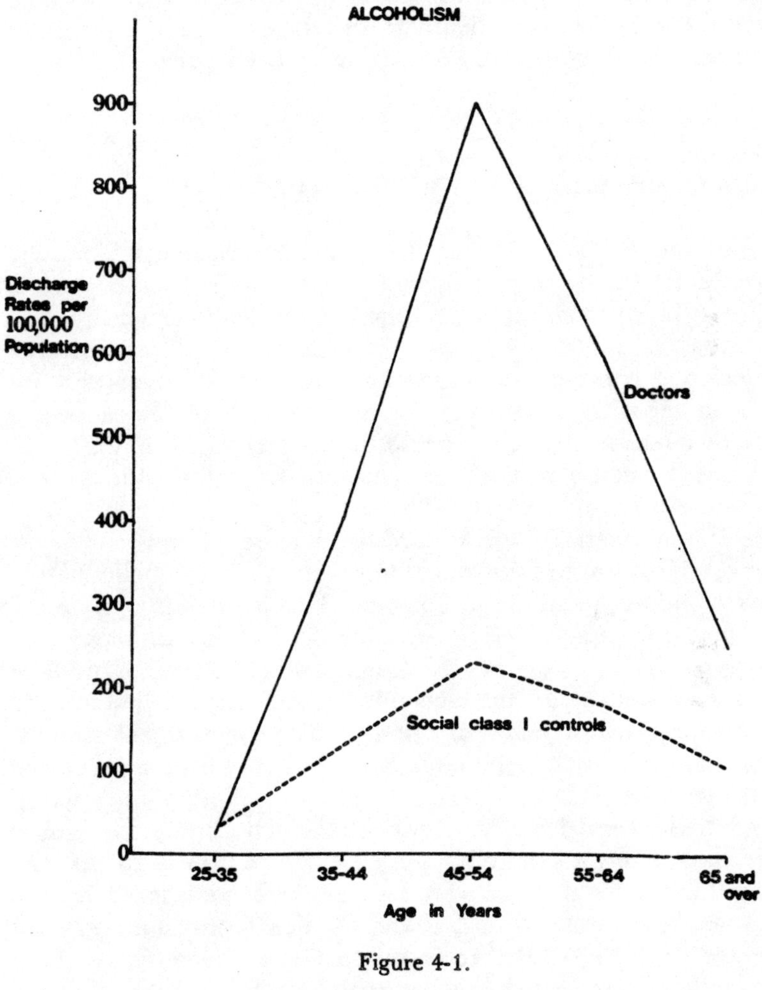

Figure 4-1.

DISCUSSION

The findings that first-admission rates for alcoholism were 2.7 times higher amongst male doctors than amongst their social and economic equals confirms the suspicions of those who have maintained that doctors are a high-risk group for alcoholism. The special position of doctors in relation to medical treatment and factors such as their greater access to psychiatrists may have contributed to their higher rates, but it is improbable that they accounted for much of the excess. Independent evidence that doctors are especially prone to alcoholism comes from an examination of their death-rate from cirrhosis of the liver. These data are not available for Scottish doctors, but over the past 50 years death from cirrhosis amongst medical pracititioners in England and Wales have been greater than expected:

	1911	*1921*	*1931*	*1951*	*1961*
Standard mortality ratio for doctors (%)	114	185	183	250	350

It is, of course, possible that cirrhosis amongst doctors may be less closely associated with alcoholism than amongst the general population. The probability of alcoholic cirrhosis is generally considered to be related to the level and length of alcohol consumption.[10] It has been tentatively suggested, however, that infection with hepatitis-B virus may be necessary for the development of alcoholic cirrhosis;[11] doctors could be more exposed to this virus. If this were the cause of the high standard mortality ratio for cirrhosis amongst doctors one would have expected nurses to have had a similarly high death-rate from cirrhosis — they do not.[9]

A larger percentage of doctors in this study were alcoholic than in previous reports of mentally ill doctors.[6] This is probably related to the fact that only male doctors were included in my investigation, and to the particular frequency of alcoholism in Scotland. a'Brook et al.[12] found a tendency for the alcoholic doctors they studied to have graduated more commonly from Irish or Scottish medical schools, and Irish and Scottish graduates are similarly over-represented amongst alcoholic doctors appearing before the Disciplinary Committee of the General Medical Council.[13] Alcoholism is the mental disorder most likely to interfere with a doctor's ability to practice competently. Of 97 doctors whose cases were considered by the Penal Cases Committee of the General Medical Council in 1974 but not referred further, 39 resulted from the abuse of alcohol; 14 of the 46 more serious cases considered by the Disciplinary Committee of the same body arose from alcohol abuse.[14] Over an eleven-year period 3.2% of the medical practitioners in one American state appeared before their professional disciplinary board on charges arising from the abuse of alcohol.[15]

Occupation is an important etiological factor in alcoholism, and two reviews[16,17] have emphasised the predisposing effects of (a) availability of cheap or free alcohol; (b) strong peer pressure to drink; (c) lack of supervision at work; and (d) separation from normal sexual or social relationships. The last factor does not usually apply to doctors, but the other three merit examination. National per-caput alcohol consumption is considerably influenced by the price of alcohol,[18] and within communities consumption may be related to disposable income. As doctors' income is well above the average for the whole community, alcohol is relatively cheap for them. Glatt[5] has already remarked on the peer pressure on medical students and doctors to drink, and since many doctors work free of close supervision they may be able to conceal their drinking more easily than those in other occupations.

Alcoholism is a preventable disorder. There are two obvious ways of altering doctors' drinking habits. The first, decreasing their available income for alcohol, is unlikely to be welcomed. The second is education to the dangers of sustained heavy drinking. The change in doctors' smoking habits sets an important precedent. Knowledge of the risk of bronchial carcinoma resulted in decreased smoking to the extent that the standard mortality ratio for lung cancer amongst doctors is now 48 percent of that of the general population.[9]

REFERENCES

1. Glatt, M. M. *Lancet*, 1974, II, 342.
2. Standing Medical Advisory Committee on Alcoholism. H.M. Stationery Office, 1973.
3. Edwards, G. *Lancet*, 1975, II, 1297.
4. Shribman, I. *ibid.* 1976, I, 88.
5. Glatt, M.M. *ibid.* p.196.
6. Murray, R.M. M. Phil thesis. University of London, 1976.
7. Heasman, M. A. *Hlth Bull.* 1968, 26, 4, 1.
8. Lockwood, E. *Br. F. prev. soc. Med.* 1971, 25, 76.
9. Registrar General. Decennial Supplements on Occupational Mortality. 1971, and also earlier supplements relating to 1911, 1921, 1931, 1951. H.M. Stationery Office.
10. Lelbach, W.K. *in* Research Advances in Alcohol and Drug Problems Vol. 1 (edited by R.J. Gibbins, Y. Israel, H. Kalant, R.E. Popham, W. Schmidt, and R.G. Smart); New York, 1974
11. Pettigrew, N.M., Goudie, R.B., Russel, R.I., Chaudhuri, A.K.R. *Lancet*, 1972, ii, 724
12. a'Brook, M.F., Hailstone, J.D., McLaughlan, I.E. *Br. J. Psychiat.* 1967, 113,1013.
13. Cargill, D. *Wld Med.* 1976, 11,22.

14. General Medical Council. Annual JReport. London. 1974
15. American Medical Association. *J. Am. Med. Ass.* 1973, 223, 684.
16. Murray, R.M. *F. Alcoholism,* 1975, 10, 23.
17. Plant, M. *Bri. F. Addiction,* (in the press).
18. Bruun, K., et al. Alcohol Control Policies in Public Health Perspective. Finnish Foundation for Alcohol Studies, Volume 25. Helsinki, 1975.

Chapter 5

THE ALCOHOLIC PHYSICIAN: A SURVEY

LECLAIR BISSELL AND ROBERT W. JONES

ALTHOUGH the problem of drug dependence in our society is receiving increased public and professional attention, information about the alcoholic physician is still relatively scarce. Seventy percent of adult Americans do drink, and of these an estimated 6 percent to 10 percent develop alcoholism (1). Assuming that physicians do not differ from their countrymen in drinking practices, then about 226,800 of our 324,000 physicians (2) are drinkers and between 13,600 and 22,600 are or will become alcoholics. The actual number is likely to fall toward the upper end of this range because of the large number of men in the physician population and because of the apparent relationship between alcoholism and higher educational attainment (3). More than four times as many men as women are alcoholics (3). The proportion of drinkers among college graduates is markedly higher than that among other educational levels, and generally, the greater the proportion of drinkers, the higher the rate of alcoholism. In addition, Glatt (4) reported an above average standard mortality rate from cirrhosis of the liver among English physicians, and many studies of physicians undergoing psychiatric treatment have reported that alcoholism is a common finding (5-12).

That alcoholism frequently precedes or underlies addiction to other drugs has been mentioned repeatedly. Vincent (13) stated that half of all alcoholic physicians eventually develop drug addiction. Modlin and Montes (14) reported that 25 physician addicts at Menninger Memorial Hospital, Topeka, Kan., all used varying amounts of alcohol, analgesics, sedatives, or ataractics in combination with narcotics. In a 1966 study of 68 physician addicts at the U.S. Public Health Service Hospital in Lexington, Ky., alcoholism, chronic

---

From LeClair Bissell and Robert W. Jones, The Alcoholic Physician: A Survey. *The American Journal of Psychiatry, 133:*1142-1146, 1976.

This work was supported in part by a grant from the Richard Ettinger Foundation, New York, New York.

The authors wish to express their appreciation to Barry Leach, Barbara Goodman, Ph.D., Jean Meyer, Judy Stires, and Elizabeth Hahn, all of whom variously worked on questionnaire design, interviewing, analysis, and typing for this study.

fatigue, and physical disease were the principal reasons given for the beginning of self-medication (15). Also frequently reported is the high incidence of alcoholism in association with physician suicides (16). Blachly and associates (17) studied 80 physicians who killed themselves during the period 1965-1967 and found that 39 percent were described as alcoholic or heavy drinkers and 19 percent were drinking at the time of their death.

Most of the available information about the alcoholic physician is drawn from observations of hospitalized patients or those under psychiatric treatment. We found only one prospective study in the literature, that of Vaillant and associates (18), who reported that in a group of 45 physicians "selected for psychologic health," self-medication with drugs or alcohol was the cause of one-third of the total time that this group spent in the hospital. Further, 36 percent of the physicians, compared with 22 percent of the control group, were categorized as being in the "high drug use" groups, which included "heavy drinking or 'trouble with control of alcohol' " (19).

The study from which this paper is drawn examined alcoholic physicians who had successfully stopped drinking, who were not institutionalized, and, for the most part, were not under psychiatric care at the time of the study. There appear to be no other studies of physicians and alcoholic populations that are not currently in treatment and in which the disease is not active.

METHOD

American and Canadian male physicians who had grown up in the United States or in English-speaking Canadian families were selected for the study. All considered themselves alcoholics, were members of Alcoholics Anonymous (AA), and had been totally abstinent for one calender year or more prior to interview. While we attempted to locate sober alcoholic physicians who are not members of AA, we were unable to find a large enough number to provide comparability.

We located the subjects primarily through the cooperation of International doctors in AA, a chapter of Alcoholics Anonymous limited to physicians and dentists which holds an annual August weekend meeting in various parts of the United States. Other subjects were found through local AA groups. We also located several men who were practicing in small towns in the Carolinas and Georgia and were known to one another. Each willingly introduced the interviewer by telephone to the next physician down the highway.

In no case did an AA member give a physician's name without first obtaining his permission to do so. It is therefore possible that some of the reports that potential subjects were away on vacation or were ill may represent their refusal to be interviewed. We made no attempt to conduct a random sampling or develop a control group. Since considerations of time and geography made it impractical to visit many western and small communities, most of the interviews were conducted in eastern urban areas, frequently during medical conventions.

A 50-part questionnaire using some items modified from a previous study (20) was administered in a face-to-face interview with each of the subjects. The interviewer recorded all of the information with the exception of a checklist of symptoms of alcoholism, physical sequelae, and social sanctions experienced, which was marked by the subject.

All interviews were conducted during the period 1968-1970 and were solicited by the study team. While only one of the physicians approached actually refused to be interviewed, three others also refused, in effect, by engaging in delaying tactics and by making it extremely difficult to contact them.

RESULTS

Characteristics of the Study Population

The study resulted in 98 usable questionnaires. Table 5-I compares the study population's distribution by field of practice to that of all U.S. physicians.

A striking proportion of the alcoholic physicians identified themselves as psychiatrists at the time of the interview, although in at least three cases the current field of practice was not the same as it had been at the time of cessation of drinking. Since the study population was not a random sample, the differences found may be related to sample variation or to differential rates of alcoholism among practitioners in the various fields. However, except for the field of psychiatry, the two groups did not appear to be distributed differently by field of practice.

Data on the study group's class standing in medical school also suggest that these physicians are not representative of the total physician population.

Of the 84 physicians who provided data on this item, 45 (53.6%) reported that they were in the upper third of their class (including 19, or 22.6 percent, who were in the upper tenth), 34 (40.5%) were

Table 5-I

Comparison of the Field of Practice of All U.S. Physicians and of 98 Alcoholic Physicians at the Time of the Interview, in Percents

Field of Practice	All U.S. Physicians*	Alcoholic Physicians
General practice	22	24.5
Internal medicine	14	13.3
Surgery	10	9.2
Psychiatry	6	17.4
Obstetrics and gynecology	6	9.2
Pediatrics	6	2.0
Radiology	3	2.0
Anesthesiology	3	4.1
Pathology	3	3.1
Ophthalmology	3	0
Orthopedic surgery	3	3.1
Other	21	12.3

*Data are from the American Medical Association (21).

in the middle third, and 5 (5.9%) were in the lower third. Fourteen physicians stated that their medical schools did not report these rankings to their graduates; we checked with the schools of four of these physicians and found this information to be accurate.

A normal distribution would obviously have produced about one-third in each level. Again, we cannot ascribe the findings to either sample variation or to differences in an alcoholic population. However, the two distributions (field of practice and class standing) do suggest that the alcoholic physician may well be different from his nonalcoholic colleagues in characteristics other than his disease.

A total of 91 subjects were working full time as physicians. Five were semiretired due to reasons of health. One had retired completely (he was well into his 70s and had been abstinent for over 20 years), and another had left active practice to become a medical writer.

Twenty-one were holding formal teaching appointments in medical schools, although the colleagues and students of only a few knew that they were recovered alcoholics. They therefore did not share their experience with their peers. Several indicated that they would like to do so but were afraid of the stigma that might follow honest disclosure.

While only 1 consecutive year of total abstinence was required for inclusion in this study, the mean period of total abstinence was 7.4 years, with a range of 1 to 29 years.

Addiction to Other Drugs

As with groups in previous studies, our study sample also reported a high incidence of addiction to drugs other than alcohol. A total of 56 (57.1%) had been addicted only to alcohol, 24 (24.5%) to alcohol and "soft" drugs, 4 (4.1%) to alcohol and narcotics, and 14 (14.3%) to all three.

We did not attempt to define "addiction" for the individual physician. If he considered himself to have been addicted to a given drug, his word was accepted. If, on the other hand, he expressed uncertainty as to whether he had merely used a drug or had actually been addicted to it, he was regarded as not addicted.

The category of soft drugs included sedative-hypnotics, tranquilizers, amphetamines, and volatile anesthetics. Codeine, whether used alone or with terpin hydrate, was included with the narcotics.

Table 5-II presents data on the drugs other than alcohol to which the physician reported addiction. It should be borne in mind that since most of these physicians stopped using other drugs at the time they stopped using alcohol and that since many had been sober for years at the time of interview, this choice of drug reflects a pattern of use probably not typical of today's active drug abuser. For example, few of our subjects mentioned diazepam, which is probably the most frequently abused drug in our present patient population, and none mentioned methaqualone hydrochloride or pentazocine hydrochloride, although both are now frequently used by self-medicating physicians.

Table 5-II

Drugs of Addiction Other Than Alcohol Among 98 Alcoholic Physicians

Drug	Number*	Percent
Narcotics	18	18.4
Barbiturates	29	29.6
Amphetamines	17	17.3
Glutethimide	11	11.2
Meprobamate	8	8.2
Chlordiazepoxide	8	8.2
Chloral hydrate	7	7.1
Ethchlorvynol	3	3.1
Diazepam	3	3.1
Bromide	1	1.0
Gas and volatile anesthetics	1	1.0

*A number of subjects reported addiction to more than one drug.

Treatment Experience

All but 22 of the subjects (22.4%) sought professional help for alcoholism or what they later recognized as alcoholism, and many sought help from more than one type of professional. They consulted psychiatrists more frequently than nonpsychiatric physicians (52 subjects, or 53.1%, versus 40, or 40.8%); in addition, almost one-third of the group (32, or 32.7%) approached the clergy.

Contrary to the popular impression that alcoholics do not remain in treatment, of those subjects who sought psychiatric help 37 (71.2%) stayed in treatment for 2 or more years and 15 (28.8%) for 8 or more years.

While many described their overall treatment experiences as helpful, they frequently complained that a professional helper had refused to identify or deal with the problem of alcoholism per se and had chosen to regard it as a symptom of some other underlying condition. Thirty-four men reported that the question of alcoholism had specifically been discussed between patient and therapist, only to have the therapist deny the fact of alcoholism. Since it is virtually impossible to arrive at a reasonable treatment plan for a disease whose existence is not acknowledged, this behavior had frequently resulted in dangerous delays in obtaining appropriate treatment.

Most of the study sample reported multiple treatment experiences as inpatients, outpatients, or both. A total of 77 (78.6%) were institutionalized one or more times, while 21 (21.4%) were not. Table 5-III presents information on all admissions to institutions for alcoholism or alcohol-related illness regardless of the diagnosis officially recorded at the time. The total time these physicians spent in institutions during their 627 admissions was just under 39 years. (If one assumes that there are in fact over 5 million alcoholics in the United States today, and if the use of health care facilities reported by these physicians is accurate and typical of other alcoholics, the drain on the health care dollar is even more staggering than previously estimated.)

Medical Sequelae

In addition to the difficulties resulting from simple physical addiction to alcohol, the physicians also reported experiencing many of the common somatic complications of alcoholism (*see* Table 5-IV). Often these conditions required hospitalization. Several of the subjects stated that they received excellent physical care during inpatient treatment of these conditions but that they and their doctors tacitly agreed not to discuss the matter alcoholism.

Table 5-III

Admissions to Institutions for Alcoholism or Alcohol-Related Illness

Type of Facility	Number of Admissions (N=627)
General hospital*	359
Psychiatric hospital	132
AA rest farm	63
Sanitarium	60
Federal hospital	7
Mission, halfway house, and municipal shelter	6

*Includes Veterans Administration hospitals.

Table 5-IV

Medical Complications of Alcoholism Reported by 98 Physicians

Complication	Number*	Percent
Gastritis	44	44.9
Peripheral neuropathy	19	19.4
Severe malnutrition	16	16.3
Fatty liver	14	14.3
Gastrointestinal bleeding	14	14.3
Peptic ulcer	10	10.2
Pancreatitis	5	5.1
Cirrhosis of the liver	4	4.1
Esophageal varices	1	1.0

*A number of subjects reported more than one type of complication.

An additional physical hazard was presented by the subjects' tendency to use other drugs in an attempt to deal with the insomnia, agitation, and depression caused by excessive drinking. (The alcoholic physician frequently confused cause and effect and believed that his problems with sleep and his nervousness caused him to drink, rather than the reverse.) As the use of other sedatives increased, frequently in a setting of increasing alcohol use, the physician often became confused as to how much he was taking. Twenty-three men reported serious sedative overdoses, most of which were not felt to have been suicide attempts.

The physicians were asked specifically about any overt suicide attempts. No effort was made to distinguish between serious attempts and gestures. If a subject reported a self-destructive episode but was unclear as to whether he was consciously attempting suicide, we did not list it as an attempt. Fifteen subjects (15.3%)

reported that they had made overt suicide attempts. Ten subjects (10.2%) had made a single attempt, one (1%) had made two attempts, and two (2%) each had made three and six attempts. Because of the criteria we used for listing a self-destructive episode as a suicide attempt, these data probably represent underreporting rather than the opposite.

Social Sequelae

Since it has been our experience that patients who are obviously seriously alcoholic often defend against diagnosis on the grounds that they are still able to work, we were particularly interested in the effect of alcoholism on the physicians' work performance.

We found that over half of the sample (53, or 54.1%) did not experience any obvious change in job status as a result of drinking. (This does not, of course, take into consideration the quality of work or volume of practice.) Among the 45 who did report work difficulties, 20 suffered periods of unemployment and five were forced to work outside the medical field altogether, one as a porter, another as a dishwasher, and yet another as a copier of blueprints. Of those who remained in medicine but reported a decline in work status, several reported that their careers were dramatically affected. For example, a chief of medicine at a major medical school took a series of locum tenens positions for general practitioners. A famous pathologist worked as little more than a laboratory technician for another physician. A neurosurgeon deprived of hospital privileges supported himself by doing routine physical examinations.

Many of the physicians experienced difficulty with the law, and many others stated that while they had never been arrested, they felt that they should have been but the police were often lenient when an erratic driver or boisterous individual was identified as a doctor. A total of 48 subjects (49%) had been arrested, 37 (37.8%) had been jailed, and 19 (19.4%) had lost their driver's license. Our sample of physicians accumulated a total of 219 arrests and 170 jailings.

Response of the Profession

Table 5-V lists the professional sanctions experienced by the alcoholic physicians. Included under "admonitions" was any statement (informal or otherwise) made by a colleague or superior to the effect that drinking was perceived as a problem. It is therefore particularly telling that in one-third of these cases, nothing whatsoever had been said.

Table 5-V

Professional Sanctions Experienced by 98 Alcoholic Physicians

Sanction	Number*	Percent
Admonished by colleague	58	59.2
Warned by medical society or licensing board	20	20.4
Lost hospital privileges	20	20.4
Lost medical license	8	8.2
Lost narcotic license only	1	1.0
Never sanctioned	33	33.7

*A number of subjects experienced more than one sanction.

DISCUSSION

These 98 alcoholic physicians were probably clearly visible to the general public and to their colleagues. The public response to their behavior, as represented by arrests, jailings, and loss of driver's license, occurred more often and with a larger number of formal indications of disapprobation than did the professional response, as represented by warnings from medical societies and licensing boards, loss of hospital privileges, and actual loss of license.

That the public was more aggressive in its response than was the medical profession raises issues about the self-regulation of colleagues by a professional group. Arrests and jailings are not actions lightly undertaken by police in response to a transient action by a physician. Police are frequently reluctant to arrest the more prominent and respected citizens of a community. Several of the subjects stated that while they had not been arrested, they felt they should have been.

It is noteworthy that many of the physicians stated that their alcoholism had never resulted in injury to their patients. Although this feeling is often shared by the colleagues of alcoholic physicians, it is a view that is difficult to accept. Since alcoholism interferes in so many ways and with such a multiplicity of functions, there can be little doubt that the patients of an alcoholic physician receive a lesser level of care than that physician is able to deliver when he is sober. The question of injury to the patient is much more subtle, although the probability that such injury occurs is much more likely than the alcoholic physician is able to recognize.

The medical field has recently (22,23) been willing to acknowledge that its members are not immune to problems of alcoholism, addiction, and mental illness and to move toward the development of legislative and administrative means to protect them from doing harm or being harmed. One hopes that other professional groups will follow this lead.

REFERENCES

1. Cahalan D, Cisin IH, Crossley HM: *American Drinking Practices: A National Study of Drinking Behavior and Attitudes,* Monographs of the Rutgers Center of Alcohol Studies, number 6. New Brunswick, NJ, Publications Division, Rutgers Center of Alcohol Studies, 1969
2. American Medical Association: *Distribution of Physicians in the United States,* 1973. Chicago, AMA, 1974
3. Efron V, Keller M, Gurioli C: *Statistics on Consumption of Alcohol and on Alcoholism.* New Brunswick, NJ, Publications Division, Rutgers Center of Alcohol Studies, 1974
4. Glatt MM: Alcoholism and drug dependence in doctors and nurses. *Br Med J 1*:380-381, 1968
5. Partlow WD: Alcoholism and drug addiction among physicains of Alabama. *Transactions of the Medical Associations of Alabama,* pp 685-691, 1914
6. Pearson MM, Strecker EA: Physicians as psychiatric patients: private practice experience. *Am J Psychiatry 116*:915-919, 1960
7. Vincent MO, Robinson EA, Latt L: Physicians as patients: private psychiatric hospital experience. *Can Med Assoc J 100*:403-412, 1969
8. Duffy JC, Litin EM: *The Emotional Health of Physicians.* Springfield, Ill, Charles C Thomas, 1967, p 55
9. Duffy JC, Litin EM: Psychiatric morbidity of physicians. *JAMA 189*:989-992, 1964
10. Simon W, Lumry GK: Suicide among physician-patients. *J Nerv Ment Dis 147*:105-112, 1968
11. Simon W, Lumry GK: Alcoholism and drug addiction among physicians — chronic self-destruction? *Drug Dependence,* July 1969, pp 11-14
12. a'Brook MF, Hailstone JD, McLauchlan IEJ: Psychiatric illness in the medical profession. *Br J Psychiatry 113*:1013-1023, 1967
13. Vincent MO, cited in *Mental illness: special risk.* Medical World News, April 25, 1969, pp 42-44
14. Modlin HC, Montes A: Narcotics addiction in physicians. *Am J Psychiatry 121*:358-363, 1964
15. Putnam PL, Ellinwood EH Jr: Narcotic addiction among physicians; a ten-year follow-up. *Am J Psychaitry 122*:745-748, 1966
16. Craig AG, Pitts FN Jr: Suicide by physicians. *Dis Nerv Syst 29*:763-772, 1968
17. Blachly PH, Disher W, Roduner G: Suicide by physicians. *Bulletin of Suicidology,* Dec 1968, pp 1-18
18. Vaillant GE, Brighton JR, McArthur C: Physicians' use of mood-altering drugs: a 20-year follow-up report. *N Engl J Med 282*:365-372, 1970
19. Vaillant GE, Sobowale NC, McArthur C: Some psychologic vulnerabilities of physicians. *N Engl J Med 287*:372-375, 1972

20. Bailey MB, Leach B: Alcoholics Anonymous: Pathway to Recovery. New York, National Council on Alcoholism, 1965
21. American Medical Association: Distribution of Physicians, Hospitals, and Hospital Beds in the US, 1966. Chicago, AMA, 1967
22. Special Report of the Medical Society of the State of New York. *NY State J Med 75*:420-423, 1975
23. Bissell LC, Mooney AJ: The special problem of the alcoholic physician. *Med Times 103*:63-73, June 1975

Drug Abuse

Chapter 6

NARCOTICS ADDICTION IN PHYSICIANS

HERBERT C. MODLIN AND ALBERTO MONTES

THE statistically "typical" narcotics addict in the United States lives in a metropolis, is unmarried, is between 18 and 25 years of age, is a member of a minority group, and comes from a low socioeconomic level (4). Because none of these specifications fit the "typical" physician-addict (9,18), by eliminating them from consideration, a survey of physician-addicts presumably should give a clearer view of the psychological factors in (1) Development of the preaddiction personality; (2) Circumstances pertinent to the onset of addiction, and (3) Responses to psychiatric treatment.

During our 15-year study, 65 persons presenting the problem of narcotic addiction were admitted to the C.F. Menninger Memorial Hospital. Thirty (46%) were physicians. Five physicians who left against medical advice before adequate evaluation could be completed were excluded from this study. The remaining 25 physicians became addicted at the average age of 38. After 3 years of addiction and an average of two-plus previous hospitalizations, at the average age of 41 they entered our hospital. Eighteen were general practitioners or general surgeons, four internists, two obstetricians, and one an osteopathic physician. None of the doctors were in salaried positions or structured institutional settings. All but one were married. Twenty-four used meperidine hydrochloride (Demerol®) as the main addicting drug; one used dihydromorphinone hydrochloride (Dilaudid®). Sedatives, analgesics, ataractic drugs and alcohol were used in combination with the narcotic drug. One patient, for example, who was periodically depressed and experienced considerable difficulties with his wife and his medical practice, used consecutively or in combinations of three or four at a time the following: Dexedrine®, codeine, barbiturates, methadone, Dolophine®, morphine, Sparine®, and aspirin.

From Herbert C. Modlin and Alberto Montes, Narcotics Addiction in Physicians. *The American Journal of Psychiatry, 121:*358-363, 1964.

Read at the 120th annual meeting of The American Psychiatric Association, Los Angeles, Calif., May 4-8, 1964

PREADDICTION HISTORY

Our emphasis in this report is upon clarifying the common denominators among our patients; individual differences are given lesser attention. Our patient population was too small to provide data amenable to standard statistical treatment. All statements in this report referring to the "typical" physician-addict apply to at least 75 percent of the persons in this project unless otherwise indicated.

The physicians generally described their fathers as stern and depriving, or passive and indifferent, or volatile and flamboyant, or irritable and withdrawn; over 50 percent were alcoholics, reformed alcoholics, or heavy drinkers. Not one patient felt himself a favorite son; and a number of them expressed the feeling that a brother was preferred. Only three highly esteemed their fathers.

Four patients spoke warmly of their mothers. The rest (84%) variously criticized their mothers as extremely nervous, pushing, demanding, dominating, depressive, perfectionistic, hypochondriacal, phobic, alcoholic, harsh, ambitious, tense, defensive, protective, cruel, distant, reserved, or "excessively religious." Four mothers suffered "psychotic" episodes; and one patient's mother, when he was 14 years of age, attempted suicide in his presence. In general, these physicians had intense feelings, both of dependency and resentment toward their mothers. To what degree their ideas and feelings concerning their parents were realistically based, or were projected distortions of their own feelings, we cannot positively say; but such attitudes undeniably represented an emotional reality for the patients (12).

Most of these patients were sickly children. Seven suffered from intestinal colic or feeding disturbances during their first six months of life, and six were enuretic. Others chronically experienced bronchial asthma, obesity, rhinitis, sinusitis, recurrent mastoid infections, repeated attacks of rheumatic fever. In adolescence, most of them were studious, ambitious, and did well scholastically. Few were interested in athletics and outdoor sports. Adolescent rebelliousness, idealism, asceticism, turbulence, and disorganization were notably absent, or of negligible extent. Most of them were reasonably compliant. Nearly all were inhibited sexually and harbored considerable guilt feelings about masturbation.

The married lives of these men were uniformly full of discord and misunderstandings. They were demanding, ambivalent, and dependently attached to their wives, seeking always proof of being loved, but frequently unable to reciprocate. Nine were married to nurses, one to a physician. Several described their wives as "motherly." About 75 percent had serious sexual difficulties with their wives, including premature ejaculation and impotence, which conditions usually became aggravated rather than lessened by their narcotic addiction. Many showed little paternal interest in their children, but were, at times in the manner of siblings, openly competitive with them for their wives' love and attention.

During the fourth year of one patient's courtship of the girl he married, her parents insisted that they either break their engagement or marry soon. Faced with the equally unwelcome horns of this dilemma, he made a show of being sick by cutting the inner aspect of his cheek and spitting blood in his fiancee's presence. Marriage plans were postponed on the assumption that he had a bleeding peptic ulcer. Remorseful, he confessed his trick; and so they were married at last. The newlyweds lived in an apartment behind his office in his mother's old home. He quickly established the routine of stopping at his mother's apartment after the day's work to eat supper with her. Upon belatedly arriving at his own apartment, he would find an angry wife; and he would respond to her demand for an explanation that he could not hurt his mother because she had given up her life for him.

Another physician described his wife as "a mother with whom I had intercourse." During convalescence from an appendectomy, he fell in love with his nurse who followed him when he moved to another state. His guilt feelings over this relationship prompted him to seek psychotherapy, and after two years, the affair was terminated; but he has had many other extramarital adventures within the five years since, especially on Sundays. He has been partially impotent with his wife and has had practically no sexual relations with her for two or three years. Despite these facts, he says he considers his marriage a happy one.

ONSET OF ADDICTION: THE PATIENT'S VIEW

The patients gave three main reasons for starting narcotics: (1) Overwork, (2) Chronic fatigue, and (3) Physical disease. These, incidentally, are the classic reasons described in the literature on physician-addicts. That these physicians were overworked seems credible, but are not most physicians? These men apparently found it difficult to put a reasonable limit on their practice. Most of them were persons of average potential with high and unrealistic aspirations. They found themselves entangled in more and more work with an inability to say "no" to patients, to referrals, to committee assignments, etc. Their overt behavior was a denial of limitations to avoid exposing their basic insecurity and vulnerable self-esteem. They apparently stayed under pressure through lack of means to escape. In a certain sense, their complaints were justified: for their particular capacities, they were indeed overworked.

The second complaint, fatigability, would seem inappropriate for 32- to 36-year-old men. When they said, "I'm tired," they actually seemed to be saying that they were tired of giving, that they felt drained of incentive by the demands of their practice. This, in itself, is not an uncommon temporary professional reaction; but most doctors have recourse to techniques for recuperation: satisfactory relationships with wife, children, and friends; participation in community activities, the medical society, the church; and a variety of avocational and recreational pursuits. The potential addict seems not to find the average physicians's fulfillment in giving of self and seeing the positive results of his services. The sense of fatigue was regularly aggravated by inner neurotic struggles which consumed a disproportionate amount of total psychic energy, leaving an insufficiency of the energy required for actually constructive work and obligations to which they had committed themselves. Many of these men, consciously or unconsciously, demonstrated a basic ambivalence toward medical practice which somehow failed to give them what they needed — oral satiety.

The third complaint, physical disease, was commonly valid. In our 25 patients, recurrent peptic ulcer was experienced by three, bronchial asthma by one, functional gastrointestinal disturbances by three, severe headache by four, and refractory insomnia by three. Two had had an acute myocardial infarction with good recovery, and one each had suffered a gall bladder operation, renal colic, postmeningeal headache, and painful arthritis of the spine. The original narcotic was prescribed by an attending physician or surgeon for 10 of our 25 addicts, who then continued self-prescription of the drug, basing their rationalization for addiction upon the past physical ailment.

ONSET OF ADDICTION: OUR VIEW

Expert opinion seems in agreement that three conditions ordinarily must co-exist to effect narcotics addiction: (1) A predisposing personality; (2) The availability of narcotics; (3) A set of circumstances which brings Nos. 1 and 2 together (12). Availability of narcotics to the practicing physician is an obviously contributing factor. The U.S. Public Health hospitals indicate that about 40 percent of their addicts are from the health professions (physicians, nurses, pharmacists) (9, 18). We were particularly impressed with the patients' magical belief in the nonaddictive properties of Demerol. They believed that, 1. "It won't hurt me," and 2. "I can stop any time I want to."

"The danger is in self-adminstration, especially in the relief of anxiety or depressive symptoms. . . . The basic problem is prevention, with adequate instruction in medical schools concerning the danger of self-medication. A vigorous anti-addictive campaign should be carried out by the medical associations"(2).

The predisposing personality in our patients is most conveniently described in terms of the psychoanalytic model. They demonstrate the characteristic stigmata of the oral character. One of our patients presented the symptoms classically diagnosed as schizophrenic; the others were variously labeled compulsive, passive-aggressive, narcissistic, and parasitic personalities. The following case vignette illustrates an example of extreme oral behavior:

> A 33-year-old physician suffered a severe intestinal infection and returned to work prematurely while he was still convalescing. At that same time, his brother, who was 10 years his senior and whom he adored, became involved in a public scandal which threatened the family reputation. Their father unexpectedly proved unequal to the role of patriarchal authority needed by the beleaguered family; and our patient felt obliged to give his miscreant older brother "fatherly" counsel and to share in and support his substantial effort to correct his behavior. In this context, the doctor began taking barbiturates at night for his insomnia, plus an occasional daytime barbiturate capsule to ease his tension. Fearing to become habituated to the drugs, he switched to highballs at night, but this did not handle his diurnal stress. He finally hit upon the expedient of giving himself 10 to 15 units of insulin. When the insulin reaction set in, he would eat a quart of ice cream or half a pie and borrow from the oral satisfaction some temporary sense of decreased tension — and peace of mind. Subsequently, he began injecting himself with Demerol and rapidly increased the dosage as tolerance developed. He eventually felt the need of a more powerful agent and gave himself two or three injections of morphine. This, however, meant to him that he was becoming a narcotic addict and, in desperation, he attempted suicide and became our patient. After a period of hospitalization, he continued in outpatient psychotherapy but soon he was drinking great quantities of beer. He voluntarily decided to stop this indulgence and whenever he craved beer, he drank a glass of milk. The measure of his self-discipline was evidenced by his consumption of a gallon of milk daily.

It is beyond the purpose of this report to document such important considerations as unconscious motivation in choosing a mate, neurotic interaction in marriage, unresolved oedipal strivings of adults, searching for a parental surrogate in a spouse. However, it should be noted that one aspect of our physician-addicts' predisposing personalities seems expressed in their invariable dependency on the emotional support of marriage even though they were uniformly unsuccessful in performing the culturally patterned role of husbands. That these men leaned heavily on their wives, needed mothering in the primitive manner of an infant, was a constant finding.

Only three of our 24 married patients appeared to have realized a relatively stable marital adjustment; the other 21 manifested heterosexual incompatibility, at least with the women they were somehow motivated to marry. In six marriages, violent conflict included physical assault. Three patients were exaggeratedly dependent and deliberately over-demanding of their wives. Two patients retained dependent relationships with their natural mothers. Ten presented case histories of severe overt sexual incapacity. Several others, while denying premature ejaculations and impotence, did confess to episodes of promiscuity. A major number of the wives were frigid or promiscuous. Even though their wives could never really meet the unrealistic expectations and demands of the patients, it is striking that they, nevertheless, remained married. The two patients who divorced, promptly remarried; and thus only very briefly lacked a wife-mother. No instance of overt homosexuality was uncovered.

THERAPEUTIC MANAGEMENT

In common with other investigators (5) we have encountered difficulties in follow-up studies, chiefly because some patients were discharged as long as 10 years ago. We collected adequate follow-up data on 15 of the 25 patients for at least three years after their release from our hospital. Five have "disappeared"; that is, our letters to them were returned marked "addressee unknown," and their names are no longer listed in the membership of the American Medical Association. Three others are known to be dead, two by suicide; and two refused to cooperate in our study.

Eleven patients accepted our recommendations for prolonged psychiatric treatment and accomplished at least two years of combined hospitalization and out-patient psychotherapy or psychoanalysis, of which seven responded well to treatment. Each of the seven completed at least two years of psychotherapy, are now practicing medicine, and claim to be cured of addiction. Two of the seven found membership in Alcoholics Anonymous beneficial. An eighth patient stopped narcotics intake, but became a severe chronic alcoholic with bouts of pancreatitis, delirium tremens, and occasional convulsions. Two of the 11 patients slipped back into the narcotics habit more than once, were rehospitalized and are still in psychiatric treatment; one of the two has been free of all drug ingestion for 18 months as his psychotherapy continues. The second has recently entered psychoanalysis and avowedly is free of the drug habit at present. Three completed treatment in psychoanalysis and are free of addiction; a fourth left psychoanalytic treatment prematurely.

We consider effective treatment to include three basic procedures: hospitalization, social casework with the spouse, and prolonged psychotherapy. Our patients had been previously hospitalized for an average of more than twice before we saw them. Most of these hospitalizations, including the ones at our hospital, were not truly voluntary, but were forced upon the patient by pressure from wife, parents, relatives, medical colleagues, licensing boards, or the Federal Narcotics Bureau. Only three came to us voluntarily.

Despite the numerous individual differences among these patients, the majority consistently denied serious addictive difficulties and shared the illusion that they could stop drugs any time they wished. Many, during hospitalization, were bland and compliant, and expressed the expectation that they would be the passive recipients of some kind of medical treatment. Most of them demonstrated a low tolerance for frustrating or anxiety-provoking experiences, and could, only with great difficulty, postpone temporary gratification. This would seem to explain why about one-third of the patients interrupted hospitalization prematurely or rejected our recommendations that they obtain outpatient psychotherapy.

Hospitalization is a necessary first step in treatment, and no compromise should be considered. The physician-addict shares many characteristics with the general addict population; his capacity for rationalization, simulation, vacillation, subterfuge, and prevarication is infinite. There is consistent agreement on this point in the literature (8,15,18). This is a disappointing finding in that the physician-addict comes from an upper socio-economic level, has an advanced education, has been imbued with the principles of medical ethics, and has a wife and children to consider. These factors supposedly should increase his motivation to seek help; we have not found this to be so.

During hospitalization, it is essential that effective work be done with the patient's wife. It is necessary to obtain historical material from her and, at the same time, to evaluate her attitude and her capacity for understanding her husband's needs. She should participate in the rehabilitative effort following diagnostic evaluation. Few of the physicians' wives have seriously considered divorce, even after many years of marital difficulty, personal abuse, and threatened loss of social position in the community. As observed of many alcoholics' wives, some women in this study, in subtle ways, abetted and encouraged their husbands' continuing psychological difficulties, including drug taking. Two joined their husbands and became addicts, and several were immoderate drinkers. In such cases, effective work with the patient depends upon involving his wife in social casework, if not in psychiatric treatment for herself.

Following a period for diagnostic evaluation and removal of the patient from all drugs, we commonly recommend continued hospitalization, usually for a minimum of 6 months. If the patient can be brought to realize the enormity of his problem, the seriousness of his self-destructive behavior, and the possibility for help, then the next step, psychotherapy, has a chance to succeed.

DISCUSSION AND SUMMARY

We hoped this clinical survey would inform as to whether or not conventional psychiatric treatment is of value to the physician-addict. We conclude that it is, if his motivation can be stimulated sufficiently that he really accepts and persists with treatment. Strictly in terms of the one presenting symptom, narcotics addiction, eight of 11 patients who conscientiously stayed with psychiatric treatment seem to have benefited, at least to the point of being able to continue in professional practice and remain free of addictive drugs. Subsequent to treatment three were divorced; one of these has a second wife.

Estimates of the incident of narcotics addiction in physicians vary from 30 (7) to 100 (25) times that in the general population; it is an occupational hazard. Reports from the United States (9,18), England (1), Germany (6,26), Holland (3), and France (22) all indicate that of the known drug addicts, about 15 percent are physicians. Another 15 percent are members of the paramedical professions, nursing and pharmacy. Previous studies of drug addiction among physicians in the United States by Wall (24), Voorhees (23), Pescor (16), Rasor and Crecraft (18), and Winick (25) have emphasized the statistics and legal problems involved, but have not evaluated the psychodynamic problems. A few psychoanalytic studies by Rado (17), Glover (8), Wulff (27), Rosenfeld (20), and Mannheim (11) have investigated the regression to and the vicissitudes of the oral drive. In this present study, based on thorough but otherwise routine clinical data, we have attempted to define some of the psychosocial factors involved in the development of addictive behavior.

Addiction in our patients was a symptom of moderately severe progressive personality disorganization. Antecedent to the present illness were the patient's disparaging view of his parents, his dissatisfaction from the relationship he experienced with them, and somatic or psychophysiological imbalance in childhood. Clustered around the onset of narcotic habituation was a four-fold complex of 1. His discouragement regarding the anticipated rewards of medical practice, 2. Disillusionment of expectations to gain succor in marriage, 3. Inability to grow into the traditional role of father and achieve satisfaction, as a parent, from the parent-child relationship, and 4. Chronic somatic or somatized illness.

Why does addiction need first appear in the mid-thirties, after five to ten years of busy medical practice? Our data seem to answer that these men are sustained in earlier life by great expectations of future satisfactions. Each move from adolescent fantasies to courtship, to marriage, to parenthood; or from college to medical school, to internship, to established practice, includes automatic transfer of dreams of glorious fulfillment into the level of realization charted next ahead. Once the final practical terminus is reached, the naive expectation of gaining a future paradise ends too; then disillusionment and reactive regression set in.

Presumably, the same basic mechanism operates in the "typical" nonmedical addict. He, however, lacking the physician's external supports, such as secure income, social position, postgraduate education, and professional status, experiences crucial disillusionment at an earlier date in his life (4).

We are still left with unanswered questions. Why do they do it? Why do they doggedly resist treatment to release them from addiction? Why are these disciples of Hippocrates, trained to preserve human life and minister to human pain, bent upon destroying themselves and hurting their intimates? The most consistent answer from the patients themselves is that they desire euphoria — a subjective sensation the addict craves and, unfortunately, can achieve (10). They seem to find this part-of-the-time feeling of complete gratification, satiation, wanting for nothing; this episodic tension-free, frustration-free nirvana worth to them whatever price they have to pay.

REFERENCES

1. Anon.: *J.A.M.A., 165:* 181, 1957.
2. Bennett, A. E. : Compulsive, Addictive Personality Problems. *Med. Times,* May, 1964.
3. Booy, Joh.: *Neder. Ti. Geneesk., 93:* 31, 2571.
4. Chein, Isidor: The Status of Sociological and Social Psychological Knowledge Concerning Narcotics. In *Narcotic Drug Addiction Problems.* Wash. D. C.: U.S. Dept. of Health, Educ. and Welfare, 1959.
5. Clark, J. A.: *J. Ment. Sci., 108:* 411, 1962.
6. Ehrhardt, H.: *Bull. Nar.,* Jan.-Mar., 1959.
7. Fox, J. D.: *J. Mich. Med. Soc., 56:*214, 1957.
8. Glover, Edward: *Int. J. Psychoanal., 13:* 298, 1932.
9. Isbell, H., and White, W. M.: *Am. J. Med., 14:* 558, 1953.
10. Kolb, L. C.: *Ment. Hyg., 9:* 699, 1925.
11. Mannheim, J.: *Int. J. Psychoanal., 36:* 166, 1955.
12. Mason, Percy: *Psychiat. Quart. (Suppl.), 2:* 1, 1958.
13. Narcotic Drug Addiction. *Ment. Health Monogr.* No. 2. Wash., D. C.: U. S. Dept. of Health, Educ. and Welfare, 1963.
14. Nyswander, M., *et al.: Am. J. Orthopsychiat., 28:* 714, 1958.
15. Osnos, R.: *N. Y. J. Med., 63:* 1182, 1963.
16. Pescor, M. J.: Statistical Analysis of Clinical Records of Hospitalized Drug Addicts. Suppl. No. 143. U.S.P.H. Reports, 1943.
17. Rado, S.: *Int. J. Psychoanal., 7:* 396, 1926.
18. Rasor, R. W., and Crecraft, H. J.: *J.A.M.A., 157:* 654, 1955.
19. Rayport, M.: *Ibid., 156:* 694, 1954.
20. Rosenfeld, H. A.: *Int. J. Psychoanal., 41:*467, 1960.
21. Savitt, R. A.: *J. Am. Psychoanal., 2:*494, 1954.
22. Vaille, C., and Stern, G.: *Bull. Nar. (U.N.), 6:* May-Aug., 1954.
23. Voorhees, W D., Jr., and Browne-Mayers, A. N.: *N. Y. J. Med., 54:* 1935, 1954.
24. Wall, J. H.: *Fed. Bull., 45:* 144, 1958.
25. Winick, C.: *Soc. Problems, 9:* 174, 1961.
26. Wolff, P. O.: *Schweiz. Med. Wschr., 87:* 443, 1957.
27. Wulff, M.: *Int. Z. Psychoanal., 18:* 281, 1932.

Chapter 7

PHYSICIANS' USE OF MOOD-ALTERING DRUGS
A 20-Year Follow-up Report

George E. Vaillant, Jane R. Brighton, and Charles McArthur

In recent years evidence has accumulated that abuse of alcohol and mood-altering drugs (narcotics, amphetamines, tranquilizers and barbituates) may be the most common sign of psychiatric illness in physicians. In a review of psychiatric admissions of physicians to the Mayo Clinic, Duffy and Litin noted that 50 percent showed dependence on either alcohol or mood-altering drugs, and 23 percent dependence on both.[1] Three other studies of psychiatrically hospitalized physicians also found drug or alcohol abuse present in roughly half of all admissions.[2-4] In a study of 66 physicians seen as psychiatric outpatients, almost a third received a primary diagnosis of either alcoholism or dependence on mood-altering drugs.[5]

There is also good evidence that in physicians in general, not just those who seek psychiatric help, narcotic abuse is more frequent than in the population at large. In 1958 the California State Board of Medical Examiners estimated that at some point in their careers 1 to 2 percent of doctors in that state abuse narcotics.[6] In a 25-year period, 0.5 percent of all physicians licensed in New York State were reported to the Bureau of Narcotic control as addicts.[7] By contrast, the prevalence of narcotic addictions among American males in the group from 20 to 50 years of age is around one in 1000, and most come from urban slums.[8]

Since most physicians are neither narcotic addicts nor admitted to psychiatric hospitals, the existing literature fails to answer two im-

---

From George E. Vaillant, Jane R. Brighton, and Charles McArthur, Physicians' Use of Mood-Altering Drugs. *New England Journal of Medicine, 282:*365-370, 1970.

Supported by a grant (MH-38798) from the National Institute of Mental Health, United States Public Health Service, and by the Grant Foundation, Incorporated.

Presented at a meeting of the American Psychiatric Association. Miami, Fla., May 5-9, 1969.

portant questions. In comparison to nonphysicians, do physicians tend to overuse drugs? If they do overuse the drugs to which they have easy access, do they use alcohol and tobacco correspondingly less? Since physicians form a group selected by both demonstrated intellectual proficiency and occupational perseverance, their use of drugs and alcohol ought to be compared with that of a nonmedical group that shares these characteristics. Finally, to obtain an accurate picture of drug abuse, subjects must be studied over long periods. In prevalence studies the relapsing patient may be counted more than once, whereas the covert user and the reformed abuser are apt to be ignored.

For all these reasons, the present study reports the use of mood-altering drugs, alcohol and tobacco in a sample of physicians selected for psychologic health 30 years previously and prospectively followed to the present. Drug use by these physicians is contrasted with that of an intellectually and socially comparable control group.

METHODS

In the late 1930s an interdisciplinary study was undertaken of a 7 percent sample of several consecutive sophomore classes at a liberal-arts college. To be accepted into the study, the student had to be considered by the college health service, the dean's office and dormitory staff members to be comparatively free of physical, emotional and academic difficulties. Of 268 men so chosen, 10 dropped out early in the project; the others have been followed until their death or to the present. Of the original sample 46 eventually became physicians, one of whom died in 1955. The 45 remaining physicians, selected for longitudinal study before firm career choice, constitute the present sample.

Over the years all the men were followed by extensive questionnaires mailed on the average once every two years and by occasional personal interview. Perhaps because the investigation began so early in their careers, and because it represented a study of normal adult development, the men have participated conscientiously and loyally. To preserve uniformity of answer, the present data are principally derived from questionnaires, but this information is supported by interview and retrospective confirmation of questionnaire answers. During times of stress some questionnaires have gone unanswered, but after 30 years, there is no evidence that any participant has given deliberate misinformation about use of drugs or alcohol.

The principal data used in the present study were the men's written answers to the following questions:

(1) "Cigarettes per day: 0/1-10/11-19/ 1 pack/ between one and two packs/two packs or more," in 1949, 1953, 1957, 1964 and 1967. (In the same years similar information about pipe and cigar smoking was collected.)
(2) "Use of alcohol; none/rarely/occasionally/few regular/many irregular/many regular" in 1949, 1953, 1957, 1964 and 1967.
(3) Whether they had trouble controlling their drinking in 1953, 1964 and 1967.
(4) Whether they increased their use of tobacco and alcohol under stress in 1954, 1967.
(5) Whether they took "any medicines or drugs" in 1949, 1957 and 1964, and more specifically if they used "sedatives" in 1951 or "tranquilizers," "sedatives" or "stimulants" in 1966-67.

If any one failed to return a designated questionnaire, but if within 3 years answered another questionnaire, the latter questionnaire was substituted. Although retrospective information was not included, if questionnaires were not available interview data and hospital records contemporary with the date of the questionnaire were used.

Ninety controls were obtained by selection, from the list of study participants, of the two nonphysicians alphabetically adjacent to each physician. Two potential controls were discarded because they had died before 1960, and they were replaced by the next alphabetically adjacent nonphysician.

Ratings of overall drug and alcohol use were made independently by two of us. In about 15 percent of cases there were minor differences in classification; such differences were resolved by discussion.

RESULTS

Table 7-I presents the results of matching doctors and controls. In terms of age, father's income on college entrance, private-school preparation, scholastic and mathematical aptitude on college entrance examinations and feeding problems during infancy, the men were fully comparable. In terms of relative psychologic soundness ratings (based on the results of intensive multidisciplinary study during college), the doctors were not significantly different from the controls. In terms of the conscientiousness over the years with which the questionnaires were returned, the doctors were slightly more

Table 7-I

COMPARISON OF 45 PHYSICIANS AND 90 CONTROLS

Group	% with Feeding Problem in Infancy	% with Private-School Education	% Whose Fathers' Incomes Were >$6,000/Yr in 1940	Mathematical Attainments Test*	Scholastic Aptitude Test*	% with Indicated Relative Psychological Soundness Rating			Average No. of Questionnaires/Man Returned†	% of Men Returning 1967 Questionnaire	Age in 1967 (Yr)
						A	B	C			
Physicians	27	60	40	550	570	47	31	22	5.8	88	46 ± 1
Control	23	59	38	550 + ‡	570 + ‡	39	50	11	5.4	80	46 ± 1

*Average score for entire college.
†Out of 7 used in study.
‡ + 0.25 SD.

faithful.

Follow-up information on the 135 men in the study was nearly complete. Prospective data were available for at least four out of the five intervals (1949, 1953, 1957, 1964 and 1967) for 89 percent of the men and for at least three of the five intervals for 97 percent. Objective information was available at two points in time and within the last five years on all but one subject.

Twenty-five years after graduation, the occupational success and physical health of the study participants was significantly superior to that of classmates not in the study. Sixty-nine percent of the physicians graduated from the five medical schools, Columbia, Harvard, Rochester, Pennsylvania and Johns Hopkins; 78 percent successfully passed their specialty boards, and almost half have held the rank of assistant clinical professor or above at a medical school. Occupational success of the controls seemed fully comparable.

Table 7-II shows the comparative use of mood-altering drugs (sedatives, tranquilizers and stimulants) by the two groups. Over-the-counter medicines are not included in the table. "Abuse" indicates use of sedatives beyond the limits usually prescribed in medical practice. The "regular-use" category referred to participants who took sleeping pills more than once a month for several months, frequent use of amphetamines (for reasons other than weight control) or daily use of prescription tranquilizers for more than a month. The "regular" use of sedatives by physicians was significantly greater than that by the controls. Twice as many physicians as controls took tranquilizers, but the difference observed was not statistically significant in a sample of this size.

It must be emphasized that the increased use of mood-altering drugs by physicians in the study is relative. Only one man, a physician, experienced prolonged social and occupational impairment because of the use of pills. Four physicians and one control combined barbiturate use with use of amphetamines, but apparently not on a daily basis. Fifty-seven percent of the controls, but only 20 percent of the physicians, were recorded as taking not more than one mood-altering pill a year. The increased use of mood-altering drugs by physicians appeared to be due to self-prescription.

Table 7-III compares the use of alcohol between physicians and nonphysicians. Category 2 — "few regular" — indicates that this was the man's reported drinking pattern on two or more questionnaires. In practice, "few regular" means 2 to 6 ounces of hard liquor daily. "Heavy drinking" indicates that on a *single* questionnaire a man reported either "many regular" or difficulty controlling his drinking. "Prolonged heavy drinking" indicates that at least two points in time

Table 7-II

MAXIMUM USER OF MOOD-ALTERING DRUGS BY 45 PHYSICIANS
AND 89 CONTROLS DURING A 20-YEAR PERIOD

CATEGORY	USE OF AMPHETAMINES (%)		USE OF TRANQUILIZERS (%)		USE OF SEDATIVES (%)	
	PHYSICIANS	CONTROLS	PHYSICIANS	CONTROLS	PHYSICIANS	CONTROLS
1-no mention of use	78	96	73	85	33	65.0
2-"occasional" use (1 mention)	18	2	9	8	27	25.0
3-"occasional" use (2 mention)	—	—	—	—	22†	4.5
4-regular use	4	2	18	7	13	4.5
5-abuse	0	0	0	0	5	1.0

*2 doctors used imipramine, 2 doctors used chlorpromazine & 1 control used chlorprothixene; all the rest used "minor" tranquilizers.

†Increased no. of physicians falling in Groups 3,4 & 5 is significant at 00.0 level of confidence (chi-square test); 1 control lost to follow-up observation.

Table 7-III

MAXIMUM USE OF ALCOHOL
DURING A 20-YEAR PERIOD

Classification	Physicians(%)	Control(%)
1 — rare or occasional	38.0	41
2 — "few regular" drinks	42.0	38
3 — heavy drinking for 1 period	11.0	12
4 — prolonged heavy drinking	4.5	8
5 — social or occupational damage	4.5	1*
Drinks more under stress	27.0	22
Ever reported problem controlling drinking	22.0	18

*Indicates man who returned no questionnaires, classified here on indirect information.

a man reported "many regular" or difficulty controlling his drinking. The table shows no difference in the drinking patterns between the two groups of men. Over the years an increasing number of men from both groups reported either "many regular" or trouble controlling their drinking — 3 percent at 28, 7 percent at 32, 9 percent at 36, 12 percent at 43, and 16 percent at 46 years of age.

Figure 7-I shows the natural history of cigarette smoking for these two groups over three decades. Over the years the percentage of smokers, per se, remained about 60 percent. Although the number of cigar or pipe smokers steadily increased, there was first a rise and then a drop in the number of heavy cigarette smokers. Two doctors and nine controls sustained regular smoking habits of two packs of cigarettes or more a day for 20 years. Only 10 percent of either group ever smoked at least a pack a day and then were able to give up cigarettes entirely. As a group, physicians included fewer heavy smokers and also fewer nonsmokers. The smoking habits of the 135 men in the study today do not differ from those of their unselected classmates. It is noteworthy that the study subjects as sophomores smoked more than sophomores at the same college 20 years later.

Table 7-IV shows the maximum use of mood-altering agents by doctors and controls. The fact that 62 percent of the doctors and only 32 percent of the controls fell in Group 3 or above is statistically significant at an 0.001 level of confidence (chi-square test). But if use

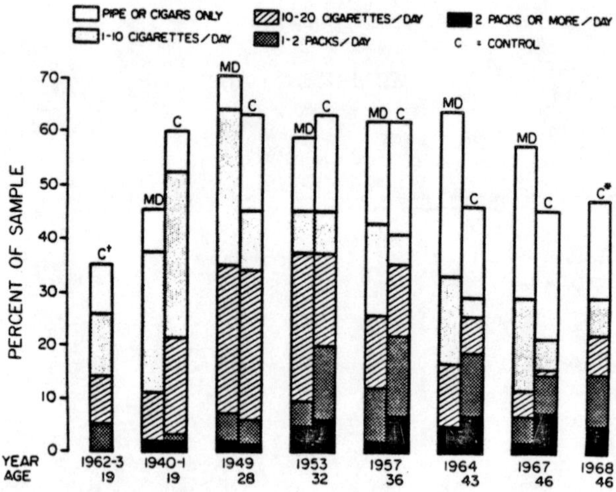

Figure 7-I. Comparison of Smoking Habits between Physicians and Nonphysicians over a 28-year period.

C + indicates the smoking habits of 443 sophomores selected from the same college in 1962-3. C* indicates the smoking habits of 623 college classmates of the study sample 25 years after graduation. One doctor and five controls were excluded because they returned fewer than four questionnaires. In 1953, 1957 and 1964 if a questionnaire had gone unanswered but the preceding and succeeding questionnaires had been answered, the average of the two answered questionnaires was substituted for the missing questionnaire. After these adjustments had been made, smoking information for any given period was still lacking for about 5 percent of subjects. In the calculation of the percentages of smokers and nonsmokers, the missing 5 percent was ignored.

of sleeping pills is excluded, only 40 percent of the doctors and 28 percent of the controls would have been classed in Group 3 or above In a sample of this size this difference is not statistically significant. In a population selected for health, then, much of the physicians' increased use of drugs is accounted for by sleeping pills.

At some point in their careers, three doctors were occupationally incapacitated by their use of alcohol or drugs, and each of these men spent about a year in the hospital. One physician required frequent short hospitalizations for alcohol but otherwise was able to keep his spree drinking and the practice of medicine quite separate. Another doctor was virtually unemployed for a decade, and the occupational efficiency of a third was impaired for five years. At last contact all three men were practicing medicine and not misusing drugs or alcohol.

Table 7-IV

MAXIMUM USE OF MOOD-ALTERING DRUGS AND ALCOHOL BY 45 DOCTORS AND 90 CONTROLS

GROUP*	PHYSICIANS(%)	CONTROLS(%)
1	11	29
2	27	39
3	31	13
4 (Drugs)	20	10
4 (Alcohol)	4	8
5	7	1

*1 – no reported use of sedatives, tranquilizers or stimulants; use of alcohol "never" to "occasional."

2 – use of tranquilizers or sedatives "occasional" (but mentioned only once): alcohol "few regular" or "varies."

3 – maximum use of alcohol reported as "trouble with control" or "many regular" (mentioned only once) or "occasional" use of pills – "occasional" means sedative use mentioned on 2 or more occasions, sedatives, more than once/mo (mentioned once), daily use of tranquiliizers for $<$ 1 mo or occasional amphetamines.

4 – (drugs) – "regular" use of pills; sedatives used "often" or "daily," amphetamines used daily, or tranquilizers used daily for $>$ 1 mo or all 3 classes of drugs used occasionally.

5 – hospitalization or clear damage to socioeconomic status owing to use of mood-altering drugs or alcohol.

Among the controls, one man drank up to a quart of whiskey a day, but was classed in Group 4 (Alcohol) because this amount of drinking impaired neither his health nor his career as a successfull creative artist. The one control in Group 5 was the only man lost to direct follow-up observation. According to a close relative, he had lost two years of employment and several jobs because of his drinking. He is currently said to be functioning effectively in a middle-management position. To our knowledge no controls were ever hospitalized for drug or alcohol abuse.

Heavy use of drugs, alcohol and tobacco occurred together. At some point all three physicians in Group 5 used drugs *and* alcohol to excess. One man (a control) classed in Group 4 (Alcohol) could also have been classed in Group 4 (Drugs); on one occasion five men in Group 4 (Drugs) – two controls and three doctors – reported alcohol use as "many regular" or trouble with control. Only 3 percent of the men classed in Group 1 or 2 (little drug use) in Table 7-IV sustained smoking habits of two packs a day for over a decade; this proportion of heavy smokers increased to 12 percent of those men in Group 3 and to 19 percent in Group 4 or 5. Over half the controls in Group 4 or 5 were trying to reduce their weight; this was true of only two of the doctors.

Neither the presence of feeding problems nor the absence of breast feeding in infancy was correlated with increased drug or alcohol use. But 40 percent of the men classed C (lowest) in psychologic soundness in college fell in Groups 4 or 5 (heavy use of drugs or alcohol); this was true of 28 percent classed B and only 13 percent classed A (highest). (This positive relation of psychologic instability in adolescence to adult drug use did not, however, account for the *differences* in drug use between physicians and controls.)

DISCUSSION

It must be emphasized that abuse of alcohol, and perhaps of mood-altering drugs, by the 135 men in the study is less than that by 45-year-old American males in general.[9,10] The paper focuses on the peak use of drugs and alcohol over a 20-year period in a group of men who have been unusually conscientious in reporting such use. But if doctors selected for health in college have less of a problem with alcohol than the general population, they do take pharmacologic agents that affect the central nervous system more than matched controls do. This increased use of mood-altering drugs is accompanied by a use of alcohol and some form of tobacco that is at least comparable to men in businesses, in which heavy social drinking may be an asset and smoking a less conscious danger. In short, doctors at the healthy as well as the pathologic end of the continuum show a relative excess of drug use.

To try to understand the results of this study, evidence will be drawn from other investigations with a larger number of drug-using physicians. Psychiatric study of physician addicts suggests that increased availability of drugs may not be enough to explain doctors' vulnerability to drug and alcohol misuse. For example, psychologically, physicians who are narcotic addicts resemble people who obtain narcotics illegally more closely than they do nonaddicted physicians.[11,12] Doctors themselves give "overwork" as the most common explanation of why they take narcotics.[11] But this explanation hides other needs. Medicine is hard work for anyone, but it is harder work for those who use the profession vicariously to give solace to others rather than themselves. In our study this was the group most prone to drug abuse. Psychiatrists who have cared for drug-using physicians are impressed by the doctor's need to be needed,[1,5] but the virtue of altruism is more taxing if it is an adaption to earlier deprivation. In our study none of the three physicians hospitalized for drugs or alcohol were literally overworked. But all three had experienced a consistent lack of support and concern from their parents that distinguished them from most other study members. All had tried to dedicate themselves to the care of others. An idealistic physician in Group 4 (Drugs) who had experienced rejection by both parents in childhood said of his practice, "A more dependent group is hard to imagine. I find this the hardest (in terms of what it takes out of me emotionally) job I have ever had."

Looking back on his career, a 47-year-old physician was quoted as saying, "I've forged the chains that now bind me . . . I think that my capacity to give at age 35 was more than it is now at 47. I'd like to have things given to me now."[13] But physicians may consider such a sentiment unseemly to express to others. Thus, after giving of himself to others, the physician may feel more than ordinarily entitled to "prescribe" drugs secretly for himself when he gets home. But a Group 4 (Drugs) physician gave up self-medication on the eve of his first vacation in years; he observed, "I am more willing now to accept my own weaknesses — I am no longer ashamed to accept pleasure for pleasure's sake."

Secondly, physicians learn to dissociate themselves from danger to be able to cope with it. For effective patient care, every physician must engender in himself the belief that "it can't happen to me." Such a credo helps the doctor's patients but creates difficulty for the doctor's own physician. At the Menninger Clinic, Modlin and Montes[11] were impressed by the doctor addicts' magical belief in the nonaddictive properties of meperidine; each thought, "it won't hurt me." The difficulty of inducing physicians to seek annual checkups, chest plates, cardiograms and the like is well known. A clinical illustration of the denial of distress in self-medicating physicians was a doctor, not in the present study, who consulted one of us (G.E.V.) because of addiction to meperidine. This doctor emphatically stated that he was not suicidal, and not depressed, and asked if he could have permission to attend to his own cure. Yet this was a practicing physician who had driven from another state for the consultation, who wept during the interview and who customarily injected meperidine into his thigh with unsterile technic while driving on a superhighway.

To mitigate the occupational hazards of drug use in physicians, several positive steps can be taken. The physicians of doctors should recognize, first of all, that their patient's tendency to deny illness will make a diagnosis difficult; secondly, the patient's virtue of not troubling his doctor may lead to the wish to self-prescribe; and, thirdly, the patient's willingness to care selflessly for others may conceal a greater than average need to be given to. The physicians of doctors should be alert to depression in their patients and must inquire directly about self-medication. Urine tests for opiates and blood tests for barbiturates may be revealing in any physician who represents a diagnostic enigma.

A frank but concerned attitude is critical for state medical societies. In seeking supervision for addicted physicians, one of us (G.E.V.) was assured by two medical societies that in their states the problem was too small to merit attention. This view may only support the addict doctor's own tendency to deny his affliction. In states like California and New York, where medical societies and boards of medical examiners have confronted the question frankly, drug abuse certainly appears to be a problem worthy of notice. In California, if they wished to retain their license, addicted physicians were required to undergo five years of compulsory supervision. The reported cure rate is 92 percent[6]; this is much higher than that reported for doctors voluntarily admitted to psychiatric-treatment centers.[11,14]

Finally, medical schools must assume greater responsibility for teaching their students that they represent a high-risk population for drug abuse, and that, unchecked, the virtues of the good physician can increase the risk. No physician, whatever his rationalization, should write a prescription for himself for a drug that will make his brain feel better, sleep better or work better. This will not be easy for the student to hear; he will use his excellent intelligence to argue that his instructor is overcautious. But in our group of 45 physicians, preselected for psychologic soundness, self-medication with drugs or alcohol was the cause of one-third of the total time that this group spent in the hospital.

REFERENCES

1. Duffy JC, Litin EM: The *Emotional Health of Physicians*. Springfield, Charles C Thomas, Publisher, 1967
2. Simon W, Lumry GK: Suicide among physician-patients. *J Nerv Ment Dis 147:*105-112, 1968
3. a'Brook MF, Hailstone JD, McLauchlan IFJ: Psychiatric illness in the medical profession. *Brit J Psychiat 113:*1013-1023, 1967
4. Small IF, Small JG, Assue CM, et al: The fate of the mentally ill physician.

*Amer J Psychiat 125:*1333-1342, 1969

5. Pearson MM, Strecker EA: Physicians as psychiatric patients: private practice experience. *Amer J Psychiat 116:*915-919, 1960
6. Jones LE: How 92% beat the dope habit. *Bull Los Angeles County Med Ass 88:*19 and 37-40, 1958
7. Bellizzi JJ: Personal communication
8. Hearings before a subcommittee of the Committee on Appropriations, House of Representatives, 89th Congress, first session, February 15, 1965. Washington, DC. Government Printing Office, 1965, pp 45-50 and 204-296
9. Cahalan D, Cisin IH: American drinking practices: summary of findings from a national probability sample. 1. Extent of drinking by population subgroups. *Quart J Stud Alcohol 29:*130-151, 1968
10. Terman LM, Oden MH: The Gifted Group at Mid-Life: 35 years' follow-up of the superior child. Stanford, Stanford University Press, 1959
11. Modlin HC, Montes A: Narcotics addiction in physicians. *Amer J Psychiat 121:*358-365, 1964
12. Hill HE, Haertzen CA, Yamahiro RS: XXV. The addict physician: a Minnesota Multiphasic Personality Inventory study of the interaction of personality characteristics and availability of narcotics. *Res Publ Ass Res Nerv Ment Dis 46:*321-322, 1968
13. Mawardi BH: A career study of physicians. *J Med Educ 40:*658-666, 1965
14. Putnam PL, Ellinwood EH Jr: Narcotic addiction among physicians: a ten-year follow-up. *Amer J Psychiat 122:*745-748, 1966

Chapter 8

DRUG ADDICTION AMONG PHYSICIANS
The Virginia Experience

ROBERT C. GREEN, JR., GEORGE J. CARROLL, AND WILLIAM D. BUXTON

As drug addiction in the general population has increased, awareness of addiction as an occupational hazard among physicians has also developed. In 1957, the US Commissioner of Narcotics estimated that one of 100 physicians was addicted, as compared with one of 3,000 in the general population.[1] In New York state alone in a 25-year period, 0.5 percent of all licensed physicians were reported as addicts to the Bureau of Narcotics Control.[2] A 1969 estimate[3] of 300 new physician addicts per year is probably now too conservative.

This communication analyzed 46 cases of drug-addicted physicians handled by the Virginia State Board of Medicine from 1949 to 1974, with emphasis on background, personality disorder, and probable causes of addiction. We also discuss the board's disciplinary, therapeutic, and rehabilitative scheme.

Our study may seem small, but the board believes these 46 cases are merely the "tip of the iceberg." Too often, the problem is handled locally, by revoking hospital privileges or by inducing the addicted physician to move to another state, without attempts at treatment and rehabilitation.

RESULTS OF VIRGINIA STUDY

From 1949 to 1960, less than one case per year was reported to the board. Since 1960, the yearly incidence increased to a peak of five cases in 1968, but has gradually declined since. One case was recorded in 1974, although two additional cases were reported but

---

From Robert C. Green et al., Drug Addiction Among Physicians, The Virginia Experience, *JAMA 236:* 12, Sept. 20, 1976.

From the Virginia State Board of Medicine, Portsmouth.

F. Juanita Mayo and Margaret P. Neville accumulated the raw data in this communication.

not included in this study (Fig 8-1).

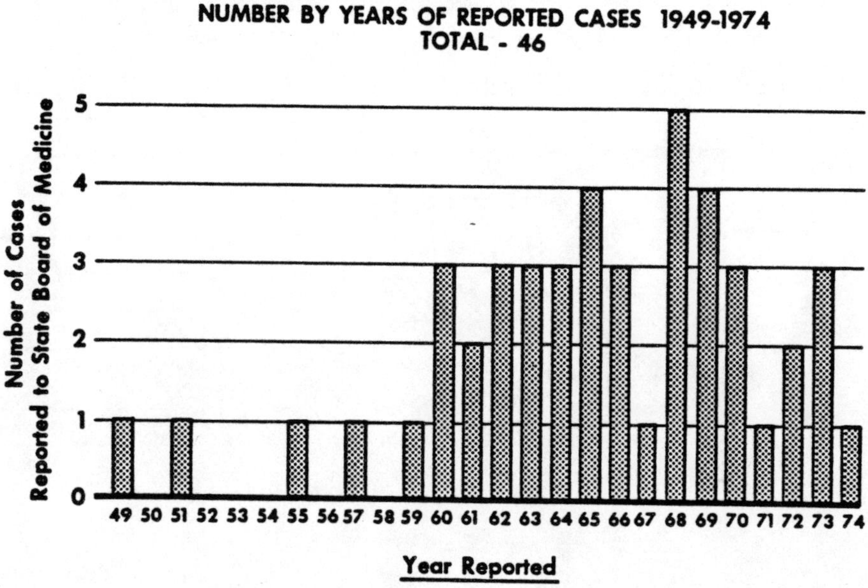

Figure 8-1.

The majority of initial reports on physician addicts in Virginia came from state and federal narcotics inspectors, with state mental institutions and hospitals the next largest source. Their distribution is as follows: state and federal narcotics investigators, 26; institutions, 10; individuals, 5; patients, 2; other state boards, 2; and Medical Society of Virginia, 1.

Regrettably, legislation passed in the 1974 Virginia Assembly no longer makes involuntary commitment of drug-addicted physicians a mandatory reportable offense to the state board. Reporting of these cases is now up to the treating psychiatrist's judgment, so there may well be fewer cases coming to the board's attention.

Physicians' ages in initial reports to the board ranged from 27 to 73 years, with a median of 45 years. It appears significant that a stair-step progression developed, peaking in the 45-to 49-year group with 13 of the 46 cases. The incidence in the older age group was markedly lower.

The number of years in practice relates directly to the frequency of addiction (Fig 8-2). Median duration of practice was 18 years, followed by a gradual decline in incidence of drug dependency.

Information on duration of addiction prior to its being reported was available in only 32 cases, but 16 were reported within a year of onset. It is noteworthy that some addicted physicians could go on for

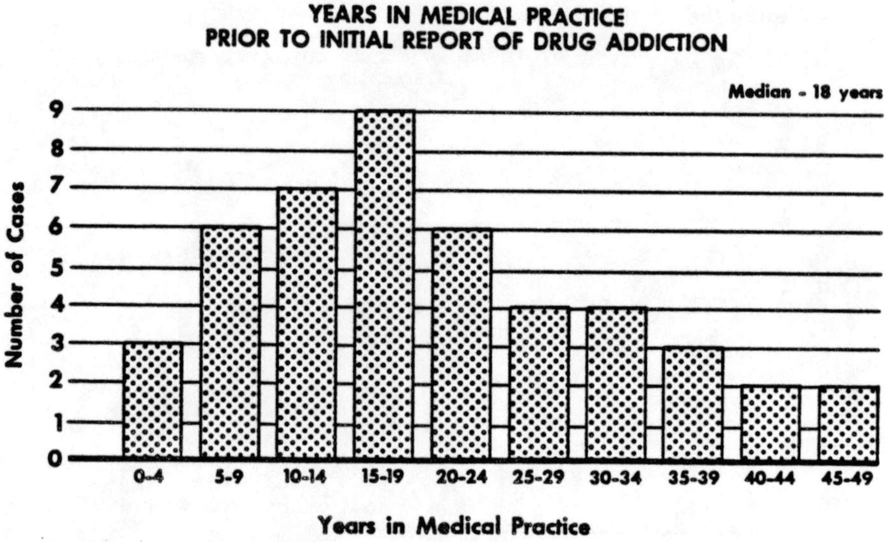

Figure 8-2.

10, 16, and, in one instance, 18 years, without being apprehended.

Median age of onset of addiction was 43 years, with seven physicians in the 45- to 49-year group (Fig 8-3). Eight physicians' ages ranged from 22 to 34 years, and two were in the 60- to 69-year span when addiction started.

Meperidine hydrochloride (Demerol) was the principal addicting drug, with morphine, hydromorphone hydrochloride (Dilaudid), and amphetamines next in frequency. Drugs most commonly used, alone or in combination were meperidine, 31; morphine, 9; hydromorphone, 8; amphetamine, 7; barbiturates, 6; pentazocine (Talwin), 3; methadone hydrochloride, 3; codeine, 2; hydrochlorides of opium alkaloids (Pantopon), 2; tranquilizers, 2; opium, cocaine, paraldehyde, and anileridine hydrochloride (Leritine), 1 each. Most of the addicted physicians used more than one drug, and often several simultaneously. Alcohol was used in ten cases, but it was never the primary addicting agent.

Precipitating factors named as significant by 22 of the 46 physicians were physical pain and illness, usually chronic, with family tragedy such as death of a wife or child, next. The third most common factor was an addicted wife. Situational stress, overwork, and marital problems were also mentioned.

A psychiatric classification, available in 31 of our 46 physicians,

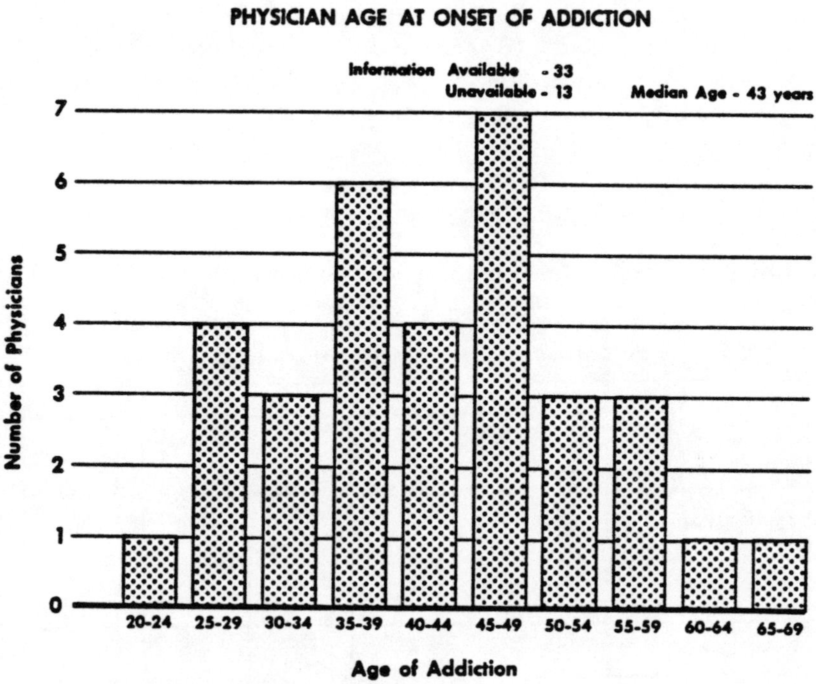

Figure 8-3.

was provided either by independent psychiatrists, mental institutions, or by the board's own Psychiataric Advisory Committee. The Psychiatric Advisory Committee consists of three psychiatrists and one psychologist, appointed by the Board of Medicine to interview and evaluate the mental status of physicians referred by the board. The committee presents its initial psychiatric evaluation and subsequent follow-up information at each physician interview with the board.

Depression, one of the most frequent psychiatric problems, occured as pure depression in 11 physicians, and in two, as manic depression. The majority of psychiatric diagnoses were listed as neurosis and personality disorders, with only nine classified as psychoses.

Of the 46 physicians, 27 returned to private practice and six remained in institutional work. Licenses were revoked in 11 cases because of repeated lapses, and two physicians left the state. The rehabilitation rate was 72 percent.

The personality profile of the drug-addicted physician would indicate that he is a graduate of the Virginia medical schools, with a specialty of general practice or internal medicine. He is white, male, and has been in practice 18 years. Age at onset of drug abuse was 43 years, and has continued one to two years until discovery. Principal drug use is meperidine. The general psychiatric diagnosis is depression.

OTHER STUDIES

Other studies[4-7] are generally comparable to our survey (Fig 8-4).

PHYSICIAN ADDICTS

Comparison of Published Reports with Virginia Study

	Authors				
	Pescor[9]	Wall[10]	Modlin and Montes[11]	Putnam[12]	Green et al (Virginia)
Year published	1942	1958	1964	1966	1976
Number of cases	47	44	25	68	46
Principal specialty	GP	--	GP IM	GP	GP
Mean age at onset	39	36	38	--	42
Mean years on drugs	13	--	3	--	3.7
Mean age of discovery of addiction	45	43	41	46	43
Principal drug	Morphine	Morphine	Demerol	Morphine	Demerol
Principal cause	Pain	Pain	Chronic Fatigue	Pain	Pain
Psychiatric diagnosis	Psychopathic Diathesis	Psychopathic Personality	--	--	Depression
Rehabilitated (percent)	"Poor"	27	28	--	72

Figure 8-4.

In view of the important implications of this problem, it is surprising that so few studies have been directed toward the psychiatric aspect of drug addiction in physicians. Winick[8] found negative attitude toward being a physician, passive personality, and feelings of omnipotence frequent traits in the 98 physician addicts he interviewed.

In a more detailed study of 36 hospitalized physician addicts, Wall[5] noted the following outstanding personality traits: sensitivity and tender-mindedness with a tendency to hypochondriasis, easy fatigability and inability to withstand stress, immaturity, inadequacy and withdrawal, neurasthenia, depression, and schizoid makeup.

Modlin and Montes[6] felt that addiction in their physician patients was a symptom of moderately severe progressive personality disorganization. Hill et al[9] employed the Minnesota Multiphasic Personality Inventory (MMPI) as a standard personality test on 42 physician addicts and found strong evidence of general maladjustment, reflected as hypochondriasis, depression, general neuroticism, and anxiety. Duffy and Litin[10] noted a high incidence of alcoholism among physician addicts, but little or no similarity between them and the street addict.

CAUSATIVE FACTORS

The basic mechanisms in physician drug addiction are difficult to define. However, it seems generally accepted that three conditions ordinarily must coexist: (1) a predisposing personality, (2) availability of narcotics, and (3) circumstances bringing (1) and (2) together.[11]

A major factor in physician addiction, aside from personality and psychiatric characteristics, is the availability of drugs and especially the drug most often selected, meperidine. This may be due to the erroneous concept that meperidine, being a synthetic derivative, is nonaddictive. Early studies[12-14] suggested that meperidine had little addictive liablility, and that its addictive properties were less than those of morphine. Also, initial manufacturers' promotions for meperidine included claims of nonaddiction. Although meperidine first became available in 1944, some physicians are still not fully aware of its addictive properties.

Another reason for physician preference of meperidine is that the drug acts more rapidly to produce greater elation, with a briefer duration of effect than other drugs, in particular, morphine.

REHABILITATION PROGRAM

The Virginia State Board of Medicine has evolved a rehabilitation program that has helped to restore 72 percent of physician addicts to medical practice. This program requires immediate surrender of the physician's nacotics license (usually for life), placing the physician's medical license on probation, and psychiatric evaluation by the board's Psychiatric Advisory Committee. The physician must then seek psychiatric and medical care. This may be of his own choosing, but must be approved by the committee. His progress and condition are monitored by the Psychiatric Advisory Committee through regular interviews, reports from the treating psychiatrist, and mandatory periodic return visits before the entire board.

When the addicted physician's treating psychiatrist, the Psychiatric Advisory Committee, and the board believe he is ready to return to practice, permission is granted to begin a limited work schedule, often in a protected environment. With constant surveillance and repeated interviews by the board and the Psychiatric Advisory Committee, the addicted physician is gradually guided back into full practice responsibility. Unfortunately, not all respond to this regimen, and relapses are frequent; ultimately, some are never salvaged.

It has been our experience, as well as that of the California State Board of Medicine,[15] that the rehabilitation of addicted physicians is best handled at the state board level for the following reasons: (1) Most general psychiatrists have limited experience in treating drug-addicted physicians, and often do not appreciate the seriousness of the problem. (2) Removing, restricting, or putting the physician's license on probation is a tremendous lever in forcing him to seek medical and psychiatric care. (3) Continued and forcible surveillance and reevaluation at periodic intervals by the board and the Psychiatric Advisory Committee help ensure against relapse. If relapse does occur, it can be properly recognized. (4) Mandatory removal of a physician's narcotics license, usually for life, helps support his abstinence from drugs.

REFERENCES

1. Anslinger HJ: Interview. *Mod Med 25:*170-191, 1957.
2. Vaillant GE, Brighton AB, McArther C: Physicians' use of mood-altering drugs. *N Engl J Med 282:*365-370, 1970.
3. Garb S: Drug addiction in physicians. *Anesth Analg 48:*1, 1969.
4. Pescor MJ: Physician drug addicts. *Dis Nerv Syst 3:*173-174, 1942.
5. Wall JH: The result of hospital treatment of addiction in physicians. *Federation Bull 45:*144-152, 1958.
6. Modlin HC, Montes A: Narcotic addiction in physicians. *Am J Psychiatry 121:*358-365, 1964.
7. Putnam PL, Ellinwood EH: Narcotic addiction among physicians: A ten-year

follow-up. *Am J Psychiatry 122:*745-747, 1966.

8. Winick C: Physician narcotic addicts. *Soc Probl 9:*174-186, 1961.
9. Hill HE, Haertzen CA, Yamahiro RS: The addict physician: A Minnesota Multiphasic Personality Inventory study of the interaction of personality characteristics and availability of narcotics: *Res Publ Assoc Res Nerv Ment Dis 45:*321-332, 1966.
10. Duffy JC, Litin EM: *The Emotional Health of Physicians.* Springfield, Ill, Charles C Thomas Publisher, 1967, p. 63.
11. *Narcotic Drug Addiction.* Mental Health monograph 2, US Dept Health, Education, and Welfare, 1963.
12. Batterman RC: Demerol, A new synthetic analgesic: Its indications as a substitute for morphine. *Conn State Med J 8:*13-17, 1944.
13. Batterman RC: Clinical effectiveness and safety of a new synthetic analgesic drug, Demerol. *Arch Intern Med 71:*344-345, 1943.
14. Noth PH, Hecht HH, Yonkman FF: Demerol, a new synthetic analgesic, spasmolytic and sedative agent: Clinical observations. *Ann Intern Med 21:*17-25, 1944.
15. Jones LE, Thompson W: How 92% beat the dope habit. *Bull Los Angeles County Med Assoc 88:*19, 1958.

Marital Discord

Chapter 9

PSYCHIATRIC ILLNESS IN THE PHYSICIAN'S WIFE

JAMES L. EVANS

FREQUENT admission of physicians' wives to a private psychiatric hospital raised the question of a possible relationship between the husbands' occupation and the occurrence and manifestations of illness in the wives. The present study was undertaken to investigate this possibility.

For the years 1960 through 1963, the first 50 cases meeting the following criteria were selected for this study: the record had been completed (patient was discharged), the patient at the time of admission was married to a physician, the illness was not definitely ascribable to organic factors (as in one case of a meningioma and another of cerebral arteriosclerosis).

Hospital records were used exclusively in this research; none of the patients was treated or interviewed by the author. Histories from 40 of the physician-husbands were obtained by the 31 different therapists who treated the patients. In addition, material presented by the patients in therapeutic sessions was recorded in their charts. Also included were copies of records obtained from other hospitals and therapists, reports of social service workers who interviewed family members and the results of psychological testing including the Minnesota Multiphasic Personality Inventory.

At the time of admission to hospital, the patients were of a mean age of 40.2 (25-62) years; the mean age of onset of illness was 33.9 (15-54), with a peak (23 patients) in the 29-35 year age-group. The onset of illness was established as the time when the first overt symptoms appeared that eventually led to psychiatric treatment.

MARITAL HISTORY. At the time symptoms became overt, patients had been married 12.8 (1-18) years and were admitted to the hospital after an average of 19.1 (2-31) years of marriage. They had been married at a mean age of 21.1 (17-33).

From James L. Evans, Psychiatric Illness in the Physician's Wife, *The American Journal of Psychiatry, 122:* 159-163, 1965.

Presented at the 120th annual meeting of the American Psychiatric Association, Los Angeles, CA, May 4-8, 1964.

Older than their wives by an average of 5.6 years, the husbands had been a mean age of 26.7 at marriage. Ten of the doctor-husbands were 8 or more years older than their wives. One of the husbands had been hospitalized for drug addiction; none of the others had a history of severe psychiatric illness. According to their wives, the husbands were undemonstrative (12), stilted or cold (12), dependent and passive (11), domineering (11), a failure at fulfilling the responsibilities of husbands and fathers (11) and stern, compulsive and perfectionistic (8).

The frequent absence of the husband was a complaint mentioned by 26 patients, and in 16 cases was specifically noted by the therapist as a precipitating factor in the patient's illness. Seven of the wives who at one time had actively participated in the husband's medical practice stated that they felt excluded and left out after the husband acquired other nursing and office help. At the time the wife's illness began, the mean age of the doctor-husband was 39.5, and, with the exception of six men, three just beginning to practice, one in residency and two who were doing poorly, the husbands were engaged in busy and successful careers.

In only nine couples were frequent and mutually satisfying sexual relations described as having existed throughout the marriage. While considerable variation was present among the remaining couples with regard to frequency and enjoyment of intercourse, in 13 of these couples relations were nonexistent, very infrequent or mutually unsatisfactory.

FAMILY BACKGROUND. There was a wide distribution of social class, religious and ethnic background in the patients studied. However, the majority were from middle class families, with only seven patients specifically described as being from upper class backgrounds and six as being from definitely lower class or poor families.

A family history of emotional disturbance was present in 31 of the wives' families. In 18 of these families, there was a history in parents or siblings of psychiatric hospitalization, suicide, or psychotic illness specified in terms of diagnostic category by the informant. This does not include statements about relatives such as "religious fanatic," "ne'er do well" or "unstable." A history of gross psychiatric symptomatology in more than one family member was present in 14 cases.

Strong negative comments about mother (78) far outnumbered the positive (19), while negative comments about father (40) were less frequent, almost equalling the positive (35). Nine of the fathers had died before the patient's 15th year, while four mothers had died before this time. Three of the patients had fathers who were physicians. The most frequently mentioned characteristics of the mother were: domineering (18), distant (11) or rejecting (10) attitude toward the patient, moody (9), demanding (9) and rigid (9). Fathers were most often seen as having a close relationship with the patient (14), and as being shy or retiring (13), easygoing (10), strict (8) and dependent (6).

ADJUSTMENT PRIOR TO ILLNESS. Of the 19 patients who were college graduates three had majored in sciences and three began but did not complete pre-medical courses. Nine had had some college education, but did not finish. Twelve were nursing school graduates and two had not completed nursing training. Eight patients had completed but not gone beyond the high school level.

Comments about the patients indicating qualities generally considered to be positive were made by informants with considerably greater frequency than negative statements, as seen in Table 9-I. Many patients had been club members, belonged to community organizations and entertained frequently. However, there was relatively little use of terms describing them as warm, accepting, affectionate, emotionally demonstrative or giving.

SYMPTOMATOLOGY. In many cases several major symptoms leading to admission were presented, such as "anxiety and muscle spasms" or "depression and excessive drinking." Depression was the most frequently mentioned of the "chief complaints" (15), followed by overuse of drugs (10) or alcohol (9), suspiciousness (8), anxiety (6), nonspecific emotional instability (6), suicidal attempt (5) and persistent pain (4). Also mentioned were withdrawal, excessive hostility, agitation, hypomania or mania and feelings of rejection.

In addition to those cases with presenting complaints of use of alcohol or drugs to excess there was a history of overuse of either alcohol (5) or addictive drugs (12) reported by informants in 17 other cases. Seven patients had sufficiently long-standing histories of overconsumption of alcohol to warrant a secondary diagnosis of alcoholism. A secondary diagnosis of drug addiction was made in the case of 11 patients, while 11 others had histories of using addictive drugs to the point of psychological and physiological dependence. These 22 patients had used one or more of the following drugs: barbiturates (7), morphine or morphine derivatives (14) and amphetamines (4).

Included in the records of 16 of these 22 patients was information on the method of acquiring the drug. Twelve women had obtained drugs from the husband's medical supplies; in these cases, five of the

Table 9-I

Characteristics of Personality Before Illness

POSITIVE		NEGATIVE	
Socially active	26	Reserved or withdrawn	11
Interested in intellectual or cultural pursuits	22	Feels inadequate	10
Outgoing, friendly	18	Attention seeking	9
Socially ambitious	14	Few close friends	8
Meticulous, conscientious	14	Overly sensitive to criticism	6
Cheerful, usually in good spirits	13	Unable to show anger	5
Good mother, homemaker	7	Somatic preoccupations	5
Driving, energetic	6	Moody	4
Affectionate, emotionally demonstrative	3	Dominating	4

husbands had either injected or given their wives medication, while four other husbands stated that they had been aware their wives were taking drugs from their bags or from office supplies. Of the four remaining cases, patients had relied primarily upon drug samples (3) and prescriptions (1). Drugs had been instituted for the treatment of somatic complaints in 15 patients (for pain in 13 cases). Use of drugs began in six patients following operative procedures.

Medical history. Twenty-eight of the patients had had from one to six previous hospital admissions because of psychiatric symptoms; many of them were admissions to general hospitals for the treatment of alcohol or drug intoxication. Hospital admissions for physical illnesses are also worthy of review, as are the general medical histories of these patients. Twenty-one had complaints of chronic or recurrent pain: eight had recurrent abdominal pain, while migraine (4), low back pain (4), severe dysmenorrhea (4), arthritis (3) and headache other than migraine (2) were also mentioned, with overlapping in several cases.

In attempts to relieve pain, ten patients had undergone the

following procedures: sacro-sympathectomy, spinal fusion and cordotomy, presacral neurectomy, pancreatic exploration (3), hysterectomy (3) and temporal artery ligation. No specific pathology was found in the above cases, in contrast to the 20 cases where definite pathology was demonstrated at operation or where the patient had other symptoms or signs, such as jaundice or fever.

Eleven patients had undergone extensive medical workups not resulting in operative procedures for symptoms of obscure etiology such as headache, dizziness, fatigue or gastrointestinal complaints, with no definitive findings.

MMPI SCORES. At the time of admission 28 patients took the Minnesota Multiphasic Personality Inventory. Highest scores for this group came in the psychopathic deviate scale, followed by hysterical, depressed and paranoid scales. (See Figure 9-1.)

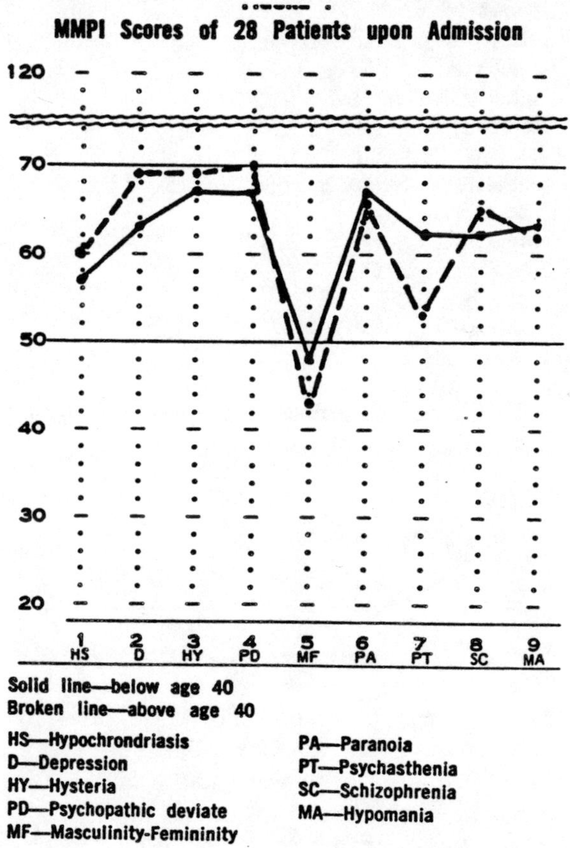

Figure 9-1.

Diagnosis. Twenty-nine illnesses were classified as nonpsychotic disorders, with 15 of these in the passive-aggressive personality category. Twenty-one came under the heading of psychotic disorders. (See Table 9-II.)

Table 9-II

Diagnosis of 50 Patients

Passive aggressive personality 15
  passive aggressive type (11)
    with drug addiction 5; with alcoholism 4
  passive dependent type (4)
    with drug addiction 2; with alcoholism 1; with depression 1
Schizophrenic reaction 12
  paranoid type (5)
  chronic undifferentiated type (2)
    with drug addiction 1
  acute undifferentiated type (2)
  schizo-affective type (3)
Depressive reaction 7
  with drug addiction 1; with alcoholism 2
Manic depressive reaction 5
  manic type (2)
  depressed type (2)
  other type (1)
Involutional psychotic reaction 2
Paranoid state 2
Paranoid personality 1 with drug addiction
Emotionally unstable personality 1 with drug addiction
Psychoneurotic reaction, other 1
Personality trait disturbance, other (hysteria) 1 with depression
Psychophysiological musculoskeletal reaction 1
Anxiety reaction 1
Obsessive compulsive reaction 1

DISCUSSION

The contrast between the reportedly good pre-morbid adjustment of the patients as a group and the severity and tenacity of their illnesses is striking. Many (41) patients had a history of repeated or protracted treatment, and were admitted to the Institute of Living only after several relapses or failure to respond to treatment. Nevertheless, prior to illness, they had been quite successful. They were well-educated and pursued a variety of intellectual and cultural activities in their leisure moments. They were able to marry men with high socio-cultural standing. As a group they had successfully weathered the difficult years of their husbands' medical and specialty training and the early years of practice. Only after an average of almost 13 years of marriage was an overt illness manifested.

By the time of admission, these women had raised families averaging almost three children, had participated in community activities and had furthered their social aims. Most patients in this group possessed enough ego strength prior to illness to achieve a superior level of social adaptation. However, the elevation of the psychopathic deviate scale on the MMPIs suggests a personality structure less mature in terms of impulse control than would otherwise have been apparent. The patients also appeared to have been overly dependent upon the environment for reinforcement of their self-concept.

With a mean age spread between husband and wife of 5.6 years, the peak age for onset of illness (early thirties) occurred at the time when most physicians, including the husbands of these women, are established and in their peak years (late thirties) of active practice. Underscoring the possibility of a relationship here is the prevalence of complaints about the increasing absence of the husband at the time when the wife's personal involvement in her husband's work is decreasing.

Informants described 14 patients as having been very close to their fathers, and the therapists of 12 patients felt that a father-daughter relationship existed between patients and their husbands. In addition, there was a mean elevation of the MMPI hysteria scale and a history of relative sexual incompatibility in at least 75 percent of the cases. Marriage to an older man, whose vocation may have been unconsciously associated with omnipotent, understanding, protective attributes may be interpreted as an attempt by many of the patients to resolve persisting oedipal conflicts. Illness developed when the equilibrium of the adjustment was disrupted by such reality factors as the increasing involvement of the doctor in his work, or a conflict between his personality characteristics and the idealized expectations of his wife.

Despite the broad variety of diagnostic categories, three symptomatic themes tend to recur: depression, drug addiction and somatization. As the doctor became increasingly involved in his work depression was precipitated by the psychological loss, which intensified the wife's ambivalent feelings. In addition, the wife, previously an active participant in her husband's career, was faced with the loss of this role. The second symptomatic theme, the use of drugs, is specifically related to the husband's profession by virtue of ready accessibility of medications. Thus, the patient unconsciously symbolized her dependency needs through the use of one of the most fundamental and gratifying resources the physician has to offer — drugs used to relieve pain.

The third theme, frequently interwoven with the previous two, appears in the history of somatic symptomatology, particularly of pain. This symptom also points to the hostile-dependent aspects of the husband-wife relationship. Pain brings a patient to the attention of the physician who, in turn, directs his energy to the alleviation of that pain. Nothing can be more frustrating, confusing or embarrassing to the physician than pain of undiagnosed etiology which he cannot relieve. It is a symptom which professionally cannot be ignored or left unattended; it must receive that attention which, in his wife's view, the doctor devotes to his patients, perhaps to the exclusion of his wife's needs.

The recorded comments of family, patient and therapist gave a number of indications that the husbands had contributed to some extent to the illnesses of their wives, a participation which extended beyond the doctor's preoccupation with his work. The physician, secure in his omnipotent role with patients who are frankly dependent upon his professional capabilities, rejected his wife's dependency strivings except when they were expressed as demands for "medical" attention. He then, without apparent cognizance of their emotional basis, gratified these needs by resorting to his professional role. A number of patients, for example, who were addicted to drugs, continued to have ready access to them even after the addiction was evident, and in several cases the drugs were furnished by the husband. Furthermore, of 17 patients who left the hospital prematurely, that is, against the recommendation of their therapists, six were withdrawn by the husband; the other 12 patients did not have any pronounced difficulty in persuading their husbands to condone this action. In many instances, the husband was unwilling or unable to set limits on his wife's behavior. This passivity, or even cooperation, in his wife's psychopathology suggests that these doctors felt guilty about their own inability to meet the emotional needs of their wives.

A number of factors should be considered in the therapeutic approach to this type of patient. First, symptomatic relief of depression and the fulfillment of dependency needs inherent in the hospital of social functioning, without necessarily effecting a change in the underlying psychopathology. The patient and her family may then conclude that she is well and ready to return home. Second, the natural desire to maintain a good relationship with a professional colleague may cause the therapist to acquiesce consciously or unconsciously to the patient's neurotic demands, for instance, to requests for intensive investigation of physical symptoms.

Third, the transference feelings of patients with a high index of hysterical fixation may be complicated and difficult to treat. They carry many of their feelings toward their physician-husbands into their relationship with the physician-psychiatrist. Fourth, because of the likelihood that the husband will continue to be absorbed in his professional commitments and can no longer serve as the principal source of gratification for his wife's dependency needs, the patient must be encouraged to establish a separate and personally meaningful role for herself.

SUMMARY

The records of 50 wives of physicians admitted to a private psychiatric hospital have been reviewed. Despite a high level of adaptation in the early years of marriage, they later developed severe psychiatric illnesses requiring repeated hospitalizations. A precipitating factor in many of these cases appeared to be a feeling of increasing exclusion from the husband's life, as he became more and more involved in his profession. Symptoms of depression, somatization and addiction were prevalent and were related dynamically and empirically to the profession of the husband.

Chapter 10

THE DOCTOR'S WIFE: MENTAL ILLNESS AND MARITAL PATTERN

JAMES E. MILES, ROBERT KRELL, AND TSUNG-YI LIN

THE marital problems of physicians may be reflected in the seemingly large numbers of their wives who present as psychiatric patients. The children of physicians, when presented for psychiatric evaluation, provide another opportunity through family assessment to study the marital patterns of physicians. The authors' experience and discussions with colleagues indicate that no matter which member of the physician's family presents as the primary patient, major marital conflict is almost invariably present. Although conjoint therapy with physician-wife couples is gratifyingly successful, all too often this is a treatment approach which is either avoided entirely or embarked upon only when the marital situation has deteriorated to such an extent that the likelihood of a successful outcome is prejudiced. Most frequently it is the wife who presents as the primary psychiatric patient, and it often appears that both the psychiatrist and the physician-husband collude to keep her in that role and avoid a conjoint approach. The referral is usually from a physician family friend who has become involved at the husband's request. The physician friend becomes aware of the emotional factors existing in the wife presenting with multiple somatic complaints, whom he investigates exhaustively and refers widely without discovering any significant organic basis for her complaints. Or the physician friend is involved in a moment of crisis, often the wife's suicidal gesture or attempt. Whether through exhaustive medical procedures or through crisis, the physician friend feels increasingly overwhelmed as the situation continues to deteriorate. Caught between his concern over the wife's condition and his reluctance to label his friend's spouse as a psychiatric patient, the family friend seizes upon the next moment of emotional crisis, often a suicide attempt, to make the psychiatric referral.

From James E. Miles et al., The Doctor's Wife: Mental Illness and Marital Pattern *Int'l J Psychiatry in Medicine,* vol. 6 (4), 1975.

These marital problems tend to be of unusual complexity and severity and show a marked similarity in the basic marital pattern. Typically, the physician's wife presents as depressed, angry and desperately unhappy. Frequently she is bewildered as to why she is experiencing such feelings. Materially comfortable, with secure social status, usually a financially generous husband, and often envied, her unhappiness and anger may seem inappropriate to her. The husband seems no less bewildered. He has "followed the rules" — worked hard, provided amply and wished the best for his family and is baffled by the turn of events which finds him with a depressed and suicidal wife and problem children. These men tend to be professionally competent and successful, but present as rigid, interpersonally distant and covertly or overtly controlling. They are extremely uncomfortable with feelings, whether of love and tenderness or hostility. They often are successful in demeaning the legitimate and meaningful feelings expressed by their wives by labelling them "emotional outbursts," and making demands for more "logical and rational" methods of problem-solving. Their need to avoid open conflict appears paramount and may, in part, explain such phenomena as:

1. Prescribing medication for the wife. Physicians, when queried about this practice, are usually defensive, and offer as excuses such statements as, "I'd do anything to keep her happy and get her off my back."
2. Increasing the amount of time spent in the practice which effectively removes him from the arena of conflict.
3. Tolerating the increasingly outrageous behaviors that his angry wife often resorts to as her needs continue to be unmet.

The poverty of communication between the marital partners is striking and they often impress the interviewer as virtual strangers, sharing only accommodation and children.

Others have noted distinctive features in emotional disorders in physicians' wives and linked these to the husbands' profession. Vaillant pointed out that physicians were more likely than matched controls to have poor marriages [1]. Evans stated, in his study of fifty physicians' wives hospitalized at the Institue for Living, that three symptomatic themes were common, namely depression, drug addiction and somatization, and related these dynamically and empirically to the husbands' profession [2]. Lewis, in a study of twenty-five hospitalized physicians' wives, noted an increased incidence of severe marital conflict as well as drug and alcohol addiction, and also related this to the husbands' occupation [3]. Harding, in an unpublished study on 107 physicians' wives hospitalized in the Harding Hospital, Columbus, Ohio, noted that 77 percent of the patients reported a "poor" relationship with their husbands at the time of admission. Eighty percent of these women stated that they felt "inferior and inadequate" in their husbands' presence. Of the seventy-six wives who gave information as to whether their husbands met their emotional needs, 92 percent indicated that these needs were not met.

METHOD

In an attempt to confirm the clinical impressions, a record review was undertaken of physicians' wives who had been in-patients in the Health Sciences Centre Hospital Psychiatric Unit, University of British Columbia, from its opening on March 1, 1969 until May 31, 1973. The Health Sciences Centre Hospital is a voluntary in-patient unit consisting of three twenty-two bed open wards, oriented to brief and intensive treatment of acute psychiatric problems. There is a major commitment to undergraduate and postgraduate training in psychiatry [4]. The orientation is eclectic, with minimal use of physical treatment methods and extensive use of medication, marital and family therapy in a milieu context. The following criteria were used for this study: the patient at the time of admission was married to a physician; the hospital stay had been completed within the above dates; the husband had been interviewed. Of the cases which met these criteria, twenty were randomly selected for this study.

The fifteen primary therapists were psychiatry residents. In all cases, the husbands had been interviewed at least once, and in fourteen of the cases there had been conjoint sessions. A majority of the patients had had psychological testing and reports from referring physicians and other hospitals were also available. Thirteen of the cases had previous admissions to psychiatric hospitals, or to general hospitals for psychiatric reasons, notably for attempted suicide. Six of the thirteen had more than one admission to the Health Sciences Centre Hospital. In this latter case the most recent admission is used as the point of reference.

RESULTS

At the time of admission to hospital, these patients had a mean age of 37.8 years (27-50), with three patients in the 20-30 years age-group, eight in the 30-40 group, and nine in the 40-50 group. Their average age at first psychiatric contact was 32.4 years (22-49). At the time of admission they had been married an average of 15.2 years (2-25), and at the time of first psychiatric contact had been married an average of 9.8 years (0-21). Thirteen of the twenty patients had paramedical training prior to marriage, eight of these being registered nurses. The average age at marriage was 22.5 years. There was an average of 2.6 children (0-4). The above figures approximate those of Evans [2].

In eleven of the twenty patients, there was a definite history of drug and/or alcohol abuse, most commonly in combination. The commonest drugs abused were barbiturates and diazepam. As Evans has noted, the husband was a frequent source of medication, either prescribing for his wife or seemingly ignoring her purloining of drugs from his medical bag [2].

Particularly striking is that eighteen of the twenty patients had expressed suicidal thoughts and thirteen had made suicidal attempts, all by overdose. It was difficult from examination of the records to determine the seriousness of the intent in all cases, but in six patients the attempt was clearly life-threatening.

In nineteen of the twenty case records, information was available on the sexual relationship. In one case this was described as satisfactory to both partners. In eighteen cases the sexual relationship was described as unsatisfactory to one or both partners. A frequent comment noted about the husband was "lack of interest."

In view of the variety of therapists involved, the diagnostic pattern is striking. Eighteen of the patients were discharged with a primary diagnosis of Depressive Neurosis, with one diagnosis of Psychotic Depression and one of Paranoid Schizophrenia. All of the patients with Neurotic Depression had a secondary diagnosis of Personality Disorder, most commonly Hysterical or Passive-aggressive Personality. Personality description contains frequent reference to such terms as "dependent, immature, histrionic, hostile and manipulative." The majority of the patients were problems in management on the ward, particularly initially when their diffuse anger and resentment were prominent features. Main described a group of twelve in-patients who "had a remarkable capacity to distress those who looked after them" [5]. These patients were severe ward management problems, and with one exception were treatment failures. All twelve patients were women and nine of them had close medical connections, for example, doctors' wives and daughters.

The description of the husbands' personality by treatment staff was, given the range of personnel recording, remarkably similar.

Only one of these husbands had been a psychiatric patient, and almost without exception they were well regarded and competent physicians, a slight majority being specialists. Such terms as "cold, distant, rigid, uncommunicative, undemonstrative" were frequent descriptive terms. A notable observation, both from the histories and records of conjoint sessions, was the extent to which the wife would go to provoke any reaction from her detached spouse. Also apparent was the urgency of the wife's need to find some explanation for her symptoms, to have the therapist see her husband as she experienced him and not as his patients and colleagues saw him. A frequent concern expressed was that "doctors stick together," and the wife feared that the psychiatrist would align himself with her husband. The husbands tended to minimize the problem, to resist any inference that they might play some role in the genesis of the wife's illness, to seek a solution for the wife's condition in medication and physical treatment methods and to avoid any psychotherapeutic approach which might involve them.

This group of women had their first psychiatric contact an average of 5.4 years prior to the reference hospitalization. Most of the patients had been seen individually, and there did not appear to have been a single serious attempt at conjoint therapy. The commonest pattern was that of a gradual deterioration in the patient and her marriage, with an increasing recourse to such avenues of escape and retaliation as alcohol and drugs, suicidal gestures or attempts and extra-marital involvement. Therapist and husband tended to become increasingly desperate, and for varying periods prior to hospitalization, the management became a series of crisis interventions. The husband and therapist often seemed to end up in an ambivalent relationship, held together by their joint impotence in the face of the wife's increasing rage and disordered behavior.

Despite the fact that independent review of the records as well as the therapists' views at the time point out in all cases the indication for conjoint therapy at least as an adjunct, in only five of the twenty patients was marital or family therapy accepted as a discharge plan, the major resistance coming from the husband.

DISCUSSION

The clinical impression of troubled physician marriages is supported by a review of hospitalized physicians' wives. It is apparent that these women experience great distress and that their marriages are deeply troubled. The basic marital pattern appears to be that of a dependent, histrionic woman with an inordinate need for affection and nurturing, marrying an emotionally detached man. The fact that he is a physician, seen by society as the ultimate in caring, may have much to do with the wife's choice of husband. The dramatic flair which many of these women have may be appealing to the rather inhibited, detached type of men the husbands in this group tended to be. The women also have a need to be "looked after" and this is complementary to some physicians' only way of relating to others, namely to "look after" them. Vaillant stated that some physicians have "painful and unstable marriages because they had married not partners but patients" [1].

As the marriage progresses, the wife appears to become progressively more resentful as her needs are not met. She becomes irritable and depressed, causing further withdrawal in her mate. His increased detachment results in an increase in her feelings of deprivation and resulting rage. Her dependency makes confrontation perilous, so there is the frequent recourse to alcohol, drugs, suicidal gestures or attempts. The husband's immersion in work, often cited as etiological, is in the authors' opinion symptomatic. It is his way of remaining detached, and also obtaining some positive reinforcement from others. These unhappy marital situations become very complex and, in spite of their obviously serious nature, satisfactory treatment approaches are often avoided.

Wherin lies the solution? Vaillant's [1] excellent study does not resort to the usual rather banal explanation of such factors as "overwork" for the physicians' emotional and marital dilemmas. He states:

> Physicians, especially those involved in direct patient care, were more likely than controls to have relatively poor marriages, to use drugs and alcohol heavily, and to obtain psychotherapy. Although these difficulties are often assumed to be occupational hazards of medicine, their presence or absence appeared to be strongly associated with life adjustment before medical school. Only the physicians with the least stable childhood and adolescent adjustments appeared vulnerable to these occupational hazards.

Medical practice itself is not the villain. Rather it may be that for some physicians the aspiration to be a doctor is part and parcel of the same personality traits which lead him to make an unsatisfactory marriage. To keep out of medical school those applicants with unstable childhood and adolescent adjustments is unworkable and indefensible.

In the authors' opinion, however, there would appear to be a need for a critical re-examination of the role of the medical school in both personal as well as professional development. It should be a positive and reinforcing experience instead of functioning as a "colossal castrator for the unwary student" [6]. Many faculty members fail dismally by not capitalizing on the potential personal growth experiences inherent in medical training. This results in a lack of enrichment for the psychologically healthy student, and helps to ensure that the vulnerable student does not get the attention he requires.

In conclusion, there is increasing evidence that significant marital conflict may be a major feature in physicians' wives presenting as primary patients. The authors would caution against treating these women in isolation, and strongly endorse conjoint therapy. The husbands' reluctance to be involved is symptomatic of the pathological marriage, and should be dealt with directly and firmly. Once engaged in marital therapy, the results are most often particularly gratifying both to the therapist and the physician-couple.

REFERENCES

1. G. E. Vaillant, N. C. Sobowale and C. McArthur, Some Psychologic Vulnerabilities of Physicians, *N. Engl. J. Med., 287:*8, pp. 372-375, 1972.
2. J. L. Evans, Psychiatric Illness in the Physician's Wife, *Am. J. Psychiatry, 122,* pp. 159-163, 1965.
3. J. M. Lewis, The Doctor and His Marriage, *Tex. Med., 61,* pp. 615-619, August 1965.
4. J. E. Miles, W. L. Maurice and R. Krell, The Student Psychiatric Ward: An Innovative Teaching Approach for Medical Undergraduates, *J. Med. Educ., 49:*2, pp. 176-181, February 1974.
5. T. F. Main, The Ailment, *Br. J. Med. Psychol. 30,* pp. 129-145, 1957.
6. M. M. Myckatyn and J. E. Miles, A Profile of Today's Medical Student, *Can. Med. Assoc. J., 109,* December 1, 1973.

Suicide

Chapter 11

SUICIDE IN MALE AND FEMALE PHYSICIANS

ROBERT C. STEPPACHER AND JUDITH S. MAUSNER

THE impression that physicians have a high rate of suidice has wide currency. The most recent report[1] indicated a high suicide rate for female physicians compared to the general female population, but no similar excess for male physicians. The current study was designed to extend available information for both sexes by expanding the period of study and by age adjusting rates. For comparison, the occurrence of suicide in another professional group, psychologists, was also investigated.[2]

In connection with the study, we reviewed the literature on suicide among physicians and other professionals. All the reports known to us that report on the frequency of suicide among American physicians since 1925 are summarized in Table 11-I. The table includes some studies that do not present directly pertinent evidence but that have been cited by others as demonstrating a high suicide rate.

Most of the reports are based on records maintained by the American Medical Association. The first investigators to utilize this source were Emerson and Hughes,[3] who found a suicide rate of 45.4/100,000 among white male physicians in 1925. In a review article, King[4] later interpreted this finding as showing that in that year suicide was approximately one and one-half times as frequent among physicians as in the general population of white males in the same age range.

This substantial excess was not found in several large-scale studies carried out over the next quarter of a century,[5-7] including one study of mortality by occupation that utilized death certificates

---

The investigation was supported by grant MH 20398 from the National Institute of Mental Health. Access to the AMA files of deceased physicians was provided by Genevieve Matanoski, M.D., and Elizabeth Elliot at the School of Hygiene and Public Health of the Johns Hopkins University.

Table 11-I.–Studies of Frequency of Suicide in Physicians (United States, 1925-Present)

Source	Yr of Report	Period Covered	Nature of Data	No. of Suicides	Suicide Rate in Study Group (per 100,000)*	Comparisons With Population Values and Remarks*
Emerson and Hughes[3]	1926	1925	AMA records	61	45.4 (WM)	...
Dublin and Spiegelman[5]	1947	1938-1941	AMA records	326	39.0 (M)	O/E=1.04
Dickinson and Martin[6]	1956	1949-1951	AMA files	191	...	O/E=1.03
Guralnick[7]	1963	1950	US death certificates Males 20-64, coded for occupation	48		O/E=1.14 (SMR=114)†
Powell[8]	1958	1937-1956	Death certificates of suicides, Tulsa, Okla for 20-yr period	5	83 (WM)	No age adjustment; rate for white males, 27/100,000
Blachly et al[9]	1963	1950-1961	Death certificates, Ore for 12 yr	8	30.3‡	Rate similar to population values; no age-adjustment
Freeman[12]	1967	1895-present	AMA obituary notices for psychiatrists	203	...	No rates calculated
Bruce et al[14]	1968	1947-1966	Deaths among ASA members from records of society	35	...	O/E=1.5
Thomas[13]	1969	1948-1964	Contemporaneous records of medical students at Johns Hopkins	14	...	No comparative figures; longitudinal study of 1,337 students
Blachly et al[15]	1968	1965-1967	AMA obituary columns	249	...	No comparison presented
DeSole et al[16]	1969	1965-1968	AMA obituary columns	291	33‡	No comparison presented
Craig and Pitts[1]	1968	1965-1967	AMA obituary columns and file folders	228	M—38.3 F—40.5	Rates calculated by authors for white males and females age 25 and over: M, 34.5; F, 11.4
Current study	1973	1965-1970	AMA obituary columns and file folders	530	M—30.9 F—33.6	M: O/E=1.15 F: O/E=3.2

*WM indicates white male; O, observed deaths; E, expected deaths.
†SMR indicates the standardized mortality ratio.
‡Sex is not indicated.

for the entire country, for men 20 to 64 years of age.[7] Interestingly, King found that for the period around 1950 the excess of suicide among physicians was much greater in England, Wales, and Denmark than in the United States.

In contrast, several reports published since 1950 have reported high suicide rates in American physicians. Powell's[8] study of death certificates for a 20-year period, for Tulsa, Okla, indicated a rate for physicians three times that of the general population of males. However, this claim is based on only five suicides, and no adjustment was made for possible differences in age distribution between physicians and the general male population. When Blachly et al.[9] studied death certificates in Oregon, they found there had been eight suicides among physicians during the 12-year period of study. They concluded that "the suicide rate among physicians, dentists and attorneys was about three times that of white-collar workers." This statement has been quoted[10,11] as indicating a high rate of suicide among physicians. However, comparison with white-collar workers may be somewhat misleading since their suicide rate tends to be lower than that of the overall population. In the study of Blachly et al.[9], the suicide rate for physicians was actually slightly lower than that for all males over the age of 19 years; it was the dentists and attorneys who had rates higher than those of the total population.

The reports by Freeman[12] and Thomas[13] imply an excessive rate of suicide in physicians but do not indicate how the numbers observed compare with those that might have been expected on the basis of rates in other groups. In contrast, after identifying 35 suicides among the members of the American Society of Anesthesiologists, Bruce and his co-workers[14] reported a frequency of suicide for that group one and one half-times that represented by US rates. A prospective study of anesthesiologists is under way to confirm this finding which is, as the investigators note, subject to several sources of error.

The last four entries in Table 11-I represent three recent studies[1,15,16] in addition to the one now being reported. All are based on information compiled by the American Medical Association; all take advantage of the fact that since May 1965 suicide has been included among the causes of death listed in the obituary notices in *JAMA*. The most detailed analysis of this information is that by Craig and Pitts.[1] They interpreted their findings as indicating no excess of suicide among men, but a fourfold excess among women when compared with overall population figures. Within the total group of physicians, several specialty groups appeared to have high rates: psychiatrists, anesthesiologists, and otolaryngologists.

In addition to the high risk of suicide among female physicians found by Craig and Pitts, there is evidence that women in other professional groups have a high risk of suicide. In a study of deaths among members of the American Chemical Society, Li[17] found that 13 of the 115 deaths in women, or 11 percent, were suicide. Powell[8] claimed that nurses have a frequency six times that of the general population, but this is based on only six deaths. In the Oregon study of Blachly et al.,[9] the rate was slightly higher for nurses than for all women over the age of 19 years; there were eight suicides. In a follow-up study of more than 25,000 student nurses, Theodore et al.[18] found that the number of suicides was almost identical to that expected. However, they suggested that this group may have had an elevated suicide rate since several deaths from barbiturate ingestion and carbon monoxide poisoning were not certified as suicide. We[2] found the suicide rate among female psychologists to be approximately threefold that in the general female population. No corresponding excess was detected for male psychologists.

METHODS

The American Medical Association attempts to maintain up-to-date information on the status of all graduates of American medical schools (except graduates of schools of osteopathy), as well as physicians who have trained elsewhere and then settled in this country. From their own correspondence with nonmembers, as well as with members of the AMA, plus local clipping services, the AMA acquires information about deaths among physicians. A file is established for each decedent, and a notification of death is published in an obituary section of each issue of *JAMA*. Along with the name of each decedent, the obituary gives information about school and year of graduation, professional activities, date and place of death, age, and cause of death. As noted, suicide has been included in the causes of death specified in the obituary section since May 1965. Further details of the AMA records and procedures may be found in the communication by Craig and Pitts.[1]

We reviewed the obituary section of all issues of *JAMA* from May 1965 through March 1971 and made a notation of the names of all those whose deaths were ascribed to suicide. In addition, the name was also transcribed if the cause of death listed suggested the possibility of suicide or if the cause had been "withheld" (i.e., possible suicides.) To allow for the time lag between the actual date of death and the publication of the death notice in *JAMA*, the 5½-year period, March 1965 through August 1970 was designated as the study period. Deaths that occurred during this interval form the basis for this report.

We selected a random sample of the deaths unequivocally identified as suicide in the *JAMA* obituary notices and checked the AMA file folders for confirmation of the classification. In all cases, the folder contained some clear evidence of suicide, either from the death certificate, or from a newspaper clipping, or correspondence. The remainder of the apparently unequivocal suicides were not verified further.

For all the "possible suicides," we consulted the AMA file folders. Some were found to contain little information; others held a copy of the death certificate, newspaper clippings, letters from family or attending physician, or all three. We used all the information in the folder to assess whether the death should be classified as a suicide. In addition, in some instances, we requested a copy of the death certificate from state authorities in order to clarify the mode of death. We also requested copies of death certificates for the women physicians reported as suicides in order to determine their marital status.

Identification of a death as suicide was done conservatively. All deaths in two categories, barbiturate ingestion and self-inflicted gunshot wounds, were accepted as suicide even without clear evidence of suicidal intent because their omission would have led to a gross underestimate of the number of suicides. Aside from this, we were quite rigorous about accepting deaths as suicide. The male and female suicide rates in our study are appreciably lower than those reported by Craig and Pitts.

For professional activity at time of death, we consulted AMA directories. Most of the physicians in our study were listed in at least one issue of the directories.

ESTIMATION OF NUMBERS OF PHYSICIANS, 1965 TO 1970. — To interpret the number of suicides among physicians over a given time period, it is necessary to calculate rates that relate the number of suicides to the total number of physicians. To estimate the number of physicians in the country during the 5½-year period of the study, we averaged the number of physicians alive on Dec 31, 1963,[19] and on Dec 31, 1971 (obtained by personal communication with the Membership Department of the AMA). The midpoint of this interval (Dec 31, 1967) coincides almost exactly with the midpoint of our study period (Jan 30, 1968).

COMPARISON OF SUICIDE RATES IN PHYSICIANS AND IN THE

General Population. — Age-specific and overall death rates from suicide were calculated separately for each sex. However, since the age composition of physicians differs from that of the general population, the number of suicides observed in the study group was compared with the number expected in a group of that size, sex, and age-composition on the basis of population rates.

The US age-specific suicide rates for white men and white women in 1967,[20] the central year of the study, were used in the calculation of expected numbers. These rates were multiplied by the number of physicians of each sex in each age group. The numbers expected in each age-sex group per year were then summed and multiplied by 5.5 (years) to yield the total number of suicides expected in each sex over the 5½-year study period. The resultant number was compared with the number actually found in AMA data. This ratio of observed-to-expected deaths is known as the standardized mortality ratio, or SMR. The frequency of suicide in male and female physicians was also compared directly, using the same technique.

RESULTS

A total of 530 suicides was identified in our study, 489 among male and 41 among female physicians.

The age distribution of suicide in the two sexes differed markedly. This is shown in Table 11-II, in which the cumulative percentage frequency by age is presented for each sex separately. A far higher proportion of the suicides in women occurred at younger ages. Almost 40% of the suicides in women, but less than 20% of those in men, occurred in persons under age 40.

Age-specific suicide rates were calculated next (Table 11-III), to permit comparison of male and female physicians with each other as well as with 1967 US population rates for white men and women. Ten-year age-groupings were used in this table to increase the stability of the rates. The population statistics show greatly higher rates for men than women for each age-group. In contrast, among physicians rates were actually higher for the women than the men below the age of 45. Above that age, rates were either similar or higher for female than male physicians.

Table 11-III also indicates that the pattern of suicide by age is different for male physicians than for the general population of white men. For the physicians, the rates were highest in middle age (45 to 64 years) whereas population statistics show the highest rates among

Table 11-II.—Suicides Among Physicians by Age and Sex

	Male		Female	
Age, Yr	No.	Cumulative %	No.	Cumulative %
<30	18	3.7	5	12.2
30-34	30	9.8	4	22.0
35-39	43	18.6	7	39.1
40-44	67	32.3	8	58.6
45-49	77	48.0	3	65.9
50-54	76	63.5	3	73.2
55-59	69	77.6	4	82.9
60-64	47	87.2	3	90.2
65-69	26	92.5	0	90.2
70-74	18	96.2	3	97.5
75+	18	99.9	1	99.9
Total	489		41	

elderly white men. For women, the rates among physicians were relatively high throughout the entire age range.

Table 11-III.—Annual Age-Specific Suicide Rates, per 100,000*

	Males		Females	
Age Group	US Whites	Physicians† (Current Study)	US Whites	Physicians (Current Study)
25-34	17.2	12.2	7.9	23.7
35-44	23.8	26.4	11.5	49.3
45-54	29.2	45.3	13.0	25.2
55-64	36.5	48.2	12.3	48.3
65-74	34.6	34.2	9.9	31.2
≥75	(48.0)†	26.7	(6.5)	17.6
Total		30.9		33.6

*Rates for US whites, male and female were from 1967. Rates for male and female physicians in the current study group cover the period 1965-1970.

†Numbers in parentheses for US whites, males and females, are approximations based on combination of rates for two age groups, 75-84, and 85 and over.

To take into account the age composition of each sex, expected numbers of deaths by suicide were calculated and compared with population value for each sex separately. The relations between observed and expected numbers of suicides are shown for male and female physicians in Tables 4 and 5. For both sexes, the number of suicides found was greater than that expected on the basis of population rates. However, the magnitude of the excess differed sharply for the two sexes. For the men, the ratio of observed suicides, 489, to the expected number, 426.4, was only 1.15. In contrast, for the women the number observed, 41, was three times greater than the 12.8 anticipated. However, the excess observed was statistically significant for both sexes.

We also utilized the observed and expected values to examine age distributions of suicide by sex, with results that confirmed the impressions given by Table 11-III. Using three age groups (under 45 years, 45 to 64 years, and 65 years and over) we found that the age distribution of suicide for male physicians (Table 11-IV) differed significantly from that of white males in the population (x^2 = 32.96, df = 2, $P<.001$), with an excess in the middle age group of physicians and fewer suicides than anticipated among the other two groups. For the women (Table 11-V), there was no such difference (x^2 = 0.92, df = 2, not significant); the excess of suicide in female physicians was distributed over the entire age range.

Table 11-IV.—Computation of Standardized Suicide Ratio for Male Physicians*

Age	Average No. in Age Group	Rate/100,000 White Males†	Expected No. in 5.5 Yr	Observed No. in 5.5 Yr
<30	31,980	16.9‡	29.8	18
30-34	39,635	17.5	38.2	30
35-39	38,632	22.2	47.2	43
40-44	36,942	25.4	51.6	67
45-49	32,906	26.8	48.5	77
50-54	28,467	31.8	49.8	76
55-59	24,298	35.7	47.7	69
60-64	19,340	37.4	39.8	47
65-69	14,000	32.2	24.8	26
70-74	9,367	37.9	19.5	18
≥75	12,237	44.0§	29.6	18
Totals	287,804		426.5	489

*O/E=489/426.5=1.15, where O is the number of observed deaths and E is the number of expected deaths; χ^2=9.205, with 1 degree of freedom; $P<.005$.
†US white males, 1967.
‡Indicates ages 25-29 yr.
§Estimated rate based on rates for three age groups.

We next calculated the number of suicides expected among female physicians on the basis of the rates among male physicians (Table 11-VI). For the group as a whole, the number of suicides among the female physicians was slightly but not significantly higher than expected. However, there was a significant difference in age distribution (x^2 = 9.71, df = 2, $P<.01$), due mainly to an excess of suicides in the young women physicians.

In view of the high proportion of suicides in female physicians that occurred at young ages, it is not surprising that more suicides

Table 11-V.—Standardized Suicide Ratio for Female Physicians*

Age	Average No. in Age Group	Rate/100,000 White Females†	Expected No. 5.5 Yr	Observed No.
<30	3,424	7.0	1.3	5
30-34	3,490	8.9	1.7	4
35-39	2,907	11.2	1.8	7
40-44	2,623	11.9	1.7	8
45-49	2,494	12.3	1.7	3
50-54	1,828	13.8	1.4	3
55-59	1,468	13.2	1.0	4
60-64	1,164	11.3	0.7	3
65-69	978	10.7	0.6	0
70-74	770	8.9	0.4	3
≥75	1,030	7.0‡	0.4	1
Total	**22,176**		**12.7**	**41**

*O/E=41/12.7=3.2, where O is the observed number of deaths and E is the number of expected deaths; χ^2=62.109, with 1 degree of freedom; $P<.005$.

†US Vital Statistics, white females, 1967.

‡Estimated rate based on rates for three age groups.

Table 11-VI.—Expected Number of Suicides Among Female Physicians Based on Rates in Male Physicians

Age	No. Males	No. Suicides in Males	No. Females	Expected No. in Females	Observed No. in Females
<30	31,980	18	3,424	1.9	5
30-34	39,635	30	3,490	2.6	4
35-39	38,632	43	2,907	3.2	7
40-44	36,942	67	2,623	4.8	8
45-49	32,906	77	2,494	5.8	3
50-54	28,467	76	1,828	5.7	3
55-59	24,298	69	1,468	4.2	4
60-64	19,340	47	1,164	2.8	3
65-69	14,000	26	978	1.8	0
70-74	9,367	18	770	1.5	3
≥75	12,237	18	1,031	1.5	1
Total	**287,804**	**489**	**22,177**	**35.8**	**41**

among the women than among the men occurred during training — i.e., among persons serving as interns, residents, or fellows. Twelve of the 41 suicides in women (29%) occurred during training, whereas this was true of only 37 of the 489 male suicides — less than 10 percent. Unfortunately, we were not able to obtain detailed tabulations of physicians by sex, age-group, and professional activity to permit separation of the effects of age from those of the training situation. Since seven of the 12 women who committed suicide while in training were already in their 30s, there would be considerable overlap in ages between those in training and those in practice.

One aspect of interest is the marital status of both the men and women who committed suicide. We have information on marital status for only a fraction of the men, since our resources did not permit us to obtain death certificates or to verify AMA files for the entire group of men. However, we did obtain death certificates for all but five of the women suicides. We found that 20 were single (never married), seven were currently married, two were widowed, and seven were separated or divorced. This seemed like a very high proportion of single women even if one takes into account the higher rate of suicide among single, widowed, and divorced persons than among those currently married. Three sets of figures on marital status were found for comparison. One comes from the 1970 census,[21] the other two from studies carried out during the 1960s on the professional activities of female physicians.[22,23]

In the census data, marital status is not given specifically for physicians, but is presented for women more broadly grouped by occupational level. Therefore, marital status of the physicians in our study was compared with that of "professional, technical and kindred workers." The two other studies of female physicians are relatively small, confined to graduates of eastern schools, and antedate slightly the period of our study. Nevertheless, they are cited since they pertain specifically to physicians. To restrict the comparisons to the women of similar age range, we included only the female suicides aged 35 to 49 years.

In all three sets of comparisons, the proportion of single women among the female suicides appeared very high (Table 11-VII). It was particularly striking that 11 of the 12 suicides in women physicians in training occurred in single women.

The methods of suicides used by male and female physicians are shown in Table 11-VIII. The findings are similar to those observed nationwide in that violent methods, especially gunshot wounds of the head, predominated in men, the use of drugs in women. However, compared with the general population, a much higher proportion of the physicians used drugs, more than one-third of male and three-fourths of female physicians. In the general population the proportion of suicides accomplished by drug ingestion is less than one in 10 for men and about one in three for women.[24]

Comment

The major finding of the study was an excess of suicides among

Table 11-VII.—Percent of Women Married

Study Group	Age Range, yr			
	25-34	35-44	45-54	35-49*
Women suicides, current study†	0 (0/9)	29 (4/14)	33 (2/6)	28 (5/18)
Professional, technical and kindred workers, US Census, 1970	65	73	70	...
Women physicians, Rosenlund and Oski[22]	...	...	...	78
Women physicians, Shapiro et al[23]	...	...	...	69

*This age range was used in the studies of Rosenlund and Oski, and Shapiro et al.
†Figures based on 36 women whose marital status at time of death is known.

Table 11-VIII.—Methods of Suicide Among Physicians, by Sex

	Males		Females	
	No.	%	No.	%
Gunshot	191	39.1	2	4.9
Drugs				
Barbiturate	139	28.4	26	63.4
Other	48	9.8	5	12.2
Carbon monoxide poisoning	16	3.3	...	...
Hanging	15	3.1	...	...
Laceration with sharp instrument	8	1.6	...	...
Jump from height	3	.6	1	2.4
Other method and unknown	69	14.1	7	17.1
Total	**489**	**100.0**	**41**	**100.0**

female physicians in comparison with the general female population, as reported by Craig and Pitts. There was a similar trend among the male physicians, but it was not as great. There was also an excess of suicides among middle-aged male physicians in comparison with the general male population, and among young female physicians in comparison with their male counterparts. However, before the implications of these findings can be considered, some general comments about sources of bias in the data and the accuracy of suicide statistics in general are in order.

We do not know what proportion of deaths among physicians are unknown to the AMA, or whether suicides are reported to them proportionately less often than deaths from other causes. Furthermore, published US suicide rates[20] come from compilations of statements about cause of death given on death certificates submitted from the more than 3,000 counties of the United States. The quality of information on death certificates varies widely. This is particularly true for suicide, where accurate diagnosis may be precluded by inadequate toxicologic and other investigation, or by dissembling in order to protect the deceased or his family. As a result, the published suicide figures are a poor reflection of the actual numbers. The true level of occurrence is probably grossly understated.

In addition, the U. S. rates may contain systematic biases. For example, it is not known whether a physician who commits suicide has an equal, a greater, or a lesser chance of being certified as having committed suicide than, say, a plumber or a teacher. It seems possible, for example, that coroners might receive pressure from the family of a physician to hide the fact of suicide. On the other hand, the public visibility of physicians and their high status in the community might lead to extra thoroughness and care in investigation of suspicious or equivocal deaths and thus, enhance the chances for detection of suicide in this group. If such inequalities did exist, then even rates based wholly on death certificates could be biased. Occupational groups might differ in published suicide rates when, in fact, no real difference existed; conversely, a true difference might be masked. This whole matter is sorely in need of investigation. Pending further clarification, it seems reasonable that only large and consistent differences in rates should be accepted as valid. This precaution seems even more important when, as here, the data are based on a mixture of death certificates and secondary data.

Despite these problems, we believe that our finding of a high rate of suicide in female physicians is genuine. First, as noted, ascertainment of deaths among physicians by the AMA may be incomplete. This fact would make one hesitate to ascribe validity to a low rate but would, if anything, bring extra weight to the finding of a high rate. Second, both male and female physicians were studied by the same methods; the same criteria were applied to each sex throughout. Yet, an appreciable excess of suicide over general population levels was found only for the female physicians. And, last, our study of suicide in psychologists also yielded a high rate for female psychologists compared to other women. In that group, the number of suicides in male psychologists was actually lower than the number expected.

The excess of suicides among male physicians in the middle years of life is of interest. It may reflect depression induced by a sense of failure to achieve early goals, of missed opportunities and constricting potential for the future. Equally interesting is the relatively low suicide rate for elderly male physicians. This may be related to the opportunities available to free professionals to continue working past the usual age of retirement.

The causes of the elevated rate of suicide among female professionals deserve more detailed consideration than is given in this report; they are discussed elsewhere.[2] One can only speculate on the extent to which the high rate may be attributed to the attraction of suicide-prone women to professional activity, to the tensions of professional training and practice, or to a combination of the two. The relative contribution of these two determinants is yet to be discovered and, in fact, may vary from profession to profession and over time and place.

The practical implications of the high rate of suicide in young female physicians relate to selection and supervision during training. As for selection, one could use the data presented here to argue against unrestricted entry into medicine for women. On the contrary, we find no support for such an argument in our data. Despite the excess, even in young women physicians, suicide is fortunately a rare event. Therefore, the increased risk should not be used to bar women from opportunities for professional careers.

However, the relatively high rate of suicide in young women in professional training should be made known to those responsible for training programs. The problem is probably more far-reaching than our figures indicate, since suicide may well represent one extreme of a spectrum of emotional distress. It seems particularly tragic that suicide should occur among people interacting daily with colleagues and supervisors. Preventive approaches other than those now practiced may be possible. The psychological climate of training programs may deserve further exploration. Perhaps unused pathways of communication could be opened. The needs of the single woman in training deserve particular consideration. There may be sources of support and assistance that are not being utilized fully at present.

A final implication of this study is that it suggests a need for research on the relation of occupation and career to the physical and mental health of women. Not only is the number of women gainfully employed outside the home now increasing, but more and more women are following careers that play central roles in their lives. the effects of such work experience on health deserves further exploration.

REFERENCES

1. Craig AG, Pitts FN: Suicide by physicians. *Dis Nerv Syst 219:*763-772, 1968.
2. Mausner JS, Steppacher RC: Suicide in professionals: A study of male and

female psychologists. *Am J Epidemiol 98:*436-445, 1973.
3. Emerson H, Hughes H: Death rates of male white physicians in the United States. *Am J Public Health 16:*1088-1093, 1926.
4. King H: Health in the medical and other learned professions. *J Chronic Dis 23:*257-281, 1970.
5. Dublin LI, Spiegelman M: The longevity and mortality of American physicians, 1938-1942: A preliminary report. *JAMA* 134:1211-1215, 1947.
6. Dickinson FG, Martin LW: Physician mortality, 1949-1951. *JAMA* 162:1462-1468, 1956.
7. Guralnick L: Mortality by Occupation and Industry Among Men 20-64 Years of Age, United States, 1950. Vital Statistics — Special Reports. National Vital Statistics Division, Public Health Service, US Dept of Health, Education and Welfare, vol 53, 1963.
8. Powell EH: Occupation, status and suicide: Toward a redefinition of anomie. *Am Social Rev 23:*131-139, 1958.
9. Blachly PH, Osterud HT, Josslin R: Suicide in professional groups. *N Engl J Med 268:*1278-1282, 1963.
10. Mentally disturbed doctors, editorial. *Br Med J 1:*643, 1972.
11. Haar E, Green MR, Hyams L: Characteristics of physicians who have had psychotherapy. *Arch Gen Psychiatry 27:*705-709, 1972.
12. Freeman W: Psychiatrists who kill themselves: A study in suicide. *Am J Psychiatry 124:*846-847, 1967.
13. Thomas CB: Suicide among us: Can we learn to prevent it? *Hopkins Med J 125:*276-285, 1969.
14. Bruce DL, et al: Causes of death among anesthesiologists: A 20-year survey. *Anesthesiology 29:*565-569, 1968.
15. Blachly PH, Disher W, Roduner G: Suicide by physicians. *Bull Suicidology* (December) 1968, pp 1-18.
16. DeSole DE, Singer P, Aronson S: Suicide and role strain among physicians *Int J Soc Psychiatry 15:*294-301, 1969.
17. Li FP: Suicide among chemists. *Arch Environ Health 19:*518-520, 1969.
18. Theodore A, Berger AG, Palmer CE: A follow-up of tuberculosis in student nurses: II, Mortality from all causes in the first decade after entering training. *J Chronic Dis 4:*111-130, 1956.
19. Theodore CN, Haug JN: *Selected characteristics of the physicians population, 1963 and 1967.* Chicago, American Medical Association, 1968.
20. *Vital Statistics of the United States, 1967.* Volume 2: *Mortality* (pt A). US Dept of Health, Education, and Welfare.
21. *US Census of Population, 1970: Marital status,* PC(2)-4C.
22. Rosenlund ML, Oski FA: Women in medicine. *Ann Intern Med* 66:1008-1012, 1967.
23. Shapiro CS, et al: Careers of women physicians: A survey of women graduates from seven medical schools, 1945-1951. *J Med Educ* 43:1033-1040, 1968.
24. *Suicide in the United States 1950-1964,* Public Health Service Publication No. 1000, series 20, No.5. National Center for Health Statistics, Dept of Health, Education and Welfare, 1967.

Chapter 12

PHYSICIANS WHO KILL THEMSELVES

K. DANIEL ROSE AND IRVING ROSOW

A PHYSICIAN'S suicide is a tragic waste of human resource. Yet it seems common knowledge that physicians are more suicide prone than other people. We critically review the evidence for this widely held notion and present data concerning the incidence of suicide among physicians and the characteristics of those suicidal physicians. In this manner we hope to identify high-risk characteristics so that preventive efforts might be facilitated.

From the abundant literature on physicians suicide, Table 12-I[1-16] summarizes existing estimates of the physician when possible, with rates for the general population. Many authors have corrected their data to insure comparison of similar age-groups, since suicide rates vary with age. The rates in this table are presented in number of suicides per 100,000 population per year. The scope is limited to studies in the United States, because physicians in other countries may experience different degrees of stress, prestige, or income and may not be truly comparable. Furthermore, "the criteria used to decide whether death is due to suicide differ between countries."[17]

Contrary to popular belief, this collection of studies indicates that physicians do not differ substantially from the general population in tendency to suicide. Physician suicide rates vary from 5.4 below to 4.6 above rates for adult men with the exception of one study involving only five cases. On closer scrutiny, however, few of the investigations withstand any degree of rigorous analysis. Serious objections can be raised on two grounds: First, the sources of data are of poor reliability in nearly every case. Second, the large statistical errors in several of the findings render them of little value.

From K. Daniel Rose and Irving Rosow, Physicians Who Kill Themselves, *Arch Gen Psychiatry*, Vol. 29, Dec., 1973.

This work was supported in part by Summer Research Fellowship AH-218-02 from the US Public Health Service and by General Research Support grants from the Langley Porter Neuropsychiatric Institute, San Francisco. We are indebted to Seth D. Rose, Ph.D. candidate, for his statistical analysis.

Harry Greenblatt and Robert Mielke, social research analysts at the Bureau of Health Intelligence, assisted in compliling data.

Table 12-I. — Studies of Physician Suicide in US

Authors	Period	Scope	No. Physician Suicides	Annual Physician Rate	Gen Population Rate	Method of Detection
Editorial[1]	1891 to 1903	US	519	39.7	NA†	Unspecified
Knopf[2]	1912 to 1921	US	398	27‡	NA	AMA records
Emerson & Hughes[3]	1925	US	61	45.4	NA	AMA records
Dublin & Spiegelman[4]	1938 to 1942	US	326§	39.0	37.6	AMA records
Public Health Service[5]	1950	US	48¶	28.7¶	24.1¶	Death certificate
Dickinson & Martin[6]	1949 to 1951	US	191	31.1#	30.3**	AMA records
Powell[7]	1937 to 1956	Tulsa Co	5	83	27.0††	Newspapers
Blachly et al[8]	1950 to 1961	Oregon	8	30.3	32.4‡‡	Death certificate
Craig & Pitts[9]	1965 to 1967	US	228	38.4	34.1‖	AMA records
Blachly et al[10]	1965 to 1967	US	249	33#	38.4§§	AMA records
DeSole et al[11]	1965 to 1968	US	291	33	38.4§§	AMA records
Thomas[12]	1948 to 1969	Hopkins	14	49.9	NA	Alumni records

* Based on physician population, 1896.[13]

† Not available.

‡ Based on physician population, 1916.[13]

§ Men, United States.

‖ White men age 25 and over, United States.

¶ Men, age 20 to 64, United States; Based on population estimates in Table A-6 of ref. 14.

\# Calculated from data supplied in text.

** White men, age-adjusted to US physician population.

†† White men, Tulsa Co, Okla.

‡‡ Men age 19 and over, Ore.

§§ White men age 20 and over, United States, 1967; based on 1,073 suicides[15] in a population of 51,422,000.[16]

Most investigators rely on American Medical Association records (*Journal of the American Medical Association* obituaries) for their source of data. The AMA learns of physicians' deaths through national newspaper clipping services: suicides that are not reported in the local papers would not be included in AMA records. Furthermore, information concerning cause of death is usually obtained from next of kin or associates and, due to the expense involved, seldom from death certificates. Recent correspondence with the Special Projects Editor of *JAMA*, whose responsibilites include preparation of the obituaries, yielded the following appraisal of their accuracy:

> The cautionary statement published in the Blachly article[10(p2)] should be reiterated, to the effect that a survey of *JAMA* obituaries would furnish descriptive data but not valid statistical data. This remains true despite the fact that in recent years we have made special efforts to obtain specific information on causes of death. [C. F. Chapman, written communication, Oct 27, 1970.]

To test the extent to which *JAMA* underreports or misreports suicide, we obtained from the California Department of Public Health a computerized list of all professional people who committed suicide in California in 1970. Among these were the names of 18 physicians for which we searched all *JAMA* obituaries from the beginning of 1970 through March 1972 (ample time for all 1970 deaths to reach print if they were ever to do so.) The list below show how *JAMA* reported these known suicides:

Definite suicide	9
Suspected suicide	1
Cause not disclosed	3
Other cause stated	4
Not include (intern)	1
Total	18

Only 50 percent of these were correctly identified: four cases were erroneously listed as pulmonary emphysema, heart attack, cancer, and hepatic and renal failure; one case was not reported at all. Therefore, studies of physician suicide that rely on records kept by the AMA may well omit as many suicides as they report. This would lead to gross underestimation of the true incidence of physician suicide.

Two studies rely on unusual sources that are difficult to evaluate: the Tulsa County newspaper obituaries[7] and records of the Johns Hopkins Alumni Office.[12] In neither instance does the author clarify the reliability of his data source, so these cannot be accepted with confidence.

Death certificates provide the most reliable source of data presently available, and two studies review such materials. The Public Health Service[5] studied many causes of death in all occupations and thereby included suicides among physicians. Unfortunately, however, men age 65 and over are excluded and, among whites, this age-group traditionally has the highest suicide rates.[18] Consequently, this physician suicide rate is almost certainly too low. Two additional limitations include the lack of an occupation entry on 6.3 percent of all certificates and the combination of "usual occupation" on death certificates with "current occupation" from census figures to calculate rates. An error in "usual occupation" would tend to lower the apparent suicide rate for physicians and others in full-employment occupations. Although these shortcomings introduce certain inaccuracies, they probably affect specific rates without gross distortions of their general magnitude. Blachly et al.[8], in their study of Oregon physicians, were not concerned with the comparability of occupational categories, the adjustment of suicide rates for age, nor with the question of how many certificates fail to show the occupation of the deceased.

In addition to a reliable means of detecting physician suicides, a sufficient number of events is required if strong conclusions are to be drawn. Three of the studies do not meet these fundamental statistical criteria. For example, the Blachly et al[8] study uncovered only eight physician suicides; the rate, stated with 95 percent confidence, is between 13 and 60 per 100,000 based on so few cases. These figures lead to two different conclusions: (1) physicians are half as prone to suicide as adult Oregon men (13/32.4), or (2) physicians are twice as suicide prone (60/32.4). Clearly such data are not definitive, for their margin of error admits completely opposite conclusions. Similar criticism applies to the studies by Powell[7] and Thomas,[12] in which only five and 14 physician suicides, respectively, were reported.

To summarize the literature, there is no compelling evidence that physicians are more prone to self-destruction than people in general. Despite a large number of investigations to date, only that by the Public Health Service[5] seems to withstand rigorous scrutiny. While it allows that physicians may be slightly more prone to suicide than the general population, these differences are comparatively minor.

Most studies have been concerned with estimations of the rate of physician suicide rather than descriptions of the characteristics of these physicians. Thus far, only Blachly et al.[10] have attempted to gather these basic descriptive data on a major scale. Reviewing *JAMA* obituaries, they uncovered 249 suicides and sent 200 detailed questionnaires to the next of kin. Since only 80 replies were received (32% of 249 deaths), the findings are limited due to the likelihood of a nonrandom response. Simon and Lumry[19] studied five physician psychiatric inpatients who committed suicide. However, this sample is too small and too biased to be of value in explaining the phenomenon of physician suicide in general. DeSole et al.[11] investigated seven physicians who committed suicide, but their findings, based on so few cases, are also of little help in identifying trends or common characteristics which distinguish suicidal physicians. At present we really have no accurate picture of physicians who are most likely to end their own lives.

METHODS

Our study is based on a computerized review of all death certificates (406,498) filed in the State of California during the 3-year period from Jan. 1, 1959, through Dec. 31, 1961. In this state all suicides are investigated by the coroner's office and physicians are required by law to notify the coroner when suicide is suspected.[20] Death records in California include information on age, sex, race, residence, marital status, occupation, and cause of death. During the study period the occupational codes on the death certificates were identical to those used by the Bureau of the Census for the 1960 enumeration.

The suicides of physicians and other selected groups were extracted on special computer runs and suicide rates were calculated on the basis of population figures in the 1960 census.[21] Information concerning the specialties of suiciding physicians was obtained from the *American Medical Directory*.[22]

COMMENT

In the 3-year period from 1959 through 1961 a total of 7,471 death certificates indicated suicide as the underlying cause of death. The occupation of the deceased could be determined in 7,351 of the 7,471 cases (98.4%): 51 physicians committed suicide during this period for an annual suicide rate of 69 per 100,000. Table 12-II adjusted suicide rates of physicians, professional-technical workers, and the general population. The comparison is limited to adult white men (age 25 and over) to eliminate any variation arising from the differing composition of the three groups. This limitation seems valid since white men represent 88 percent of the state's physicians[21] and 94 percent of their suicides.

It is evident from the table that physicians are twice as prone to suicide as either of the other groups and the difference is highly significant statistically ($P < .0005$). Stated with 95 percent conficence, physicians are 1½ to 2½ times as suicide prone as the other two groups (based on 48 cases). This constitutes compelling evidence for an increased suicide risk among physicians. Although suicide is generally more common in California than in the whole United States, the higher California rates do not affect patterns among groups within the state. Hence, we would expect these same relationships to apply elsewhere.

Table 12-III compares physicians with people of similar class standing, i.e., professional-technical workers. The data are controlled for age and sex, although the variable of race could not be eliminated for lack of detailed census figures. Table 12-III shows a wide variation in the rates for these occupations of similar income, education, and status: from six for social workers to 120 for chemists. Physicians are exceeded only by chemists, dentists, pharmacists, and non-medical technicians in tendency to suicide.

A striking and significant pattern emerges from the table: of the four highest suicide rates, three occur in the three principal professions concerned with the delivery of health care: pharmacists, dentists, and physicians. Table 12-IV focuses exclusively on medical and health workers within the professional-technical group. Adjustments of the rates for age and race are not possible, again for lack of adequately detailed population figures. Nevertheless, one can see that among both men and women the tendency to self-destruction is

Table 12-II.—Age-Adjusted Suicide Rates For Selected White Men, 25 and Older, in California*

Group	Suicides 1959 to 1961	Population† April 1960	Annual Rate No./100,000/yr
Physicians	48	22,290	77
Prof-Tech	553	462,730	36
General Population	4,606	4,008,763	38

* Age-adjusted by indirect method, $\chi^2 = 38.6$ (method described in ref 23), $P < .0005$. General white male California population is the standard.

† Source: ref 21, Tables 17 and 123; white and nonwhite are included in the physician category for lack of more detailed figures. Nonwhite male physicians account for only 4% of total male physicians and the effect is negligible.

twice as great among health care workers as it is among others of similar social class. It is painfully evident that suicide is a general problem of major proportions for physicians and health care workers who, ironically, have dedicated their lives to caring for others.

Table 12-III.—Age-Adjusted Suicide Rates for Male Professional-Technical Workers, 25 and Older, California*

Occupations	Suicides 1959 to 1961	Population† April 1960	Annual Rate No./100,000/yr
Chemists	18	6,359	120
Dentists	20	8.174	83
Physicians	49	22,290	79
Account, audit	73	39,386	68
Social sci	7	4,384	65
Auth, edit, rept	18	11,194	61
Lawyers, judges	26	16,540	54
Architects	5	3,829	50
Engineers	127	118,311	45
Natural sci	5	6,776	33
College fac, admin	5	12,940	15
Total Professional	**353**	**250,183**	**55**
Pharmacists	21	6,729	104
Non-med technicians	26	13,942	88
Musicians	16	8,528	70
Med & dent tech	10	7,243	53
Artists	8	8,643	37
Other technicals	90	97,521	37
Design, draft	15	23,913	28
Teachers	18	45,929	18
Clergy	3	11,927	9
Social workers	1	6,989	6
Total Technical	**208**	**231,364**	**36**
Total Prof-Tech	**561**	**481,547**	**46**

* Age-adjusted by indirect method, $\chi^2 = 181$ (method described in ref 23), $P < .0005$. General white male California population is the standard.

† Source: ref 21, Table 123.

Our data do not explain why physicians are so prone to suicide. We can, however, identify some concomitants of physician suicide, factors that are associated with increased risk within the physician group. Age, sex, race, marital status, and specialty area are examined in order to specify these high-risk characteristics.

Age-specific suicide rates for white male physicians and the general population are shown in Table 12-V. Physicians age 65 and over have the highest suicide rate, while the 45 to 54 age-group experiences the single greatest number of suicides. Indeed, half of these deaths occur during the most productive phase of a physician's life — age 35 to 54. This finding only serves to emphasize the social cost that suicide exacts.

Table 12-IV.—Suicide Rates for Health Care, Prof-Tech Workers, All Ages, California

Group	Suicides 1959 to 1961	Population* April 1960	Annual Rate† No./100,000/yr
Men			
Health care‡	124	56,228	74
Other prof-tech	461	479,592	32
Total§	585	535,820	36
Women			
Health care‡	82	82,207	33
Other prof-tech	109	190,240	19
Total‖	191	272,447	23

* Source: ref 21, Table 120.

† Not age-adjusted rates; the magnitude of the correction introduced by age-adjustment seldom exceeded 10% (in rates where these calculations were possible), so the bias from not age-adjusting here would be quite small.

‡ Category as defined by US Bureau of the Census, except psychologists were excluded and grouped with social scientists (Other prof-tech). Included are chiropractors, dentists, dietitians, healers, medical and dental technicians, nutritionists, optometrists, osteopaths, pharmacists, physicians and surgeons, professional nurses, student professional nurses, therapists, and veterinarians. Source: ref 21, intro, P XXXII.

§ $\chi^2 = 71.4, P < .0005$.

‖ $\chi^2 = 14.8, P < .0005$.

Both physicians and the general population show the customary increasing suicide rate with increasing age. But the rate of increase is drastically different for the two groups. In the general population, men of retirement age are three times more suicide prone than those age 25 to 34 (61/20). Among physicians, however, this ratio jumps to 12:1 (247/20). Physicians seem to have a greater age-sensitivity to suicide than the population in general.

In the general California population, men are 2½ times more prone to suicide than women (Table 12-VI). Among physicians, no statistically significant difference was observed. This does not mean that both have the same suicide rate; rather, there are too few female suicides to demonstrate a difference.

Whites in the general population are 1.8 times more prone to self-destruction than nonwhites (Table 12-VII). Again, due to the small number of cases, a statistically significant difference could not be established between the races within the physician group. The observed rate difference is easily accounted for by chance alone.

Marital status, however, is an important factor in suicide (Table

12-VIII). Similar patterns of proneness to suicide exist among physicians, professional-technical people, and the general population. Married men appear least prone, single and widowed are next, and divorcees are most inclined to take their own lives. However, here the similarity ends. While divorcees in the general population are three times as suicide prone as married men (82/25), divorced physicians are 13 times more likely to kill themselves than their married colleagues (662/52). This sensitivity to divorce is likewise demonstrated by professional-technical people (347/29). The foregoing data indicate that suicidal factors operating in the general population are intensified among physicians and other high occupational groups.

Table 12-V.—Suicide Rates by Age for White Male Physicians and General Population, California*

Group, Age	Suicides 1959 to 1961	Population† April 1960	Annual Rate No./100,000/yr
Physicians‡			
25 to 34	3	5,027	20
35 to 44	8	7,875	34
45 to 54	17	5,328	119
55 to 64	11	2,843	129
65 and over	9	1,217	247
Unknown	0		. .
Total	48	22,290	72§
General Population‖			
25 to 34	591	971,908	20
35 to 44	905	1,040,095	29
45 to 54	1,106	830,441	44
55 to 64	951	588,862	54
65 and over	1,051	577,457	61
Unknown	2	. . .	. . .
Total	4,606	4,008,763	38§

* For entire table, $\chi^2 = 43.3$, $P < .0005$.

† Age-adjusted by indirect method, $\chi^2 = 38.6$ (method described in ref 23), $P < .0005$. General white male California population is the standard.

‡ $\chi^2 = 32.5$, $P < .0005$.

§ Not age-adjusted rates.

‖ $\chi^2 = 680$, $P < .0005$.

Although suicide rates in the various specialties have received much attention in the literature, there is no evidence to suggest that one specialty is more prone to suicide than any other. Blachly and associates'[10] review of *JAMA* obituaries concluded incorrectly that "specialty seems to be a highly significant variable" and proceeded to label psychiatrists as the most suicidal group. A simple x^2 test of their data reveals that the differences they observed between specialties could easily have arisen from chance alone ($P < .20$). Craig and Pitts[9] reviewed *JAMA* obituaries from the same period and found no

Table 12-VI.—Age-Adjusted Suicide Rates by Sex for Whites, 25 and Older, California*

Group	Suicides 1959 to 1961	Population† April 1960	Annual Rate No./100,000/yr
Physicians‡			
Men	48	22,290	77
Women	1	1,970	18
Total	49	24,260	. . .
General Population§			
Men	4,606	4,008,763	38
Women	2,056	4,216,572	16
Total	6,662	8,225,335	. . .

* Age-adjusted by indirect method, $\chi^2 = 38.6$ (method described in ref 23), $P < .0005$. χ^2 calculated by Mantel Haensel method described in ref 24.

† Source: ref 21, Tables 17 and 123. White and nonwhite are included in the physician category for lack of more detailed figures. Nonwhite male physicians account for only 4% of total male physicians and the effect is negligible. Nonwhites account for only 6% of total female physicians.

‡ $\chi^2 = 1.93$, $P < .20$.

§ $\chi^2 = 1157$, $P < .0005$.

difference among specialists, except perhaps for otolaryngologists.

Freeman[27] investigated suicide among psychiatrists by reviewing *JAMA* obituaries, journals, and newspapers over the 70 years from 1895 to 1965. He fails to calculate rates or to include adequate material for the reader to do so. Although asserting that they are highly suicidal, he presents no evidence that psychiatrists are unusually prone to self-destruction. Bruce et al.[28] studied causes of death among anesthesiologists during the 20 years from 1947 to 1966 and uncovered 35 suicides. From data supplied in the article, one calculates an average annual rate of 31 per 100,000, a figure not unlike existing estimates for physicians in Table 12-I.

Our data on suicide by specialty area are presented in Table 12-IX. No adjustment of the rates for age, sex, or race is possible due to the absence of detailed population figures. One can see from the table that general practitioners account for the single greatest number of suicides. However, there are no statistically significant differences between the suicide rates of the specialties ($P < .30$). Chance alone accounts for the minor differences observed, and greater numbers are required before one must give up this position. Interestingly psychiatrists, purported by Blachly to have the highest

Table 12-VII.—Suicide Rates by Race for California Men Age 25 and Older

Group	Suicides 1959 to 1961	Population* April 1960	Annual Rate† No./100,000/yr
Physicians‡			
White	48	21,677	74
Nonwhite	1	892	37
Total	49	22,569	72
General Population§			
White	4,606	4,008,763	38
Nonwhite	210	334,508	21
Total	4,816	4,343,271	37

* Ref 21, Tables 17 and 122.

† Not age-adjusted rates; the magnitude of the correction introduced by age-adjustment seldom exceeded 10% (in rates where these calculations were possible), so the bias from not age-adjusting here would be quite small.

‡ $\chi^2 = 0.472$, $P < .50$.

§ $\chi^2 = 75.6$, $P < .0005$.

suicide rate, experienced no suicides during the study period. Thus, there is no evidence that propensity to self-destruction and one's specialty area are particularly related.

In addition to information concerning the characteristics of suicidal physicians, data were gathered on the methods of suicide used (Table 12-X). Physicians have a marked preference for drug ingestion (55%) and a marked distaste for firearms (12%) in the suicidal act. This differs from the other two groups, where firearms are the method of choice (32, 37%) and drugs are used less frequently (29, 21%). The differences are highly significant statistically ($P < .0005$ for comparisons between groups). It has been suggested that access to drugs and knowledge of their use prompts physicians to use this method in preference to others. However, dentists and pharmacists do not show this same propensity (35% and 40%, respectively, from data not shown in Table 12-X). Hence, suicidal physicians demonstrate a unique attraction to this means of self-destruction.

In summary, we have found compelling evidence showing that physicians and other health care workers are exceedingly prone to suicide. Clearly we record the minimum number of suicides, for one

Table 12-VIII.—Age-Adjusted Suicide Rates by Marital Status for Selected California White Men Age 14 and Older*

Group	Suicides 1959 to 1961	Population† April 1960	Annual Rate No./100,000/yr
Physicians‡			
Divorced	6	259	662
Widowed	3	327	188
Single	4	1,742	97
Married	36	20,241	52
Unknown	0	...	...
Total	49	22,569	...
Prof-Tech§			
Divorced	74	6,686	347
Widowed	38	4,629	184
Single	86	73,036	60
Married	375	429,984	29
Unknown	3	...	...
Total	576	514,335	...
General Population‖			
Divorced	583	188,882	82
Widowed	441	151,131	61
Single	851	1,239,890	40
Married	3000	3,520,670	25
Unknown	103	...	...
Total	4,978	5,100,573	...

* Age-adjusted by indirect method; χ^2 calculated as described in ref 23. Due to limitations of our data base, this table includes persons age 14 and older instead of the preferred 25 and older age range.

† Source: ref 21, Table 105 for general population. Calculated for others by applying the percent marital and age distributions of US physicians and prof-tech to corresponding California population (source: ref 25 and 26, Tables 3 and 5, respectively).

§ $\chi^2 = 821, P < .005$.

‖ $\chi^2 = 960, P < .005$.

cannot be certain how many suicides go unrecognized and are reported as accidental falls, automobile and firearm accidents, and so on. Whether relatively more physician suicides are concealed by sympathetic colleagues, one cannot say.

Considering the magnitude of this problem, further study seems mandatory. Follow-up interviews of next of kin of verified suicides could provide useful information about the private lives of suicidal physicians. Detailed psychiatric examination of physicians who unsuccessfully attempt suicide also would provide further understanding. A large prospective study based on psychological testing of present medical students may identify specific traits of those who later suicide. Finally, physicians should become alerted to the existence of this problem and be more attuned to a colleague's "cry for help."

Table 12-IX.—Suicide Rates by Specialty Area in California

Group	Suicides 1959 to 1961	Population* July 1960	Annual Rate† No./100,000/yr
Surgical subspecialties‡	16	5,603	95
Internal medicine	6	2,926	68
General surgery	4	2,186	61
General practice	14	9,264	50
Medical subspecialties§	4	3,490	38
Psychiatry	0	1,218	0
Retired, unknown	7	...	...
Total‖	51	24,687	69

* Source: ref 29.

† Not age-adjusted rates; the magnitude of the correction introduced by age-adjustment seldom exceeded 10% (in rates where these calculations were possible), so the bais from not age-adjusting here would be quite small.

‡ Includes otology, laryngology, rhinology, anesthesiology, pathology, gynecology, neurosurgery, ophthalmology, obstetrics, orthopedics, plastic, proctology, thoracic, and urology.

§ Includes allergy, aviation, bacteriology, cardiovascular, dermatology, gastroenterology, administrative, legal, neurology, occupational, pediatrics, public health, pulmonary, and radiology.

‖ $\chi^2 = 7.1$, $P < .30$.

Table 12-X.—Method of Suicide Used by Selected Groups in California*

Method	Physicians, %†	Prof-Tech, %‡	General Population, %
Drugs	55	29	21
Poisons	14	9	6
Gas	4	12	12
Hanging	6	8	13
Drowning	0	1	2
Firearms	12	32	37
Cutting	8	3	2
Jumping	0	3	4
Other	2	3	3
Total, %	101	100	100
No. suicides	51	776	7471

* For entire table, $\chi^2 = 111$, $P < .0005$.

† $\chi^2 = 108$, $P < .0005$.

‡ $\chi^2 = 749$, $P < .0005$.

§ $\chi^2 = 7{,}206$, $P < .0005$.

REFERENCES

1. Suicides of physicians and the reasons, editorial. *JAMA* 41:263-264, 1903.
2. Knopf SA: Suicide among American physicians. *NY Med J* 117:84-87, 1923.
3. Emerson H, Hughes HE: Death rates of male white physicians in the United States, by age and cause. *Am J Public Health* 16:1088-1093, 1926.
4. Dublin LI, Spiegelman M: The longevity and mortality of American physicians, 1938-1942. *JAMA* 134:1211-1215, 1947.
5. *Mortality by Occupation and Cause of Death,* Vital Statistics Special Reports, No.3. Government Printing Office, Department of Health, Education, and Welfare, Public Health Service, 1963, vol 53, p 157.
6. Dickinson FG, Martin LW: Physician mortality, 1949-1951. *JAMA* 162:1462-1468, 1956.
7. Powell EH: Occupation, status, and suicide. *Am Social Rev* 23: 131-139, 1958.
8. Blachly PH, Osterud HT, Josslin R: Suicide in professional groups. *N Engl J Med* 268:1278-1282, 1963.
9. Craig AG, Pitts FN: Suicide by physicians. *Dis Nerv Syst* 29:763-772, 1968.
10. Blachly PH, Disher W, Roduner G: Suicide by physicians. *Bull Suicide* 1-18, 1968.
11. DeSole DE, Singer P, Aronson S: Suicide and role strain among physicians. *Int J Soc Psychiatry* 15:294-301, 1969.
12. Thomas CB: Suicide among us. *Johns Hopkins Med J* 125:276-285, 1969.
13. *Historical Statistics of the United States, Colonial Times To 1957.* Government Printing Office, Bureau of the Census, 1960, p 34.
14. *Mortality by Occupation and Industry,* Vital Statistics Special Reports, No. 2. Department of Health, Education, and Welfare, Public Health Service, 1962, vol 53.
15. *Vital Statistics of the United States, 1967.* Government Printing Office, Department of Health, Education, and Welfare, 1967, vol 2, part B, Table 7-6.
16. *Current Population Reports,* .series P-25, No. 441. Government Printing Office, Department of Commerce, Bureau of Census, 1970.
17. *Prevention of Suicide,* Public Health Papers No. 35. Geneva, World Health Organization, 1968, p 32.
18. *Suicide in the United States, 1950-1964.* Department of Health, Education, and Welfare, Public Health Service Publication No. 1000, series 20, No. 5, p 16.
19. Simon W, Lumry G: Suicide among physician-patients. *J Nerv Ment Dis* 147:105-112, 1968.
20. *Dering's California Codes: Government Code Annotated,* State of California, Adopted April 13, 1943. San Francisco, Bancroft & Whitney, 1962, Sec 27491.
21. *US Census of Population 1960.* Department of Commerce, Bureau of Census, 1963, vol 1, part 6. Washington DC, 1963.
22. *American Medical Directory 1958,* ed 20. Chicago, American Medical Association, 1958.
23. Armitage P: *Statistical methods in Medical Research.* Oxford, England, Blackwell Scientific Publications, 1971, pp 373-375.
24. Ipsen J, Feigl P: *Bancroft's Introduction to Biostatistics,* ed 2. New York, Harper &

Row Publishers, 1970, pp 135-137.
25. *US Census of Population 1960, Subject Reports: Characteristics of Professional Workers,* Final Report PC(2)-7E. Government Printing Office, Department of Commerce, Bureau of Census, 1964.
26. *US Census of Population 1960, Subject Reports: Marital Status,* Final Report PC(2)-4E. Government Printing Office, Department of Commerce, Bureau of Census, 1966.
27. Freeman W: *The Psychiatrist.* New York, Grune & Stratton Inc, 1968, pp 274-284.
28. Bruce DL, et al: Causes of death among anesthesiologists. *Anesthesiology* 29:565-569, 1968.
29. *Directory Report Services,* No. 108. Chicago, American Medical Association, 1960, vol 14.

Etiology I: Stress

Chapter 13

ANXIETY IN MEDICAL PRACTICE — THE DOCTOR'S OWN ANXIETY

W. A. CRAMOND

INTRODUCTION

THE stereotype of the doctor as seen by the patient would, I suggest, be that of a man or less usually, a woman, dedicated to the healing art. Adjectives such as kindly, wise, understanding, busy, skillful and knowledgeable would commonly be used, particularly if the patient were ill at the time. The need for an omnipotent, all caring parent is obvious. Such paragons do not know frailty or doubt; anxiety has no place here unless it is in the concern of the physician as he awaits the outcome of his ministrations while wondering if he has been called in time.

None of us has escaped the unpleasant tension introspectively and physiologically felt which we call anxiety. We have known realistic situational anxiety when faced with a new critical diagnostic or therapeutic dilemma. A number of us will have experienced the unease of free floating anxiety, or the tension of the phobic state. Doctors being human, must accept the human condition. Our patients, if pressed, would I have no doubt, agree that doctors could be expected to become anxious but would be unwilling to admit that the doctor's anxiety could affect them directly. Yet I believe that the doctor's anxiety, whether reality based or conflictually generated, has very real implications for the patient, his treatment and its outcome.

My awareness of this problem was kindled many years ago, when as a new young assistant in general practice I was over-stimulated by a young mother's graphic description of her 4 weeks' old baby's vomiting. "Yes doctor, right across the room, as sure as I'm sitting here." My anxiety, born of inexperience, caused the mother and baby an 80 mile journey in wintry conditions. I was reassured

---

From W. A. Cramond, Anxiety in Medical Practice — the Doctor's Own Anxiety. *Aust N Z J Psychiatry 3*: 324, 1969. Reprinted by permission.

The author would like to thank the doctors in South Australia for their cooperation in this study and Ms. G.M. Mainelis for her work in processing the material.

that there was no pyloric stenosis but had to treat a severe chest cold in the infant which resulted from the unnecessary referral. The resolution of my anxiety undoubtedly endangered that particular patient's health.

It is all too easy nowadays to allay our anxiety by sending patients for further investigations. I believe it was a physician at one of the Melbourne hospitals who talked of the menace of the ball point pen and as Schimmel (1964) has so convincingly shown, our investigative procedures carry a risk of injury to the patient. He studied the occurrence of hospital-induced complications on a university medical service at New Haven, Connecticut, in a prospective investigation of over a thousand patients admitted over an 8-month period; 20 percent of the patients admitted to the medical wards experienced one or more untoward episodes and 10 percent had a prolonged or unresolved episode. The severity of the 240 episodes was minor in 110, moderate in 82 and major in 48, of which 16 ended fatally. The risk of having such episodes seemed directly related to the length of time spent in the hospital. While Schimmel discusses such hazards as severity of sickness, drug reactions and investigative procedural difficulties he does not suggest that the doctor's own anxiety may be a factor in recommending injudicious diagnostic and therapeutic measures — one wonders however.

Working closely with the surgical and medical members of a Renal Unit as they developed their skills and expertise in haemodialysis and homotransplantation, I have been aware of how the doctor's own unspoken anxiety is communicated to the group of patients under care. Florid psychiatric disturbance was not infrequent in the first 18 months or 2 years of work, but is now rarely seen.

This appears to have a direct relationship to staff morale and confidence. Similar observations were made by the cardiac surgeons at the Mayo clinic who noted in the early days of closed heart surgery that psychotic disturbances in patients were not uncommon. After a period, they all but disappeared only to reappear again when open heart surgery and valve replacement became the new technique.

We know from personal experience that the work is stressful and anxiety-provoking, but is it more so than in other jobs? Reference to the literature shows that anxiety in doctors is not a subject that is much discussed. The late Gregory Zilboorg drew attention to the "beginning psychiatry training syndrome" and later Merklin and Little in 1967 wrote a descriptive anecdotal paper on this theme.

They described the new resident's anxiety and some of his methods of coping with it. The pressures leading to anxiety and shared with other medical residents included competition within the peer group, formation of a satisfactory relationship with authorities, assumption of increased medical responsibility and the adjustments necessary between home and hospital life. Halleck and Woods in 1962 had earlier referred to anxiety in psychiatric residents and the almost complete lack of information as to the incidence of anxiety attacks, depression, suicide, psychosis or serious acting out. Indeed, they suggested that the failure to study these problems perhaps reflected the guilt among the supervisors, arising from a sense of responsibility for these casualties, from anxiety about the nebulous qualities of selection procedures and from a sense of inadequacy about successfully meeting the resident's emotional reactions.

A 1968 paper by Davies, Mowbray and Jensen showed that the incidence of psychiatric symptoms as ascertained by their survey of Australian medical students is of the same order as noted for other groups of medical students in the United Kingdom and that medical students give lower indications of psychiatric symptomatology than other types of student and other groups of young people. The symptomatology includes anxiety and Mowbray and Davies (1968) measured anxiety directly on the Eysenck Personality Inventory and found it to be lower for medical students. Adcock (1965) had previously confirmed Bendig's (1962) view that the neuroticism factor of Eysenck corresponds with the anxiety factor of Cattell's scales.

I mention this point here since this latter was the scale used in this present study. From these previous studies of Mowbray and Davies we might expect doctors to be less anxious than others in the community.

METHODOLOGY

In an attempt to obtain some basic information, our department recently conducted a survey of all practising doctors in South Australia. This survey had its origins rather fortuitously in a seminar organised by the Australian College of Pathologists in 1968 on screening methods in medicine. Mr. John Court, Lecturer in Clinical Psychology took part in this seminar and invited the participants to complete the Neuroticism Scale Questionnaire (N.S.Q.) devised by Scheier and Cattell in 1961. This group of pathologists were predominantly laboratory workers and non-clinical medical people. Anxiety as measured by the N.S.Q. was normally distributed and not significantly different from the normative

American sample. With this as a starting point, could it be shown that clinicians were more anxious than their non-clinical peers?

In collaboration with our Visiting Professor, Professor Malcolm Miller of the University of Aberdeen and with others in the department, a questionnaire was devised. It was decided that to obtain cooperation and a good response the questionnaire would require to be short and non-threatening. It was tried first on a pilot group of general practitioners and took an average of 15 minutes to complete. Arrangements were made for the completed questionnaire to be returned anonymously, but respondents who wished to know their personal scores could identify themselves if they so wished. The questions to be answered covered such items as age, sex, religion, length of time since first qualification, where this was taken, the type of practice engaged in, whether or not the respondent considered he or she was more or less anxious than average. There was also included a series of 15 common anxiety provoking situations in clinical medicine to which the respondent was invited to reply, indicating which, if any, caused anxiety. Along with these general items was included the N.S.Q. of Scheier and Cattell. It is derived from their better known 16PF test and consists of 40 items, claiming not only to discriminate between neurotic and normal controls, but also to give measures on four other scales — a tough/tender-minded dimension, a depressive/happy-go-lucky dimension, a submissive/dominance dimension and fourthly, anxiety. For the purpose of this paper I shall be reporting only on the anxiety scale of the test. The advantages of the N.S.Q. in this study were that, in addition to the American population samples upon which the test was validated, results with a normal population sample had also been reported from Scotland by Colwell (1965) while we also had the Australian pathologists' group who had been shown to be no different from the other two overseas groups.

RESULTS

All practitioners whose names appeared in the 1968 edition of the South Australian Medical Register and whose address was given as being in South Australia were circulated. The total was 1589. 912 replies were received of which 810 were effective. The 102 rejected came from doctors who had retired, had left the State or who were for one reason or another not currently in practice or had left no forwarding address. The response rate of 54.5 percent was considered high — for doctors — to this type of questionnaire. Only three hostile letters of reply were received. Of great interest was the fact that 577 doctors chose to give their names, i.e. 72.9 percent of the effective responders. There was no significant difference in the anxiety scores between the anonymous group and the group revealing identity. From this it would seem reasonable to assume that the non-responders were not likely to be any different to the responders.

Were the doctors honest? A comparison of their subjective assessments of anxiety with the N.S.Q. anxiety scale was highly significant (beyond the 1 in 1,000 level or $P<0.001$). This suggests that either the doctors were honest in their personal appraisal or that the N.S.Q. scale for anxiety measures what it sets out to measure, or both. At any rate, it can I believe be assumed with a high degree of confidence that the questionnaire findings are valid.

When compared with the American and Scottish normative samples, the total South Australian medical clinical population, male and female, was significantly more anxious ($P<0.001$). When compared with the non-clinical group of pathologists the difference in anxiety was also significant ($P<0.05$).

In general then, it would appear that south Australian clinicians in all fields are more anxious than normal overseas populations and more particularly, since there is less chance of a cultural bias, are more anxious than a non-clinical Australian sample of doctors.

Our sample showed no significant difference between the sexes in terms of anxiety, although the female sample was not significantly different from normal populations either, so that the female medical sample lies somewhere between the male doctors and the controls in terms of anxiety.

If we chart relative anxiety levels derived from various psychological tests (see Fig. 13-1) we can see quite clearly that male South Australian doctors report more anxiety than the other groups. Of great interest is the difference between the anxiety reported by medical students and the practitioners.

A comparison of the distribution of medical anxiety scores, male and female, with normal controls clearly shows the skew in the direction of higher medical anxiety (see Fig. 13-2). This anxiety appears greater than simply the degree of anxiety required for alertness and drive in a demanding profession.

The 154 country doctors are not more anxious than the 654 urban practitioners. There is no significant difference for age in our sample, nor for religion or place of qualification, whether overseas or in Australia. When the different specialties are compared with Cattell's normative, American sample general practitioners, surgeons

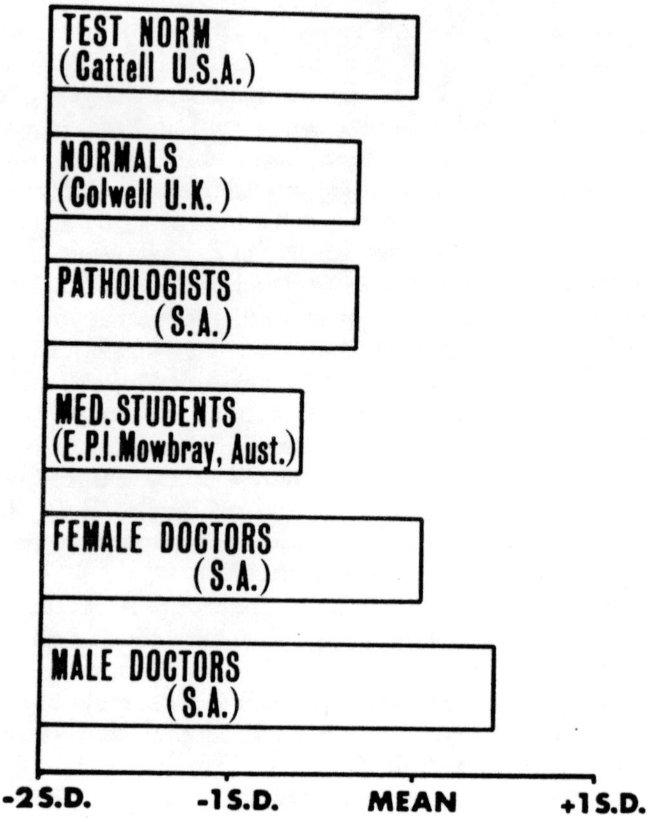

Figure 13-1.

and those carrying out two types of practice, e.g. general practitioner *cum* surgeon, or general practitioner *cum* anaesthetist, are significantly more anxious at the <0.001 levels of confidence respectively. General practitioners and surgeons are indistinguishable from each other but those with two specialties were the most anxious (see Fig. 13-3).

Physicians, obstetricians, anaesthetists, psychiatrists and other specialists grouped together were not significantly more anxious than the American samples. There were representative returns from each of these specialist groups.

What are the clinical situations the doctor sees as particularly anxiety provoking? (See Tables 13-I and 13-II).

For the total group and for family doctors the greatest problems are to be found in obstetrics, the failure of treatment, in the death of the young, in diagnostic difficulties and in the impact the work has

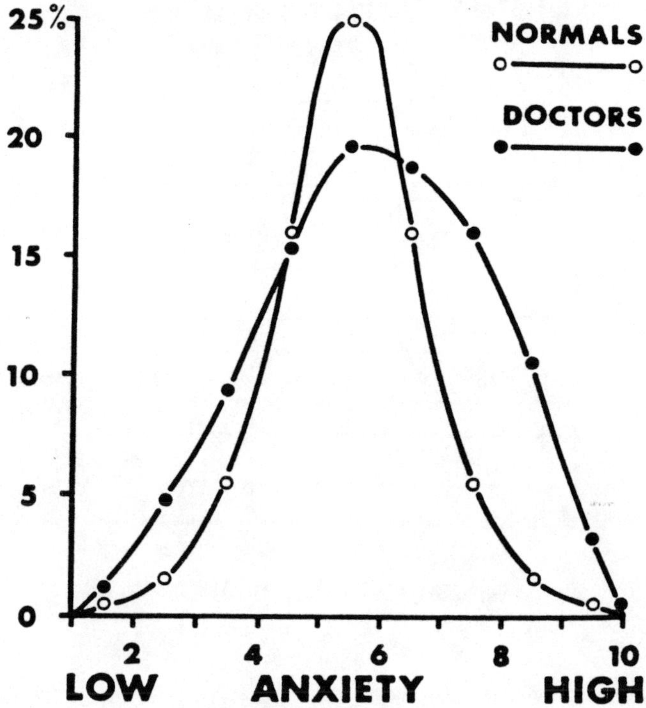

Figure 13-2.

on the doctor's own family life.

Included in the questionnaire, as an additional means of tapping anxiety, was a section inviting comments on aspects of work which either irritated, embarrassed, were burdensome or were satisfying. The respondent was also invited to indicate how he dealt with or thought he dealt with anxiety. The material here did not lend itself to statistical analysis but an overall profile was obtained. Relatively few mentioned recourse to drugs or alcohol or reported psychosomatic symptomatology. Denial, suppression and displacement of affect were commonly recognised ego defences.

Discussion

Allowing for the methodological difficulties of questionnaires, and the possible cultural differences in N.S.Q. ratings of anxiety, it appears from this study that South Australian clinicians are significantly more anxious than nonclinicians and more anxious than normal population samples. Male doctors show a trend towards higher anxiety than females. This may be a reflection of

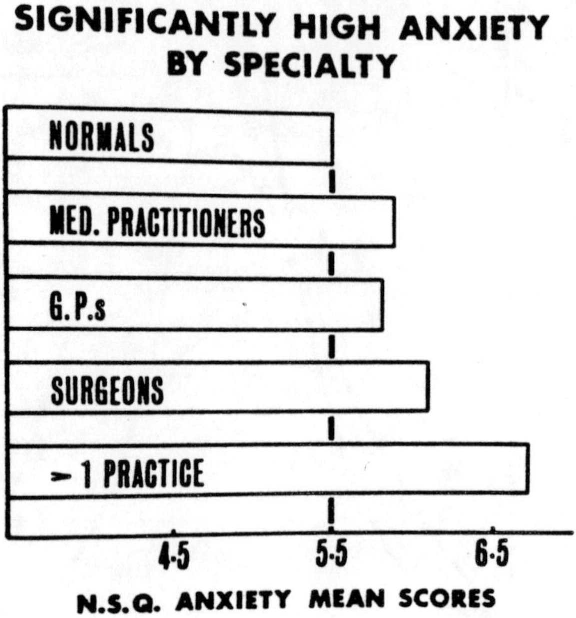

Figure 13-3.

responsibility as the ultimate home providers, since 52 of the 78 female respondents were married and presumably were not the sole providers at home.

General practitioners, and particularly those combining this with a specialty, and surgeons are more prone to anxiety than doctors in other specialties. As well-recognised causes of anxiety we have therapeutic failures, diagnostic difficulties especially in obstetrics, the death of young patients and the impact of professional on family life. Very few doctors admitted to indulgence in alcohol or in drugs as a means of coping with their anxiety. Very few saw excessive investigation of illness as coping device although large numbers referred or discussed difficult cases, which may imply some further investigation. A large group of doctors reported long-term patients presenting as social or emotional problems as irritating, burdensome or embarrassing. This seemed to arouse in the doctors the anxiety of helplessness. As Davis (1964) has said, "when anxiety is felt, mental activity . . . is disorganised in greater or lesser degree. This disorder and the disorder of skill should be regarded not as cause and effect, but as complementary aspects of a disorder of the reaction to complex psychological dangers, which the individual perceives to be pre-

Table 13-I

Reported frequency of sources of anxiety among doctors (N = 782)

1.	Failure of Treatment	347
2.	Diagnostic Difficulties	272
3.	Impact of Work on Family Life	263
4.	Death of Children	259
5.	Obstetric Difficulties	237
6.	Emergencies	201
7.	Looking after Colleagues and Family	121
8.	Night Calls	122
9.	Practice Management	92
10.	Medical Competition	90
11.	Chronic Illness	55
12.	Death and Dying	51
13.	Death and Dying in the Elderly	23
14.	Publication of Practice Standards	15
15.	Looking after Colleagues' Patients	9

Table 13-II

Reported frequency of sources of anxiety among G.P.s (N = 355)

1.	Obstetric Difficulties	194
2.	Failure of Treatment	144
3.	Death of Children	136
4.	Impact of Work on Family Life	130
5.	Diagnostic Difficulties	109
6.	Emergencies	103
7.	Night Calls	76
8.	Looking after Colleagues and Family	53
9.	Practice Management	46
10.	Medical Competition	24
11.	Death and Dying	21
12.	Chronic Illness	20
13.	Death and Dying in the Elderly	9
14.	Publication of Practice Standards	9
15.	Looking after Colleagues' Patients	4

sent in his environment, and which he cannot immediately remove."

Miller and Rice (1967) in discussing anxiety in air crew suggest that the glamour with which our society invests the pilot especially, provides him with insulation against stress and that it is institutionalised within the flight organisation. Similarly they speculate that in medicine glamour has helped to defend doctors against anxiety. They note that in the United Kingdom outbursts from the British Medical Association about pay and conditions of work may be seen as a reaction to declining status. Despite the image presented by television and other fictional build up, general practitioners are increasingly perceived by the public as writers of simple prescriptions. More importantly, they suggest that the profession as a whole increasingly glamourises and raises the relative status of the specialist, to the point where the work of the general practitioner is in reality denigrated. The resulting rise in anxiety in a group in danger of losing status can therefore be forecast. Their interesting theory is not supported by this work. Surgeons and general practitioners who enjoy very high social status in our community show the highest levels of anxiety. It could be argued that some of the anxiety at least stems from the need to retain that status and from the competitiveness of the working conditions.

If this present work and that of Mowbray and Davies in Melbourne on medical students' anxiety is valid, we have a situation where a group of people experience a significant rise in anxiety levels presumably on the assumption of clinical responsibility. The doctors themselves identify situations that consciously cause anxiety. In addition they recognise a large group of social and emotional problems that arouse feelings of helpless frustration. Can doctors burdened with this degree of anxiety gain much satisfaction in their work? Their own health would appear to be in danger of suffering. Russek (1962) has already shown that doctors in stressful conditions of work have a higher incidence of coronary artery disease than doctors in non-stressful work situations.

What can be done to help? Two possible lines of action suggest themselves and both courses are, so far as I can see, being slowly evolved as a reaction to felt need. Firstly, to cope with the anxiety aroused by diagnostic and therapeutic difficulties more comprehensive opportunities for continual ongoing postgraduate training are necessary. To do this effectively and on the scale required, significant imaginative financial support and Goverment backing will be critical.

Secondly, to cope with the conflict between professional duties and family responsibilities, to help deal with the admittedly heavy and protracted social and psychiatric problems, team and group approaches in medical practice will be more and more essential. It must be emphasised that the team will include workers other than medical, e. g. social workers, clinical psychologists, mental health visitors. All have a very significant part to play and as Miller has said, "the great advantage of having non-medicals in the team is to counteract that degree of professional omnipotence that often goes before a fall. I think that almost any purely medical organisation can be too rigid and its members therefore, too vulnerable to sudden change."

Unfortunately in our questionnaire I omitted to ask for information as to whether the respondents were working in group or single handed practice. However, a number of doctors spontaneously commented on partnership problems. These appeared to stem from financial contractual obligations and different attitudes to medicine; but both led to recognised tension and anxiety. So that while the days of the single handed practitioner are surely numbered, the financial problems of group practice may require attention. At any rate the high levels of anxiety we have recorded here may be too high a price to pay for rugged individual freedom.

Finally, it is suggested that whatever action may be taken, study group should be organised to investigate its effectiveness. The high number of doctors who chose to give their names in this questionnaire suggests not only a personal interest but a wide awareness of the need for further helpful research and action.

REFERENCES

Adcock, C. J. (1965). A Comparison of the concepts of Cattell and Eysenck, *Brit. J. E. Psychol.*, 35: 90.

Bendig, A. W. (1960). Factor analyses of anxiety and neuroticism inventories. *J. Consulting Psychol.*, 24: 6.

Burgess, G. N., Kirklin, J. W., and Steinhilber, R. M. (1967). Some psychiatric aspects of intracardiac surgery. *Mayo Clin. Proc.*, 42: 1.

Davies, B., Mowbray, R. M. and Jensen, D. (1968). A questionnaire survey of psychiatric symptoms in Australian medical students. *Aust. & N.Z. J. Psychiat.*, 2: 46.

Davis, D. R., (1964). Psychological mechanisms in pilot error. In *Aviation Psychology*, A. Cassie, S. D. Fokkema and J. B. Parry (Eds.). The Hague and Paris: Mouron. pp. 12-23.

Halleck, S. L. and Woods, S. M. (1962). Emotional problems of psychiatric residents. *Psychiatry*, 25: 339.

Kear-Colwell, J. J. (1965). Studies of the I.P.A.T. Neuroticism Scale Questionnaire (N.S.Q.). *Brit. J. soc. clin. Psychol.*, 4: 214.

Merklin, L. and Little, R. B. (1967). Beginning Psychiatry training syndrome, *Amer. J. Psychiat.*, 124: 297.

Miller, W. M. (1969). Personal communication.

Miller, E. J. and Rice, A. K. (1967). *Systems or Organization* – the control of task and sentient boundaries. Tavistock publications. pp. 201-215.

Russek, H. I. (1962). Emotional stress and coronary heart disease in American physicians, dentists and lawyers. *Am. J. Med. Sci.*, 243: 116.

Scheier, I. H. and Cattell, R. B. (1961). Handbook for the Neuroticism Scale Questionnaire, "The N.S.Q." Champaign, Illinois: Institute for Personality and Ability Testing.

Schimmel, E. M. (1964). The hazards of hospitalisation. *Ann. Int. Med.*, 60: 100.

Chapter 14

SATISFACTIONS, DISSATISFACTIONS, AND CAUSES OF STRESS IN MEDICAL PRACTICE

BETTY HOSMER MAWARDI

THE practice of medicine offers many satisfactions, but there have been increasing sources of stress in the profession and increasing signs of stress-related problems among physicians.

For the past decade, the careers of alumni of Case Western Reserve (CWR) School of Medicine have been studied in projects supported in part by the Commonwealth Fund. The objectives were to see what the graduates are doing now, how they like what they have been doing, and how they feel about the education they received at CWR.

The first study[1,2] (*Medical World News,* March 25, 1966, p 114) concerned the graduates of 1935 through 1945, who had a traditional type of medical education. The current study focuses on the careers of approximately 180 alumni in nine different specialties selected randomly from the classes of 1956 through 1965, the first decade after the curriculum at CWR was revised in 1952.

The format consists of an interview in the physician's own office and a written set of short-answer questions. One part of the questionnaire concentrates on the satisfactions, dissatisfactions, and stresses in their careers in medicine.

The alumni are, as a whole, content with their practices and their lives. They report more satisfactions than dissatisfactions, and only two or three of either group interviewed so far have said that they would have chosen a different career if given a second chance. What is increasingly apparent, however, as the more recent graduates are interviewed, is that physicians today are reporting some stresses that are quite different from those found in the previous study.

From the Division of Research in Medical Education, Case Western Reserve University School of Medicine, Cleveland, OH.

LIKES AND DISLIKES

In both studies questions were posed about what types of patients they liked and did not like, what types of medical problems they preferred to work with, and what aspects of practice they found particularly satisfying.

The graduates of 1935 through 1945 said that being needed gave them the greatest satisfaction as physicians. They also enjoyed the successful management of difficult cases where they could save a patient's life or make him more comfortable. They did not like treating patients whom they could not help appreciably. Another source of pleasure was the development of personal relationships with patients and their families. Some said they liked doing well financially; others remarked that they had enjoyed making money when they were first in practice, but time off was now more important.

Time, the lack of leisure time and time pressures of work, presented the biggest source of stress. Too many patients to see in too short a time, too large a case load, and too much time on call were mentioned repeatedly.

Table 14-I shows the satisfactions that were named most frequently by private practitioners. Accurate diagnosis and successful therapy were first, with service to humanity and a good physician-patient relationship following closely. The figures add up to more than 100 percent since more than one response could be given.

Not all the physicians in the earlier study were in full-time private practice; one group was composed of medical school faculty, and another was hospital based. The faculty, although representing many specialties and engaging in some private practice, held full-time appointments in medical schools and had teaching and research commitments. The full-time hospital personnel (anesthesiologists, pathologists, and radiologists) technically might have been in private practice, but they were hospital based. Together these two groups were called non-office-based, and their most frequently named satisfactions are shown in Table 14-I.

Table 14-I illustrates dissatisfactions named by the private practitioners and non-office-based practitioners. Private practitioners suffered most often from time pressures. Paperwork was a major anathema, and therapy failures, when encountered, were major frustrations. The non-office-based practitioners were mainly dissatisfied because of too much administrative work, time pressures, office detail and paperwork.

Table 14-I.—Satisfactions and Dissatisfactions*

	% of Private Practitioners	% of Non-Office-Based Practitioners
Satisfaction		
Accurate diagnosis and successful therapy	53	33
Service to humanity and good physician-patient relationship	50	17
Respect and appreciation from patients and community	29	19
Teaching	9	31
Research	1	42
Administration	...	6
Dissatisfaction		
Time pressures†	47	25
Therapy failure and patient-related problems	26	11
Office details and paperwork	24	17
Problems with other physicians	9	11
Financial considerations	8	6
Insufficient medical facilities	7	6
Isolation due to specialization	3	...
Personal limitations in knowledge or ability	3	3
Administration and committee work	2	25
Limits of science	2	8
Academic politics	...	8
Aspects of teaching	...	6

*Percentages reflect several responses from some of the physicians.

†Includes too little personal free time, continuous on-call responsibilities, and pressures of the work load.

CAREER SATISFACTION

The participants in the study were also given career satisfaction tests (a modified version of the Brayfield Job Satisfaction Blank)[3] because some objective criterion for career satisfaction was needed. The overall job satisfaction was examined to see which physicians were at the top and at the bottom of the scale. Then the types of satisfactions and dissatisfactions that were most often named by those who were either extremely happy or unhappy with their professions were examined. Satisfaction with providing successful therapy was approximately the same for those with overall extremely high or low scores on job satisfaction. Dissatisfactions were different, however. The people who scored highest on job satisfaction were most bothered by the changes in the image of the physician and by not being able to get beds for their patients in their hospitals. The physicians who had the lowest job satisfaction scores disliked being disturbed in the middle of the night and the lack of leisure time for hobbies and family.

The findings indicated that full-time medical school faculty members were the most satisfied with their careers. Of the private practitioners, the general surgeons were the most satisfied. They had strong identities as physicians, they usually saw the results of their interventions quickly, and they had the highest incomes. Some physicians had qualms about their identity. Said one psychiatrist, "I feel I'm getting further and further away from the practice of medicine. I don't think I could do a physical anymore if I had to. I'm practicing something that's not in the mainstream of medicine."

Many internists were unhappy because they handled too many minor illnesses and believed they served as general practitioners rather than as specialists. This was particularly true for the internists practicing in large cities; in medium-sized towns or cities, they were able to practice more as specialists on referrals from the general practitioners. General practitioners, as a group, scored next to the lowest in job satisfaction; pediatricians scored the lowest. The latter group did not complain about their patients, but they did not like dealing with the parents, particularly mothers. Table 14-II shows the average scores for the groups of physicians on the job satisfaction test; possible scores ranged from a low of 18 to a high of 90. Confirmation of these findings is found in such alumni statements as "It's obvious that general practitioners have a hard job and the pediatricians are always complaining about the mothers. No wonder we have so many surgeons and so few general practitioners."

SUICIDE AND CAREER SATISFACTION

As analyses were being completed on the graduates' satisfaction with their career choices, articles[4–6] began appearing on the high rate of suicide among physicians. The exact rates varied, but all articles seemed to indicate that the rates for physicians were higher than for the public at large or for most other professional groups. Some authors (*Medical Tribune,* April 5, 1967, p 15) said that the rate for physicians may go as high as 88 per 100,000, or eight times the rate for the general population. Within medical specialties the rates also vary, from a high of 61 per 100,000 for psychiatrists to a low of ten per 100,00 for pediatricians.

We examined our data to see if the suicide rates bore any rela-

Table 14-II.—Ranking of Physician Groups and Satisfaction With Profession*

Profession	Satisfaction Score	Suicide Rate†
Full-time medical school faculty	80.18	47
Surgeons	79.36	34
Psychiatrists	76.89	61
Internists	75.12	34
Obstetrician-gynecologists	74.26	36
Full-time hospital physicians (anesthesiologists)	73.87	52
Full-time hospital physicians (pathologists, radiologists)	73.87	25, 27
General practitioners	72.94	34
Pediatricians	69.85	10

*Test scores are contrasted with suicide rates. Suicide rates are from Blachly et al.[4] Scores are averages for each group and are from the modified Brayfield[3] Job Satisfaction Blank. A higher score indicates greater satisfaction.

†Per 100,000.

tionship to the CWR graduates' expressed degree of career satisfaction. No direct correlation existed between suicide rates for the various specialties and the job satisfaction scores of the CWR graduates (Table 14-II). Psychiatrists were the epitome of high career satisfaction with high suicide rates, and surgeons represented high career satisfaction with low suicide rates. Full-time hospital-based physicians were prime examples of those with low career satisfaction and high suicide rates, while pediatricians were the best example of low job satisfaction with low suicide rates. Physicians need more than continuing medical education to keep them up to date with the latest techniques and medical advances. They need support to cope with the stresses and strains inherent in the practice of medicine today.

The articles concerning physician suicide brought the topic of stress out in the open. In the last six or eight years, national attention has been directed toward the problems of physician alcoholism, drug addiction, and divorce rates. The American Medical Association has sponsored at least two programs on these topics, including a major half-day symposium at their medical education meetings in 1973. No one at those meetings will forget the statement[7] that the

United States loses the equivalent of graduates from seven entire medical schools (approximately 700 physicians) per year due to suicide, drug addiction, and alcoholism. At a time when one hears so much about physician shortages, it is essential to preserve the physicians there are.

It is therefore important to understand the stresses and career dissatisfactions facing physicians. As described earlier, Table 14-I lists the dissatisfactions that came from the first career study of 1935 through 1945 graduates at CWR. Time pressures and factors related to it were the major stresses. As the second study progresses with alumni from the classes of 1956 through 1965, many of the same stresses emerge, especially the time aspects. An interesting point about the time pressures was the influence that the new medical curriculum has had on the graduates in the present study. The revised curriculum allowed the students free time each week; many of these graduates now said that they still attempted to include some free time in their schedules.

NEW STRESSES

A number of new stresses appeared that were not mentioned in the earlier study. In the first study, only the graduates in California mentioned malpractice suits as a problem. Malpractice is on all of the graduates' mind today. The majority of the physicians interviewed in the study have been named in malpractice suits. Often the suit was not brought against them personally; they were named in a suit against an entire group or hospital.

One alumnus had given a list of three consultants to a friend. The friend did not like what the consultant did and sued the physician for recommending him. The suit had been a tremendous stress for the physician, and he said he would give up medicine if he ever had another one. Another graduate described poignantly the impact on his entire family and career when he was sued for malpractice. His children were taunted on the way to school with cries that their father was a quack. Dinner invitations were mysteriously postponed and then never rescheduled. Patients canceled their appointments. He went on to explain that being sued for malpractice was such a traumatic experience that he would have preferred being accused of any violent crime. Another graduate said, "In a country where you're supposed to be innocent until proven guilty, you're not when you're accused of malpractice." The graduates have usually coped with the malpractice threat by paying the higher insurance rates. In some cases the physicians have required patients to sign agreements to submit to compulsory arbitration in case of dispute, or they have joined in protective group arrangements. Some have contemplated giving up the practice of medicine.

A second new stress relates to the malpractice situation but is manifested by a change in the content of a physician's practice or the style with which the practice is carried out. A physician colleague described the situation as one in which physicians are "doing less because the risks are too tough to run." They are using laboratory techniques and new machines more for verifying diagnoses, for practicing defensive medicine, or for economic reasons while they themselves are doing less and withdrawing more from certain portions of health care management.

Kern[8] spoke of this proliferation of tests in his 1976 presidential address to the American Gastroenterological Association. He noted: "Society pays us much more handsomely for performing a procedure than for a careful, critical history, physical examination, and a thoughtful, discriminating formulation of diagnosis and management, even though the latter requires far more training and experience and much more extensive knowledge and understanding." The physician's values come into play as he assesses the stress of the risk taking involved. Often it is a question of legal risk or moral risk, and deciding which risk to assume is a stress. In one instance the risk factor provided such a stress that a surgeon in the study decided to give up the trauma work that had been so satisfying to him for many years earlier in his career. Medical care that patients need is often not being provided by the qualified and willing physicians who receive satisfaction from carrying out that kind of medical assistance because of stress attached to the risk in performing certain types of procedures.

The third new stress expressed in the study came as a surprise. It had not been heard at all in the first study and was repeated more than once in the present one. One could scarcely believe it when it was learned that physicians feared violence against themselves and their families from disgruntled patients. Fortunately, these instances are few, but this fear has become a new or more prevalent stress on physicians. Shortly after the first physician in the study reported this stress, an article appeared (*New York Times,* Feb 27, 1976, p 14) entitled, "Death Threats to Boston Doctors Stir Worry Among Physicians Nationally." The article described the alarm among physicians after a Tewksbury, Massachusetts, physician and his family had been killed and other physicians had been threatened. Later in the study, others reported this same fear.

The fourth new stress is related to the realm of peer review and to ensuring continued competency of physicians. Hitherto, physicians who were aware that one of their colleagues did not have a steady hand, or was woefully behind in his field, or appeared at the hospital after drinking, covered up for the erring physician. They may have ceased to refer their own patients to him, but they had a policy of live and let live. Soon this may no longer be possible because of the system of peer review. It is stressful to report a colleague; it is reminiscent of the honor systems at many colleges where students are supposed to report their friends for cheating.

It is impossible to say whether or not these four new causes of stress will be important when the study is finished. To date a little more than three-fourths of the interviews have been completed, and, while the sources of satisfaction are similar in the two studies, the dissatisfactions and causes of stress are different. Though time, or the lack of it, is a major dissatisfaction for physicians in both studies, there are new stresses and new dimensions to the old ones. The earlier practitioner, primarily in solo or partnership practice, found the time pressures often beyond his capacity to cope and knew no way out because there was often no other person available. Today many believe that the physician in the city who is completely overwhelmed by the time factor is so because of his own ego. The physician's narcissism keeps him from ever saying no or believing that his patients can get along for a day without him. It is true that the inundation of paperwork has increased severalfold, but it is usual for most groups to have specific personnel to handle the multitudinous forms exclusively. With more of the physicians in the present study practicing in large or small groups, it is possible to go out in the evenings, to get away on weekends, and to take regular vacations. The group organization alleviates the time and overload factors in ways not available to such a large degree to physicians in the earlier study. The groups also provide colleagueship that helps dispel the professional loneliness previously expressed by the solo practitioner. The rural practitioner still faces some of these same dissatisfactions, although more of the small-town physicians are also joining in groups.

On the other hand, many of the new sources of stress that are being heard today relate to a breakdown in the traditional physician-patient relationship. Some believe this breakdown may be due to the lack of one and the same physician's being able to spend sufficient time with the same patient during a period of years. Good physician-patient relationships, as other relationships, take time to develop. On an office visit today, the patient may spend more minutes with technicians, assistants, or laboratory personnel than with the physician. This can be a factor responsible for precipitating some of today's new sources of stress such as malpractice suits or threats. Similarly, the facts of peer review have broken down the previous pattern of physicians' inter-relationships. Certainly the results of the present career study so far and the incidence of new stresses seem to point out how the practice of medicine has changed and how many of the problems that physicians will have to face in practice are often impossible to foresee and predict in medical school.

REFERENCES

1. Mawardi BH: A career study of physicians. *J Med Educ* 40:658-666, 1965.
2. Mawardi BH: Relation of student learning to physician performance. *JAMA* 198: 767-769, 1966.
3. Brayfield AH, Roth HR: An index of job satisfaction. *J Appl Psychol* 35:307, 311, 1951.
4. Blachly PH, Disher W, Roduner G: Suicide by physicians, in *The Bulletin of Suicidology*. Chevy Chase, Md, National Clearinghouse for Mental Health Information, 1968, pp 1-18.
5. Craig AG, Pitts FN Jr: Suicide by physicians. *Dis Nerv Syst.* 29:763-772, 1968.
6. Ross M: Suicide among physicians. *Dis Nerv Syst* 34:145-150, 1973.
7. Casterline RL: Deviant behaviour in physicians. Read before the 69th Annual Congress on Medical Education of the American Medical Association, Chicago, Feb 9, 1973.
8. Kern F Jr: Gastroenterology — 1976: Good news and bad news. *Gastroenterology* 71:537-541, 1976.

Chapter 15

PERCEIVED SOURCES OF STRESS AMONG FIRST-YEAR MEDICAL STUDENTS

DAVID COBURN AND AL V. JOVAISAS

THE process of medical education can be a highly discomforting experience. At no time is this more true than in the first year of medical training, a period in which the budding physician is faced with an intense, concentrated program of study, generally in the basic rather than the clinical sciences. The overwhelming amount of material to be absorbed, the social isolation, the pressure of examinations, and the discrepancies between expectations and reality all can be anticipated to bring psychological stress (used here as a synonym for feelings of discomfort, tension, or distress). In fact, McGuire (1) has described the characteristic state of the individual medical student as one of anxiety.

> He is anxious while in pre-med training, wondering if he will be able to meet the competition and achieve high enough grades; he is anxious when he applies, feeling that his whole future is about to be decided within a few short weeks or months; and he is anxious when he begins his training. He displays a variety of anxieties during the next four years, and except for a certain amount of short-lived relief when he receives his diploma, he is still anxious when he graduates.

Evidence from a number of studies suggests that the stresses of medical school may have undesirable consequences. Adsett (2) and Gottheil and his colleagues (3), for example, report that dropouts do not differ in ability (measured by Medical College Admission Test scores and/or college grades) from those who graduate; that is, it is not necessarily the intellectual capacity of the student that decides whether he will continue or drop out. Adsett also notes that in 1968 at the University of Oklahoma 13 percent of all medical students received counseling for psychological problems each year and a much higher percentage were seen for somatic complaints in which emotional conflicts played the major etiological role. Furthermore, it was first-year students who were the most frequent patients. Hunter and his colleagues (4) reported in 1961 that 18.3 percent of medical students at McGill University sought help for emotional problems. They also claimed that 60 percent of these problems were attributable to the process of medical education itself rather than to preexisting conditions. And, as these authors recognize, visits to university facilities provide only minimal estimates of the actual occurrence of emotional disturbances.

The approach to the question of stress in medical school in the present study is (*a*) to identify perceived sources of stress, (*b*) to investigate the uni- or multi-dimensionality of stress, (*c*) to examine the relationships between background factors and felt stress, and (*d*) to briefly consider some possible outcomes of perceived stress.

METHODS

Two-thirds of the way through the first medical year (1973-74) at the University of Toronto, each student in four randomly selected laboratories (from a total of 15) was asked to complete a questionnaire. Fifty-two of the 55 students in the laboratories (from a class of 240) completed the questionnaire. In comparison with age/sex data from the class as a whole, the sample is fairly closely representative, although older students and female students are somewhat overrepresented in the sample.

FINDINGS

In the questionnaire, in addition to background data, 19 potential sources of stress were described (drawn mainly from Boyle and Coombs [5]), with students being asked to label these as not stressful or as highly stressful on five-point scales. Sources of stress were divided into "current" sources (that is, characteristics of the present situation of the students) and "anticipated" sources (that is, those conditions likely to be encountered during later life as a physician). Table 15-I lists the 11 current sources in order of magnitude of mean perceived stress.

The top four characteristics all relate to academic aspects of medical training and to doubts concerning scholastic ability. Examinations are viewed as particularly stressful (31 percent of respondents gave the examination item the highest stress rating possible). In spite of the overall tendency for academic factors to be felt as highly stressful, a few students (8 to 19 percent for items one

Table 15-I

CURRENT SOURCES OF STRESS FOR FIRST-YEAR MEDICAL STUDENTS

Sources of Stress	Mean† Stress Score
1. Entering a final examination in an important course	3.48
*2. Fear of inability to absorb all the course material	3.15
*3. Fear of getting bad grades	3.08
4. The number of hours one has to study in order to keep up	3.04
*5. Limited recreational and social outlets	2.65
*6. Lack of sexual outlets	2.44
*7. Loneliness	2.36
*8. Initial dissection experience with the cadaver	1.98
9. Talking to instructors in a social situation	1.92
*10. Other sexual problems	1.92
11. Talking to instructors about course subject matter	1.90
*12. Long-term conflict over being in a helpless and dependent role	1.80

*Questions similar to those used by Boyle and Coombs to characterize areas of student stress (five-point items).

†Ns = 52 except for item 11, N = 51.

to four) rate these areas as sources of very little stress.

Next to academic sources of stress are factors referring to the inadequacy of social contacts, although in a sense these are again a reflection of academic work load. Dissection of the cadaver, often assumed to be a particularly traumatic experience, ranks fairly low on the list. The four low stress items are seen as being little or not at all stressful by 50 to 57 percent of the students.

Regarding anticipated sources of stress (Table 15-II), there is a large gap in mean scores between the first three and the last four items. The most salient anticipated sources of stress deal with patient death, chronic illness, or diagnostic error. Students show far less concern with physical examinations or talking with patients about marital or sexual problems (42 to 58 percent of respondents anticipated little or no stress regarding sexual aspects of the doctor-patient relationship — the last three scores).

The rank-order correlations of the means for both the current and anticipated areas between Boyle and Coombs' students and the present sample are almost identical (Spearman's rho = .93 for cur-

Table 15-II

ANTICIPATED SOURCES OF STRESS FOR FIRST-YEAR MEDICAL STUDENTS

Sources of Stress	Mean* Stress Score
1. Death of a patient	3.58
2. Fear of error in diagnosis or treatment	3.33
3. Dealing with a patient with a chronic and helpless disease	3.21
4. Fear for personal health in contact with the sick	1.98
5. Talking to patients about marital and sexual problems	1.96
6. Carrying out physical examinations with patients	
Opposite sex	1.88
Same sex	1.69

*Ns = 52 except for item 6, N = 51. All items are similar to those used by Boyle and Coombs (five-point alternatives).

rent and .94 for anticipated sources of stress).* For the total 14 similar items the rank order correlation is .65, the main discrepancies being due to the higher rank given by the Toronto students to "death of a patient"† and "dealing with a patient with a chronic and hopeless disease" and the much higher rank given by American students to "long-term conflict over being in a helpless, dependent role."

Boyle and Coombs formed an index of total stress by combining replies to all 14 items. There is, however, a prior question: Are sources of stress unidimensional or multidimensional?

Possible sources of stress have already been divided into current and anticipated areas (because the two refer to qualitatively different areas of experience). An oblique factor analysis was carried out within these two areas separately (oblique rather than orthogonal because it would be unrealistic to contend *a priori* that sources of stress are completely independent of one another). The factor analyses produced four separate factors in current stress and two regarding anticipated stress.

The first two current factors accounted for 71 percent of the total variance and are the only ones in that area considered here (the two

*There were eight similar items in the two samples regarding current stress and six concerning anticipated stress.

†Perhaps because their course in behavioral science included films and lectures on aging and death.

"talking to the instructor" items were the only ones loading highly on Factor 3; the only item loading highly on Factor 4 was the dissection experience question). The items with high loadings on Factor 1 all concerned social sources of stress; those with high loadings on Factor 2 related to academic stress. Two factors emerged from the anticipated stress item pool. Items loading highest on the first concerned physical examinations and talking to patients about marital or sex problems; the second related to death, serious illness, or diagnostic error.

Four indexes were constructed from the highest loading items on the two current stress and two anticipated stress factors.* A total stress index was also formed by summing responses to all 19 current and anticipated sources of stress.

The intercorrelations of these indexes (Table 15-III) indicate that social stress is slightly negatively related to academic stress but is independent of both anticipated stress indexes.† Students who are discomforted by the social situation are likely not the same type of persons as those troubled by other facets of medical education. Possibly there is a trade-off here between social and academic life, those highly engaged in social activities feel less social but more adacemic stress and vice-versa. Academic and patient stress do go

Table 15-III

INTERCORRELATION OF STRESS INDEX
(Pearson *r*)

Stress Areas*	Academic	Anticipated		Total
		Patient	Sex	
Current				
Social	-.134	-.022	-.066	.431
Academic		.369	.100	344
Anticipated				
Patient			.314	.636
Sex				.493

*Items and weights are as follows (items numbers from Tables 1 and 2): Social—6(1), 7(.98), 10(.85), 5(.82); Academic—2(1), 3(.71), 1(.50); Patient—1(1), 2(.72), 3(.59); Sex—7(1), 6(.82), 5(.78).

*Items were weighted proportionately to the highest loading item (for weights see Table 15-III).

†Because of the possible influence of skewed distributions on the intercorrelations, two other types of correlation coefficients were calculated (Kendall's tau and phi). The correlation matrices in both of these instances showed a pattern highly similar to that of the Pearson correlation matrices.

together, however, indicating a possible common component, that is, doubt regarding one's own capacities or competence.

BACKGROUND FACTORS

Sixteen background factors were correlated with the four stress indexes (Table 15-IV). Twenty-three of the 80 correlations reached at least the .10 significance level and 16 at least the .05 level. The three variables most closely associated with academic stress are the stress felt in everyday life (high), years spent in Toronto (low), and birth order (later born). The variables most highly correlated with social stress are marital status (single), sex (male), and birth order (later born). In six instances a variable significantly positively related to academic stress is negatively correlated to social stress or vice versa (another indication of the separateness of these stresses).

Higher social class (two items), familiarity with the university (three items), academic preparation (two items), and being single, male, and born in Canada are all related to lower academic but higher social stress (although these trends are not necessarily particularly strong ones).

Four variables are related to all the stress indexes in the same direction. Students with older siblings, younger students, those high in everyday stress, and Catholics and Jews show higher stress across the board than do their classmates.

CONSEQUENCES

Previous writers have hypothesized or implied that the number of dropouts and the incidence of illness are likely consequences of perceived stress. The relationships between the five stress measures (academic, social, patient, sex, and total) and two presumed correlates or effects of stress were calculated (although without knowing which factors are temporally prior to which, any assumption of causality is highly tentative). Table 15-V indicates that although the stress indexes are not statistically significantly related to frequency of thinking about dropping out or to number of days off school because of one's own illness, in every case the direction of the relationship is that hypothesized. In each case students high in stress are more likely to have thought about dropping out and a higher proportion of them have taken three or more days off school because of their own illness than is the case with low-stress students.

Table 15-IV

CORRELATIONS BETWEEN BACKGROUND VARIABLES AND STRESS SCORES
(Kendall's tau)

	Stress Indexes				
	Academic	Social	Patient	Sex	Total
Social class (high)					
Father's occupational status (high)	−.14†	.17‡	−.10	.20‡	.03
Subjective social class (high)	−.06	.02	−.17	.09	−.10
Demographic					
Age (young)	−.08	−.04	−.06	−.10	−.18‡
Sex (male)	−.11	.22§	−.14†	.01	.09
Marital status (single)	−.05	.24§	−.04	.11	.10
Religion*	.27	.29	.25	.21	.26
Born in Canada (Yes)	−.09	.11	−.12	−.22	−.12
Familiarity with Toronto (high)					
Attended U of T or premed (Yes)	−.05	.02	−.15	−.02	−.08
No. of years in Toronto (high)	−.19‡	.01	−.13†	−.02	−.12
Size of high school town (large)	−.15†	.17‡	−.06	−.01	.05
Academic preparation (high)					
Self-assessment (high)	−.11	.15†	−.03	−.02	−.04
Surprised to be accepted (No)	−.03	.05	−.02	−.18	.02
Birth order					
Birth order (first-born)	−.17‡	−.21‡	−.11	−.16‡	−.30§
Current pressures (high)					
Close to/apart from classmates (apart)	.04	.09	−.03	.28§	.23§
Family pressure for good grades (high)	.10	.09	.08	0	.18‡
Stress felt in everyday life (high)	.24§	.06	12†	.14	.32§

*Cramer's V. None of the correlations for religion are significant (chi-square).
† $p<.10$.
‡ $p<.05$.
§ $p<.01$.

DISCUSSION

Toronto students rate future performance as a physician higher as a stress factor than do students in at least one U.S. medical school. On the whole, however, first-year medical students in two schools, one in the United States and one in Canada, show remarkable agreement as to what is stressful and what is not.

Table 15-V
FREQUENCY OF THINKING ABOUT DROPPING OUT AND THE INCIDENCE OF ILLNESS FOR HIGH VERSUS LOW STRESS MEDICAL STUDENTS*
(In Percent)

Sources of Stress	High Stress		Low Stress		Percentage Difference
	Percent	No.	Percent	No.	
			Dropout†		
Academic	36.4	(11)	10.0	(10)	26.4
Social	20.0	(10)	18.2	(11)	1.8
Patient	25.0	(12)	20.0	(10)	5.0
Sex	25.0	(16)‡	11.8	(17)	13.2
Total	30.0	(10)	12.5	(8)	17.5
			Illness†		
Academic	18.2	(11)	10.0	(10)	8.2
Social	30.0	(10)	9.1	(11)	20.9
Patient	33.3	(12)	10.0	(10)	23.3
Sex	12.5	(16)‡	11.8	(17)	0.7
Total	40.0	(10)	0.0	(8)	40.0

* None of the full tables are statistically significant (chi-square) at beyond the .10 level.

† Have you every contemplated dropping out (for any reason whatsoever)—frequently, occasionally? How many days have you missed from medical school due to your own illness (since September)—three or more?

‡ A higher N because of skewed distribution.

Students are obviously concerned with possible inability to grasp and absorb all the material being presented to them. This is reflected not only in their ratings of the item directly referring to this area but also in their fears of taking final examinations and receiving poor grades. In addition, it may be supposed that fear of failure to absorb course materials might be producing feelings of stress concerning later performance, that is, making an error in diagnosis/treatment or death of a patient.

One of the chief findings in the present study then is the importance of students' fears concerning their own inadequacy or incompetence. In this respect the findings support those of Rosenberg (6), who concludes from his own study that "the violence done to the self-image of the medical student is the most serious consequence of his educational program."

In addition to academic life certain factors in the student's social milieu are also sources of stress. There is, of course, an interaction between academic and social sources of stress — the necessity to spend long hours studying leaves little time for social activities.

Dissection of the cadaver is ranked low as a source of stress by both the Toronto and the Boyle and Coombs samples. These findings are supported by McGuire (1), who notes that Becker and his colleagues (7), despite a great deal of searching, failed to detect evidence of stress among students in the dissection room.

An alternative explanation is that students may have experienced a great deal of tension during the initial dissection experience but have had time in the intervening months to work through or come to terms with their distress. A third possibility may be that the cadaver seems "not human" because, during dissection, it is only partially unwrapped and because of the effects of preservatives on the appearance of the cadaver.

It is quite evident from the factor analysis and from the correlation matrices that there are several distinct sources of stress. A student feeling high stress in one area may or may not feel stress concerning other facets of life as a medical student. This is particularly true for social versus academic factors.* The independence of academic and social stresses is emphasized when their relationship with background variables is examined. A number of factors positively related to academic stress are negatively related to social stress and vice-versa. Being a member of a small subgroup within medical school or being outside of or different from the mainstream of medical students (for example, being from a lower social class background unfamiliar with Toronto, female, or married) is associated with higher academic but lower social stress. Why is this so?

It is assumed here that most medical students are academically oriented, that is, that acquisition of knowledge and high performance as evidenced in grades are viewed as being important. It seems likely that subgroup students are much less sure than their mainstream classmates of their academic ranking or competencies. This may be because they actually are lower in ability (and get lower

*One must wonder then what "total stress" indexes are really measuring. Total stress scores seem more an index of "trait" than of situation specific stress. Variables related to total stress measures thus may reflect only those factors associated with stress proneness. Furthermore, in looking at the possible precursors or consequences of stress, indexes encompassing various types of stress might obscure rather than clarify possible relationships.

grades), because they are higher in the need to achieve, or because they have had less chance to compare themselves with their peers than mainstream students. Mainstream students, because of their previous experience in premedical education at the University of Toronto, their better (or at least more conventional) academic preparation, and their current statuses (predominantly male and single), are relatively more stressed by their restricted social lives than by academic matters.

In support of the more indirect findings of previous writers, it was found that stress is related to such diverse matters as student thoughts about dropping out and illness patterns. Perceived stress thus may be an important conceptual link relating student-medical school interaction to student attitudes and behavior.

Even given the limited nature of the data, the findings presented raise a number of questions concerning the process of medical education during the first year. The impression, strongly held by students, of the limitless boundaries of knowledge to be acquired is stressful. Is this perception a necessary one, or should student expectations be made more structured and limited? Does the competition between medical school departments encourage unnecessary demands being made on students? If stress is to be used as a motivator of performance or as a predictor of those able to withstand the stresses of medicine as a profession, should not optimal regions of stress be consciously defined? Finally, what types of preparation or supports might aid students (especially those whose backgrounds predispose them to feel greater stress than the average) to cope with the stresses they encounter?

REFERENCES

1. McGuire, F. L. Psycho-Social Studies of Medical Students: A Critical Review, *J. Med. Educ.*, 41:424-445, 1966.
2. Adsett, C. A. Psychological Health of Medical Students in Relation to the Medical Education Process. *J. Med. Educ.*, 43:728-734, 1968.
3. Gottheil, E., Thornton, C. C., Conly, S. S., Jr., and Cornelison, F. S., Jr. Stress, Satisfaction, and Performance: Transition from Universtiy to Medical College. *J. Med. Educ.*, 44:270-277, 1969
4. Hunter, R. C. A., Prince, R. H., and Schwartzman, A. E. Comments on Emotional Disturbances in a Medical Undergraduate Population. *Can. Med. Assoc. J.*, 83:989-992, 1961.
5. Boyle, B. P., and Coombs, R. H. Personality Profiles Related to Emotional Stress in the Initial Year of Medical Training. *J. Med. Educ.*, 46:882-888, 1971.
6. Rosenberg, P. P. Students' Perceptions and Concerns During Their First Year

in Medical School. *J. Med. Educ.*, 46:211-218, 1971.

7. Becker, H., Greer, G., Hughes, E., and Strauss, A. *Boys in White: Student Culture in Medical School.* Chicago: University of Chicago Press, 1961.

Etiology II: Personality

Chapter 16

SOME PSYCHOLOGIC VULNERABILITIES OF PHYSICIANS

GEORGE E. VAILLANT, NANCY CORBIN SOBOWALE, AND CHARLES MCARTHUR

THREE symptoms suggestive of psychologic vulnerability are frequently seen in physicians. These are bad marriages, drug abuse and tendency to use psychotherapy. These symptoms are frequently dismissed as occupational hazards of medical practice. In the first place, medicine is a jealous mistress. Poor marriages can be chalked up to long hours and the demands of patients. Secondly, the fact that physicians tend to abuse drugs elicits a ready explanation. Physicians have increased access to drugs and fall innocent victim to their privileged position. The drug-abusing physician offers a different reason. Only through drugs can he overcome the long hours and fatigue that threaten his occupational efficiency. Thirdly, the fact that physicians are heavy users of psychotherapy is explained by the fact that doctors are less self-conscious than nonprofessionals in seeking this avenue of help.

Are the generalizations cited above adequate? Comparison of physicians with their socioeconomic peers suggests that only a minority of physicians experienced the difficulties under consideration and that their vulnerability antedated entrance into medicine. This possibility has often been suspected by physicians who care for other physicians.[1-4] Increased understanding of these vulnerabilities seems important if we are to offer our colleagues the help they deserve.

METHODS

The selection of the sample and the matching of the physicians with controls has been described in detail elsewhere.[5,6] Thirty years

---

Supported by a research scientist development award (MH-28798) from the National Institute of Mental Health, U.S. Public Health Service, and by Grant Foundation, Inc.

Presented at the eleventh symposium of the Carrier Clinic, Belle Meade, N.J.

ago 268 college sophomores were chosen for intensive study by a university health service. They were selected for reasons of having no easily detectable health problems (mental or physical), and for easily meeting the academic demands before them. The subjects were not selected by volunteering. Of these 268 men, 47 attended medical school, and 46 graduated. These 47 men were compared to a control group of 79 men (not physicians) who by chance were selected from the larger sample. All the men have been followed prospectively by questionnaire and occasional interview for the past 30 years. All the controls and 16 of the physicians, also selected by chance, have been personally interviewed for two hours by one of us (G.E.V.). Thus, the controls are, in fact, the more intensively studied sample. Aside from death, attrition from this prospective study has been less than 5 percent.

Each man's marital history was assessed over 30 years of prospective follow-up observation. In 1954 and 1967, each man was sent questionnaires asking specifically about his marriage, and in 1967, with his consent, a questionnaire was sent to his wife. Much additional information was gleaned from the questionnaires that the men returned roughly every two years for three decades.

The drinking and drug history was determined both from interview data and from prospectively gathered questionnaires. Most questionnaires inquired about alcohol and drug use. Although at times of serious drug misuse, the men often withheld questionnaires, a reliable pattern could be obtained by pooling of all available data.

The childhood of each subject was evaluated by a researcher (N.C.S.) who was blind to the course of the men after 18 years of age. She had notes of a home visit to each boy's parents when he was in college. These included a discussion of each boy's early developmental and medical history. The rater also had a summary of each boy's attitude toward his parents that was derived from eight research interviews with a psychiatrist.

The blind researcher assigned each subject a score from 0 to 20 derived in the following manner. Each man received two points for each of the following: if his early developmental history was without problems; if his childhood health was good; if the mother-child relation and, again, if the father-child relation seemed warm, encouraging, and conducive both to autonomy and to self-esteem; if the home atmosphere was warm and cohesive; if he was close to at least one sibling; and if he did well in school both academically and athletically. For any clearly negative item he received no points. For each item that was ambiguous or for which inadequate data existed he received one point. Then, making a global evaluation of the subject's childhood, the researcher gave 0 points if his early environment seemed worse than the average, three if it seemed average, and six if it seemed like one of the warmer and more nurturing environments in the study.

Several clinical assessments were made. Of necessity, these were subject to observer bias. When the men were in college each man was rated on overall psychologic "soundness." Thirty-seven percent were A, 45 percent B, and 18 percent C. Each control and the 16 interviewed physicians were rated on his use or nonuse during his adult life of 18 mechanisms of defense (e.g., projection and sublimation). Mechanisms of defense were identified by observation of each man's behavior and his style of adapting to crises and important events during his life.[7] In 50 cases, these ratings were made independently by three raters. Rater reliability — depending on the defense — ranged from 60 to 90 percent agreement. Men were also rated on the traits of self-doubt, pessimism, passivity, and dependence.

RESULTS

In terms both of socioeconomic status on college entrance and of intellectual aptitude there were no differences between the physicians and controls. Sixty-nine percent of the physicians attended the following five medical schools: Columbia; Harvard; Johns Hopkins; Pennsylvania; and Rochester. Seventy-eight percent of them passed their specialty-board examinations; all but one received his M.D. degree. All are gainfully employed.

Almost certainly, this sample of physicians is skewed in the direction of health. Yet almost half have had bad marriages, and a third sought relief from drugs, and a third from psychotherapy. Table 16-I suggests that the differences from controls are probably significant.

In general a bad marriage meant that the couple did not consider the marriage "stable," sexual adjustment was "not as good as wished" or worse, and divorce had been at least casually considered. A definition of good marriage meant that over the years, the subject had considered his marriage to be "stable," sexual adjustment was rated "satisfying" or better, and divorce had not been seriously considered. Fourteen percent of the controls and 20 percent of the doctors had been divorced. "High drug use" meant that on two or more occasions in time the man had reported heavy drinking or "trouble

Table 16-I. Relative Occurrence of Difficulties Often Associated with Medical Practice.

Difficulty	Physicians (%)	Controls (%)	Significance*
Poor marriage or divorce.	47	32	$p < 0.1$
High drug use	36	22	$p < 0.1$
10 or more visits to psychiatrist	34	19	$p < 0.1$
2 or more of above difficulties	36	18	$p < 0.05$
Psychiatric hospitalization	17	6	NS†

*Chi-square statistical test used. †Not significant.

with control" of alcohol, or that he "often" used sleeping pills, used amphetamines daily or had used tranquilizers daily for more than one month. In four doctors and one control, drug or alcohol misuse had actually interfered with employment or family relations.

However, the three "symptoms" under study appeared to depend much more upon preadult psychologic status than upon the choice of a medical career per se. Table 16-II shows that if the physicians and controls are pooled, among men with the most supportive childhoods (scores of 10 or more on the Childhood Adjustment Scale) only 15 percent experienced two or three of the symptoms under consideration. Whereas, almost half those with relatively poor childhoods (score of 6 or less) experienced two or more symptoms.

The same relation held true if the men were judged by their relative psychologic soundness in college. Of those who were considered most psychologically sound in college, only one-ninth experienced two or more of the symptoms in adult life. Almost half the men judged least sound in college reported such symptoms.

If the presence or absence of a given "symptom" is controlled for, the childhood scores of the physicians and controls are quite similar. Table 16-III shows that men who experienced any given symptom received a lower average childhood score than those without such a symptom. Ever having been hospitalized in adult life for psychiatric illness was associated with a dramatically lower mean score for childhood adjustment.

Two questions arise. The first is whether all the differences between the doctors and controls can be entirely accounted for by the

Table 16-II. Relation between Childhood Adjustment and Poor Marriage, Drug Abuse and More than 10 Psychiatric Visits.

No. of Symptoms	Adjustment Ratings (%)			
	childhood*		college†	
	top 1/3‡ (55)§	*bottom 1/3¶ (38)*	*top 2/5‖ (45)*	*bottom 1/5** (26).*
0-1	85	53	89	58
2-3	15	47	11	42

*Childhood associated with outcome, $p < 0.001$, chi-square test of significance.
†College adjustment associated with outcome, $p < 0.01$, chi-square test of significance.
‡Rating of 10+.
§Figures in parentheses represent no. of subjects.
¶Rating of < 7.
‖Rating of "A."
**Rating of "C."

Table 16-III. Mean Childhood Scores for Doctors and Controls with and without Individual Symptoms.

Status	Mean Childhood Scores	
	doctors	controls
2-3 symptoms	6.7*	7.1*
No symptoms	9.6	10.5
Divorce or bad marriage	7.2*	8.8
No divorce or bad marriage	9.4	9.5
10+ psychiatric visits	6.9*	7.0*
Few or no psychiatric visits	9.2	9.8
Regular drug use or alcohol abuse	7.7	6.75*
No drug use or alcohol abuse	8.8	10.0
Psychiatric hospitalization	5.9	4.2

*Mean childhood score of men with symptom significantly < mean score of men without that symptom at level of $p < 0.05$ (student's t-test used to determine statistical significance).

effect of childhood. Secondly, do doctors come from less happy homes than their college classmates?

Table 16-IV suggests that easier access does affect physician's use of psychiatrists. Whether a physician came from a good or a poor childhood, he was still twice as likely as a control to have seen a psychiatrist 10 or more times. However, if a physician or a control had come from a poor childhood, he was twice as likely to have seen a psychiatrist as if he had come from a good childhood environment. Poor marriages and high drug use were still more strongly associated with the quality of childhood. Neither quality of marriage nor drug use differed in controls and physicians who had enjoyed similar childhood backgrounds. It can be seen from the Table 16-IV that 39 of 79 (49 percent) of the controls and only 16 of 47 (34 percent) of the physicians received childhood scores of 10 or above ("Good"). Although these differences are not statistically significant, they appear to account for the differences in symptom frequency observed between physicians and nonphysicians.

There were some types of physicians whose childhoods did seem significantly worse than those of the controls. Table 16-V contrasts the nonsurgical, actively practicing physicians with the surgeons, administrators and researchers. The physicians whose careers were not those having primary responsibility for patient care had both psychiatric symptom patterns and childhoods very similar to those of the controls. It was the internists and psychiatrists, the obstetricians and pediatricians who were significantly different from the other groups, in terms of both emotional difficulties during adulthood and instability of childhood. The division of specialties is somewhat arbitrary. The differences and the numbers are both small. Thus, the finding must be taken as only suggestive. However, the implication of Table 16-V might be that some physicians may elect to assume direct care of patients to give others the care that they did not receive in their own childhoods.

Table 16-IV. Effect of Controlling for Childhood and Occupation on Relative Occurrence of Psychiatric Symptoms.

Childhood	10+ Visits to Psychiatrist (%)	Drug Use (%)	Poor Marriage (%)
Good:			
Doctors (16)*	31	25	13
Controls (39)	15	10	28
Poor:			
Doctors (15)	60	53	53
Controls (23)	35	48	48

*Figures in parentheses represent no. of subjects.

Of 18 defense mechanisms studied, at least five seemed to be used to a significantly greater or lesser degree by physicians than by controls (Table 16-VI). At times of adult life crises, hypochondriasis and turning against the self, i.e. masochism and passive aggressive

Table 16-V. Number of Symptoms (Drug Use, More than 10 Psychiatric Visits, Bad Marriage) Present in Different Occupational Groups.

Group	Symptoms Present (%)			Mean Childhood Score
	0-1	2	3	
Controls (79)*	82	13	5	9.3
Doctors in administration, surgery & research (21)	76	24	0	9.9
Nonsurgical practicing doctors (26)	54	11	33	7.2†

*Figures in parentheses represent no. of subjects.
†Difference between nonsurgical practicing doctors & each of the other 2 groups significant at $p < 0.05$ (student's t-test).

behavior, were seen twice as often among the physician sample as among controls. Physicians in the sample were also twice as likely to use reaction formation — that is, a vehement aversion to some instinctively gratifying behavior and often the substitution of opposite behavior. Some physicians seemed almost phobic about asking for help.

Table 16-VI. Difference in Observed Frequency of Coping Mechanisms between 16 Physicians and 79 Controls.

Coping Mechanism	Adaptive Episodes/Man*		
	Doctors	Controls	Significance†
Hypochondriasis & turning against self	2.4±2.9	1.1±1.6	$p < 0.01$
Reaction formation	3.0±1.6	1.5±1.7	$p < 0.01$
Altruism	1.6±1.5	0.8±1.3	$p < 0.05$
Suppression	1.7±1.7	3.5±3.7	$p < 0.001$

*Mean ± SD; during 30 yr of the adult life of each subject every time an adaptive vicissitude that illustrated a coping mechanism was noticed, it was recorded—admittedly, quantification of clinical judgment is imprecise, & since many men were never noted to use the mechanism in question, SDs are large.
†Student's t-test used as statistical test.

Altruism, closely related to reaction formation, was also used twice as often by physicians as by controls. In contrast, the controls used roughly twice as much suppression and somewhat more repression than the doctors. (By repression, we mean that by personality style and by profession, the nonphysician is often permitted to remain exceptionally naive about illness and the facts of life.) During interviews nonphysicians frequently repressed critically painful events in their lives. In contrast, physicians told us in detail about their medical symptoms.

By suppression, we mean that the nonphysicians were sometimes very difficult to interview. They took Pollyannish attitudes toward the difficulties in their lives; they successfully denied depression and minimized distress. In contrast, the physicians gave remarkably vivid histories. At the risk of oversimplifying, it was as if the controls said, "There is really very little wrong with me," whereas the physicians said, "There is a lot wrong with me, but I will not inconvenience anyone else."

DISCUSSION

Other clinical observations supported the finding that doctors might be expected to have more problems with their marriages and with drug misuse than matched controls. The physicians in the study were statistically more likely to exhibit the traits of dependency, pessimism, passivity, and self-doubt. (These traits are clinically associated with addiction.) Terman's prospective study of 800 gifted men confirmed our impression that feelings of inferiority are relatively more common among physicians.[8] To a statistically significant degree, doctors tended to have mothers and fathers who were overprotective; normal rebellion from parental ties sometimes failed to take place. For example, the interviewer wrote of one college sophomore, "Fred has never spent but one night away from his family . . . mother and son seem to enjoy doing things together." Thirty years later, as a doctor, he still spent as much time with his parents as with his wife; his marriage did not benefit.

In situations of conflict, physicians were more likely to turn their anger against themselves than to strike out at the environment. One physician's mother had said of him, "As a child, Sam always did things the hardest way; the other children call him the martyr in the family." The mother of another doctor reported, "When they were roughly two, I made them go and get the switch and switch themselves."

But if some doctors have trouble expressing aggression, this difficulty is of great benefit to humanity; it is not "bad," "sick," or maladaptive per se. However, such a difficulty must be fully appreciated by the doctor's doctor. Gandhi's passive resistance was a tremendous boon to the world, but it led to his being a difficult medical patient and having a very painful family life.

If it is clear that a doctor's vulnerabilities extend beyond the demands of his profession, how may that alter his medical care? In the first place, medicine becomes a strain only when the physician asks himself to give more than he has been given. The long hours, the demanding patients, the ready access to narcotics were not a problem to the doctor whose childhood had been happy and who appeared psychologically sound by the time he reached college. Similarly, a doctor from an unhappy childhood may gain comfort and strength from appreciative patients. Medical-school admission committees must realize that excellent clinicians can come from very troubled families. Rather, it is when the physician from a barren childhood becomes overly burdened by the demands of his dependent patients that trouble arises. He, not the literally overworked doctor, resorts to drugs to alleviate fatigue.[9] In our study it was not the physician who worked late who got divorced. But some physicians worked late in response to unhappy marriages. Other physicians experienced painful and unstable marriages because they had married not partners but "patients."

Secondly, this paper's discussion of coping mechanisms may be applied to the clinical care of physicians. Altruism is no problem, for, by definition, it involves getting pleasure by giving to others. Reaction formation is a problem. However, it is possible to interpret reaction formation to the physician or to work tactfully around it. But defenses can never be interpreted without an offer of something in their place. To an underloved, overworked physician, it would be of little service to point out that he was trying to give his patients what he had never received and that he was rigidly depriving himself in the process. Doctors need permission to cherish themselves and admit that they, too, have needs. One might ask a self-medicating colleague, "Dr. Jones, if a favorite patient came to you who had trouble getting to sleep and was so busy that he could never catch up, what would you suggest?"

Rather than try directly to relieve the hypochondriacal physician's complaints, his physician must realize that the uncomfortable, compaining patient needs something that he is often unable to request. This may be a variant of tender, loving care. More than one hypochondriacal doctor in the study was relieved by a regimen of bed rest, intensive psychotherapy (probably providing as much support as insight) and vacation by prescription.

In summary, the care of other people rather than of oneself is a superb form of adaptation — but only if the self is also cared for. The adage, "Physician heal thyself," is callous; physicians often heal others in hopes that they, too, may be healed. Physicians of physicians should be alert to this possibility.

REFERENCES

1. Duffy JC, Litin EM: *The Emotional Health of Physicians.* Springfield, Illinois, Charles C Thomas, Publisher, 1967
2. a'Brook MF, Hailstone JD, McLauchlan IEJ: Psychiatric illness in the medical profession. *Br J Psychiatry 113:*1013-1023, 1967
3. Vincent MO: Doctor and Mrs: their mental health. *Can Psychiatr Assoc J 14:*509-515, 1969
4. Small IF, Small JG, Assue CM, et al: The fate of the mentally ill physician. *Am J Psychiatry 125:*1333-1342, 1969
5. Heath CW: *What People Are: A study of normal young men.* Cambridge, Harvard University Press, 1945
6. Vaillant GE, Brighton JR, McArthur C: Physicians' use of mood-altering drugs: a 20-year follow-up report. *N Engl J Med 282:*365-370, 1970
7. Vaillant GE: Theoretical hierarchy of adaptive ego mechanisms: a 30-year follow-up of 30 men selected for psychological health. *Arch Gen Psychiatry 24:*107-118, 1971
8. Terman LM: Scientists and non-scientists in a group of 800 gifted men. *Psychol Monogr 68:*1-44, 1954
9. Modlin HC, Montes A: Narcotics addiction in physicians. *Am J Psychiatry 121:*358-365, 1964

Chapter 17

PERSONALITY TRAITS OF FIRST YEAR MEDICAL STUDENTS: TRENDS OVER SIX-YEAR PERIOD, 1967-1972

J. Parlow and A. I. Rothman

MOTIVATED by similar considerations as those underlying the AAMC Longitudinal Study as described by Hutchins (1964), the University of Toronto medical school has been administering a battery of psychological tests to its students, both on arrival and at intervals thereafter. The data have been used for several purposes: cross-sectional description of selected candidates, comparison of selected versus rejected applicants, and longitudinal description of cohorts as they progress through the medical school environment. Use of the data for prediction remains a distant but eagerly sought objective.

The principal purpose of this study was to examine changes in the entry characteristics of medical students over the six-year period during which the current test battery has been used, and to consider the implications of these changes for selection policies. A secondary purpose was to compare entering medical students at the University of Toronto with (a) general arts and science students at this university, and (b) general university students across North America. A particular concern was whether data on cognitive and noncognitive measures would support recent proposals (Gee, 1959; Caughey, 1967; Erdmann, *et al.* 1971) that the latter be given more emphasis in medical student selection.

METHOD

The cognitive data reported are from Raben's *Advanced Progressive*

From J. Parlow and A.I. Rothman, Personaltiy Traits of First Year Medical Students: Trends Over Six-Year Period 1967-1972, *Brit J of Medical Education, 8:* 8-12, 1974.

This study was supported by the Province of Ontario Department of Health Grant PR-81.

The cooperation of Professor Joan Preston in collecting the arts and science data is gratefully acknowledged.

Matrices (1965); the non-cognitive data were obtained by administering the short version of Jackson's *Personality Research Form Manual* (PRF) (1967). Medical students were tested with both instruments on the first day of classes in all six years reported. Participation was not mandatory; overall, 86 percent of the accepted students participated. The arts and science students were intact classes in their second and third years, tested as part of the requirements of their psychology courses. The Raven was administered to one arts and science class of 233 students in 1970; the PRF was administered to a class of 60 in 1969 and a class of 34 in 1970.[3] While the medical classes averaged only 17 percent women, the arts and science classes had roughly equal sex distributions. The PRF North American norms presented have been weighted to correspond to the sex composition of the medical classes. Sex differences reported in the PRF manual were considered in interpreting the arts and science data.

RESULTS

Fig. 17-1 presents mean scores on the cognitive measure (Raven's *Advanced Progressive Matrices*) for the six medical classes and the arts and science class (no North American college norms are available for the advanced form of the Raven). Analysis of the medical scores

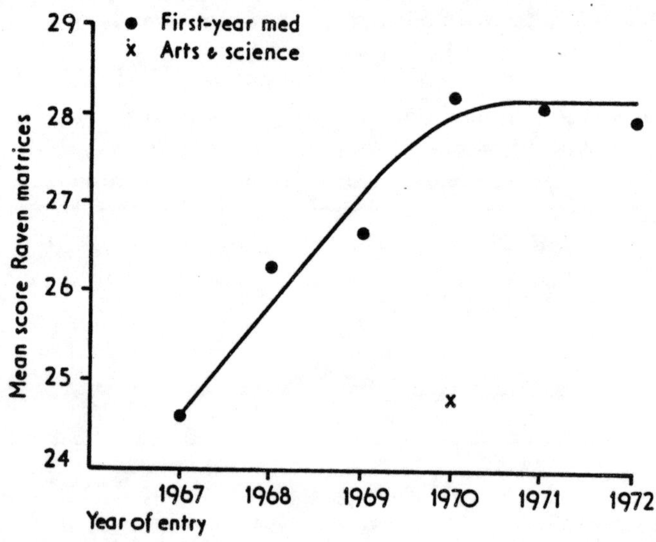

Figure 17-1. Mean scores on Raven Advanced Progressive Matrices.

shows significant linear ($P<0.001$) and quadratic ($P<0.01$) trends, confirming the apparent increase in the first four years, and subsequent levelling off. A linear comparison of the pooled means confirms that over all six years together, the medical students scored significantly higher than the arts and science students ($P<0.001$).

The noncognitive measures were 14 scales of the *Personality Research Form* (PRF). Table 17-I presents mean scores for the six medical classes. Previously, multivariate analysis of variance of the first four medical classes' data indicated significant ($P<0.001$) changes in terms of all 14 PRF scales taken together (Parlow and Rothman, 1971). In the present study, regression analysis of individual scale scores over six years revealed linear changes in the following individual scales: achievement, endurance, impulsivity, and nurturance.

Table 17-I. *Trends of six successive first-year medical classes on personality research form (PRF) scales*

PRF scale	*Year of entry* 1967 (158)[2]	1968 (165)	1969 (169)	1970 (135)	1971 (190)	1972 (209)
Achievement[1]	13·7	14·4	14·2	14·9	14·8	15·0
Affiliation	14·6	14·8	14·3	14·9	14·9	14·5
Aggression	5·4	5·4	6·3	5·4	5·5	4·8
Autonomy	9·0	8·8	9·3	9·0	9·4	8·8
Dominance	9·3	10·3	10·2	10·4	10·2	9·8
Endurance[1]	11·9	13·1	13·0	13·6	13·2	14·5
Exhibition	9·1	9·1	9·2	8·8	8·9	8·8
Harm avoidance	8·1	8·8	8·6	8·9	8·4	9·1
Impulsivity[1]	9·1	8·6	8·3	8·0	8·4	6·9
Nurturance[1]	13·9	14·0	13·8	14·1	14·8	14·9
Order	12·3	12·2	11·5	11·2	11·5	12·2
Play	10·6	9·8	9·7	9·8	10·1	9·8
Social recognition	8·8	9·5	8·8	9·0	8·8	9·1
Understanding	13·8	14·7	14·1	14·6	14·8	14·0

[1]Significant linear change over 6 years ($P<0·01$).
[2]Numbers in each group.

Comparisons of the pooled medical means with the means for (a) the arts and science group and (b) the North American norms (Table 17-II) showed nine differences for the former and 13 for the latter. Those scales on which the medical students either exceeded or were lower than both the other groups ($P<0.01$) are plotted in Fig. 17-2 and 17-3. The plots are best fits by least-squares estimation.

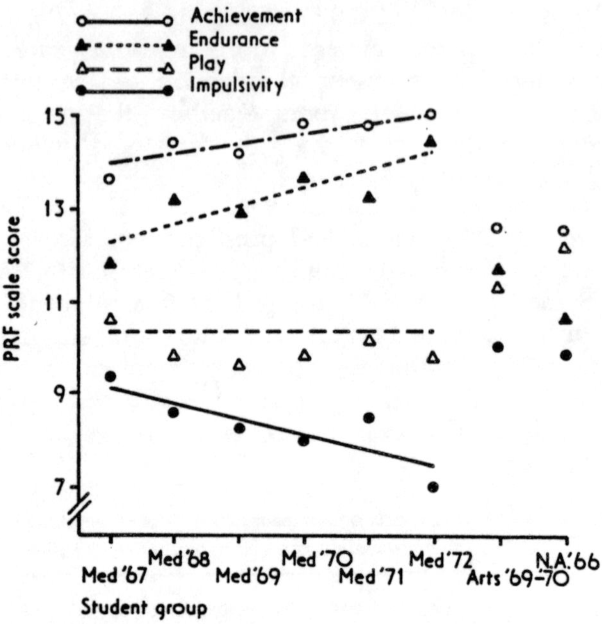

Figure 17-2. Mean scores on achievement-related Personality Research Form (PRF) Scales.

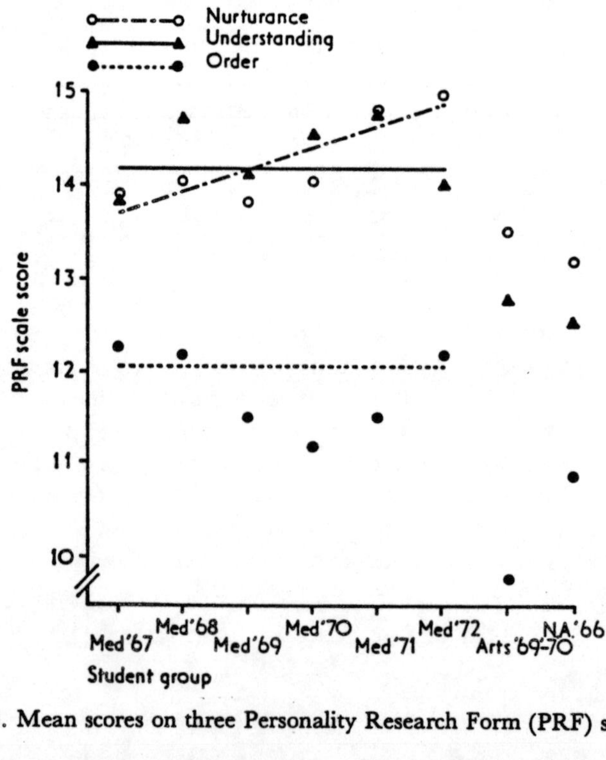

Figure 17-3. Mean scores on three Personality Research Form (PRF) scales.

Table 17-II. *Mean scores for three student groups on personality research form (PRF) scales*

PRF scale	*First-year medicine 1967–72 pooled (877)*[2]	*Arts and science 1969–70 pooled (not sex-weighted) (94)*	*North American College norms 1966 (sex-weighted) (2031)*
Achievement	14·5	12·6[1]	12·5[1]
Affiliation	14·8	13·7[1]	15·2
Aggression	5·5	5·9	7·6[1]
Autonomy	9·1	9·9	8·4[1]
Dominance	10·1	9·8	10·7[1]
Endurance	13·1	11·6[1]	10·6[1]
Exhibition	9·0	9·0	10·6[1]
Harm avoidance	8·7	10·6[1]	8·0[1]
Impulsivity	8·3	10·0[1]	9·9[1]
Nurturance	14·4	13·5[1]	13·2[1]
Order	11·8	9·7[1]	10·8[1]
Play	10·0	11·2[1]	12·1[1]
Social recognition	9·1	9·7	11·8[1]
Understanding	14·4	12·7[1]	12·5[1]

[1]Differ from medicine ($P<0·01$).
[2]Numbers in each group.

DISCUSSION

Raven's *Advanced Progressive Matrices* test is considered a culture-reduced measure of aptitude for abstract reasoning and spatial perception purporting to reflect general intellectual ability. Entering medical classes at this university since 1967 show an increase in Raven scores for four years, levelling off at a high value as compared to arts and science undergraduates in this university, and as compared to a British population for whom a score of 24.0 was at the 95th percentile. This pattern of increasing intellectual performance is not confined to this medical school, but is occurring generally as the ratio of applicants to available places rises. Dubé, Johnson, and Nelson (1973), reporting on medical school applicants in North America, show increased scores on three of the four MCAT subtests, from 1967 to 1971. These data are consistent with the notion that increased competition for places in medical school, and use of grades as the primary criterion for admission, assures a student input of very high intellectual ability. At the same time, the substantial difference between medical students and general students on this cognitive measure suggests that they probably differ in other respects.

Such differences emerge clearly in the non-cognitive measures. As Table 17-II indicates, medical students differ from both groups of general students on seven of the 14 personality measures. Fig. 17-2 demonstrates this for a group of PRF scales related to need achievement. A brief definition of these scales follows.

Achievement (ACH): striving, driving, competitive.

Endurance (END): persistent, relentless, zealous.

Impulsivity (IMP): rash, impetuous, spontaneous.

Play: fun-loving, gleeful, carefree.

Medical students are sharply higher in need for achievement and endurance, and lower in impulsivity and play, than either of the other groups. On all but the play scale, the six-year trend is toward greater divergence from the norms. Compared to general students, medical students are very sober, purposeful, and disciplined — predictable from the grades-oriented selection criteria.

Fig. 17-3 displays trends and group comparisons for the remaining personality scales on which there are clear differences or changes. Some defining adjectives assigned to these scales are:

Nurturance (NURT): sympathetic, consoling, assisting.

Order (ORD): systematic, consistent, methodical.

Understanding (UND): analytical, rational, inquisitive.

Of these traits, the most germane to medical practice is nurturance, on which our medical students rank higher than the other groups, and have been increasing progressively. These findings are comparable to some reported by B. H. Mawardi (personal communication, 1972) at Case-Western Reserve, showing a radical shift by recent entering medical classes toward values characterized as 'kind, sympathetic, and unselfish' and 'interest in people as individuals.' Turning to another finding in the present study, the high score on order indicates an emphasis on careful organization. Relatively high scores on understanding are maintained over the six-year period. All these findings appear to reflect on selection policies, though the scores on nurturance are attributable to other factors such as social change or self-selection.

Table 17-III presents data on two scales which have been administered to only one medical class, in 1972. Adjectives used to describe these scales follow.

Change: flexible, adaptive, innovative.

Cognitive structure: avoids ambiguity, rigid, needs structure. The medical students score lower on a measure of flexibility-adaptiveness (change) than the other groups, and also score lower on ability to tolerate uncertainty (cognitive structure). Convergent validity on the cognitive structure scale may be inferred from the order scores; medical students were seen to have a greater need to be methodical, that is, to require structure. This trait (high need for certainty) also seems incompatible with a fundamental characteristic of clinical practice, the high degree of uncertainty associated with many diagnostic and therapeutic situations. The comparatively low preference for change underscores concerns such as those voiced by Bruhn (1971) on the need for "sweeping changes in the health care system."

> What is critically needed is an increasing number of individual advocates who will actively resist conformity and produce ideas for change which will materially alter the structure of institutions which are no longer responsive to the changing needs of man.

Table 17-III. *PRF scale means for three groups*

PRF scale	*First-year medicine 1972*	*Arts and science 1969 and 1970*	*North American college norms 1966 (sex-weighted)*
Change	11·38	12·20[1]	12·02[1]
Cognitive structure	12·28	10·06[2]	10·77[2]

[1]Differ from medicine ($P<0{\cdot}05$.)
[2]Differ from medicine ($P<0{\cdot}01$.)

How can this profile of traits result from a traditional selection system? Predictably, admitted students would have high intellectual ability, and achievement-related personality traits. But Caughey and others have argued that the large pool of high-ability applicants who now wish to enter medical school assures us of students whose intellectual capacity is more than adequate to meet the requirements of the profession; it is the noncognitive, nonachievement components of clinical excellence that are lacking. In the present study, the traits most relevant to these concerns are those labelled nurturance, order, understanding, cognitive structure, and change. It seems probable that students who are highly achievement motivated have become accustomed to, and therefore prefer, a stable, structured, predictable environment, accounting for the high scores on need for order and cognitive structure, and the low scores on tolerance for change. The high understanding score apparently reflects the 'rational' rather than the 'inquisitive' aspect of this trait; perhaps these are separable dimensions. The high nurturance and low change scores suggest a hypothesis: that students selected via traditional criteria of academic performance, if highly motivated to a career in medicine, see themselves as helping patients, rather than changing the system. Years of deference to the demands of teachers and grades make for clinicians not social activists. To test this hypothesis, medical schools employing appropriately different selection criteria could compare performance of admitted students on these two scales, and subsequently on their behaviour in clinical and community settings. This would require that methods be found to extend measurement from the self-report instruments used in this study, to behavioural situations in practice.

Finally, the results of the study constitute construct validation of the relevant PRF scales. The selection criteria in use result in admission of medical students who score exceptionally on the noncognitive scales called achievement, endurance, impulsivity, play, order and understanding, as well as on cognitive measures; and this exceptional performance has characterized entering students over a considerable time.

Summary

The Faculty of Medicine, University of Toronto, has administered a battery of psychological tests to its entering students each year since the autumn of 1967. These data have been used for several purposes: cross-sectioned description of entering students, comparisons of selected versus rejected applicants, and longitudinal description of student cohorts as they proceed through medical school.

The principal purpose of this study was to examine changes in the entry characteristics of medical students over the six-year period 1967-72, during which the current test battery was used and, in addition, to compare the entering students with general arts and science students at the University of Toronto, and general university students from North America.

Measures used in this study were Raven's *Advanced Progressive Matrices* and Jackson's *Personality Research Form* (PRF).

The results revealed that entering medical classes at the University of Toronto had increasing mean Raven scores for the years 1967-70; in the past two years the scores levelled off at a value high relative to general University of Toronto arts and science undergraduates and a British sample of students. In addition, the medical students differed from the general arts and science students on seven of the 14 scales of the PRF. Finally, trends over the six-year period on seven of the PRF scales were described.

In conclusion the authors discussed the possible implications of the results of this study to selection policies.

REFERENCES

Bruhn, J.G. (1971). On social responsibility. *Journal of Medical Education,* 46, 166-168.

Caughey, J. L., Jr. (1967). Nonintellectual components of medical education. *Journal of Medical Education,* 42, 619-625.

Dubé, W. F., Johnson, D. G., and Nelson, B. C. (1973). Study of U.S. medical school applicants, 1971-72. *Journal of Medical Education,* 48, 395-420.

Erdmann, J. B., Mattson, D. E., Hutton, J. G., Jr., and Wallace, W. L. (1971). The medical college admission test: past, present, future. *Journal of Medical Education,* 46, 937-946.

Gee, H. H. (1959). Differential characteristics of student bodies — implications for the study of medical education. In *Selection and Educational Differentiation.* Center for the Study of Higher Education, Berkeley, California.

Hutchins, E. B. (1964). The AAMC longitudinal study: implications for medical education. *Journal of Medical Education,* 39, 265-277.

Jackson, D. N. (1967). *Personality Research Form Manual.* Research Psychologists press: Goshen, New York.

Parlow, J., and Rothman, A. I. (1971). Personality traits of first-year medical students: trends over the four-year period 1967-70. Paper presented at the Annual Meeting of the Association of American Medical Colleges, Washington, D.C., October.

Raven, J. C. (1065). *Advanced Progressive Matrices, Sets I and II.* H. K. Lewis: London.

Chapter 18

THE BENT TWIG: PSYCHIATRY AND MEDICAL EDUCATION

HENRIETTE KLEIN AND EMILY MUMFORD

PSYCHIATRY has been accused of taking on too many roles and inappropriate tasks. However, in one situation where it should be an integral part of the system, psychiatry has been relatively inactive: this is the selection, monitoring, and nurturing of students in medical schools.

Medical college faculty do not believe they have the perfect solution for the selection and development of student physicians. The Medical College Admission Tests (MCATs) are studied annually and their predictive power assessed. Current recruitment and screening procedures are adequate for selecting students who have the cognitive skills to master required material (1-3), but as Korman and Stubblefield noted, "Insofar as they select systematically, such variables as MCATS and premedical GPA [grade point average] identify smart, achievement-oriented, rather aloof individuals who know how to get good grades" (1, p. 409).

Thus, although medical schools can boast of considerable success in screening for cognitive skills, there is little evidence that present methods work equally well in the selection of personal attributes.

One survey of admissions committees (4) found that psychiatrists were generally underrepresented in selection processes and were called in only when a non-psychiatrist had some question about possible psychopathology in an applicant. Psychiatrists are also underrepresented in research on admissions variables and predictors of later performance as physicians.

It is hoped that the recent increase in psychiatrists' interest in studies of their own residents will lead to increased interest in selection and prediction (5). Holt and Luborsky's selection study of psychiatric residents (6) demonstrated the discriminatory potential

From Henriette Klein and Emily Mumford, The Bent Twig: Psychiatry and Medical Education, *Am J Psychiatry, 135:* 3, March, 1978.

This is a revised version of a paper presented at the 130th annual meeting of the American Psychiatric Association, Toronto, Ont., Canada, May 2-6, 1977.

of psychological tests, but few American schools put much reliance on such screening. Such studies as that by Carter (7) provide promising leads for more efficacious selection of residents. Extension of such studies could also be applied to selection of medical students.

An article in the *Journal of Medical Education* stated,

> For some years now, we have been hearing from medical school admissions officers and committees and from medical faculty members . . . about unusually high quality of the applicants who appear annually in great numbers at the doors of these professional education centers . . . However, one notes a strange silence about all this superlative manpower four years later (8, p. 123).

Average Medical College Admission Test scores of students have risen, and now a "totally new" test, twice as long as the 30-year-old one, has been developed "to eliminate racial and sex bias." This concentrated attention suggests a commitment to the notion that if students are bright enough, all will be well. Unfortunately, personal attributes that are highly desirable for physicians do not scale along with cognitive test performance. Further, there is far more to the successful development of physicians than selection of applicants.

PROJECTED PERSONAL QUALITIES

The personal qualities of the physician may be crucial in determining what patients do with medical advice, and evidence from studies is not reassuring (9-13). In a carefully drawn sample of 576 households, Kasteler and associates (13) found that almost half (48%) of the upper-income and more than one-third (37%) of the lower-income families had changed doctors because of personal dissatisfaction. In this study as in others, ability and fees were rarely mentioned as the reason for changing physicians. The respondent's evaluation of the doctor as a person seems to be more closely related to "doctor shopping" than does the patient's socioeconomic status (13).

Within medical schools, there is immediate evidence for the need to attend more to personal attributes in the education of physicians. Medical educators decry the excessive destructive competition of medical students, which leads to cheating and to vandalism in libraries and laboratories. This hints that all is not well in either the selection or the medical education process. Evidence that increasing proportions of medical students are seeking psychiatric help cannot be assumed to be an indicator of faulty selection (3): indeed, awareness of the need for help may be an encouraging sign.

However, the phenomena of severe psychopathology and of disaffection should be studied. Students' complaints about the deleterious impact of excessive competition on their image of the medical career also deserve attention.

Edwards and Zimet concluded their survey of medical students with the comment, "This personal warmth and caring, once the hallmark of the physician, appears to be unavailable to the young doctors who have been so severely deprived in the very area during their years of study and training" (14, p. 625).

Physicians are considered to be a high-risk population for suicide, drug addiction, and alcoholism (14-20). According to Coombs (21), physicians' wives are also at risk for the same set of problems. The common tendency toward self-medication by doctors is said to begin in medical school and to be particularly marked during internship and residency (22-24). Clinical studies of addicted and alcoholic physicians report that many began to assume early in their careers that their special knowledge of drug action and addiction made them less prone than laymen to habituations and addictions.

Thus there is evidence in the medical school years and afterward of an abundance of those very problems which fall within the realm of psychiatry for assessment, possible prediction of at-risk individuals, and socializing students who are still in medical school.

It is not that psychiatric skills have proven to be irrelevant in the few studies that have addressed the issue. For example, a study of 1,198 medical students at Johns Hopkins University provided a wide range of material that is available for all medical students (24). The researchers then pulled out the material on nine students who had committed suicide and selected two matched controls for each of them. These 27 protocols were then submitted to a psychiatrist who was blind to the number of suicides and controls. He was able to identify the nine suicides from the available material (24).

Several factors outside psychiatry contribute to inattention to variables that psychiatry should be well able to study in order to improve medical education. Competition for a space in medical school has become fierce, sometimes unfair, and viewed with disfavor by both sides of the medical school admission process. In 1961-1962, there were 14,381 applicants for 8,483 places; in 1974-1975, there were 46,624 applicants for 14,703 places (25). In one state medical school, well over 5,000 qualified applicants sought admission for 216 available spots. The numbers of people hurling themselves at the gates of medicine may abate; indeed, the number was down slightly in 1976 (26). However, there is every indication that medical colleges will continue to have an abundance of bright and determined applicants in the near future.

Compounding the problems that each medical school faces are the multiple applications that candidates submit in the hope of increasing their chances for admission. This takes up the valuable time of over-worked admission committees and as a result the interview, while still a semi-standard part of the admissions procedure, may be cursory. Further, interviews are not necessarily conducted by individuals who have good interviewing skills. Consequently, because it is often frequently misused, the interview has not been shown to be a powerful tool in predicting later performance in medical education (27-31).

Applicants' determination to gain the prized admission to medical school aggravates the tendency for faculty to cling to selection criteria that are considered both "proven" and legally unassailable. At times students do invoke "civil rights" and legal proceedings to support their demand to be admitted to or to stay in medical school. Once a student has been admitted, the mystique of an "inalienable right" appears to float like a fog over consideration of ultimate sanctions throughout the medical career. Reinforcing the tendency to retain students, even in the face of contraindications, is the understandable perception within the profession that medicine is the *only* career. Thus, expelling a student is viewed as an act of aggression, even when it might in fact be an act of long-term wisdom for the student who has made an unwise career choice. Moreover, there is the factor of the large investment that is made after the selection. The cost of educating a physician is breathtaking: one medical economist has estimated that "the cost to society of taking one high school graduate and turning him into a physician now exceeds $100,000" (32). In this context, reluctance to expel a student or to take a chance on new selection criteria is understandable. Grade point averages and scores on the Medical College Admission Tests are viewed as reassuringly "objective" or "scientific." They are also relatively easy to use defensively should a student decide to initiate litigation. Such factors inhibit admissions committees from experimenting with "unproven" criteria and create a "Catch 22" situation, since there can be very little improvement without experimentation.

THE BENT TWIG HYPOTHESIS

The bent twig hypothesis, which states that the important shaping of the physician takes place before entry into medical school, supports the present patterns of action in medical education. If the hypothesis were true, then more informed and carefully evaluated selection would be imperative. The extreme reluctance to expel students suggests a misplaced faith in the wisdom of present selection procedures. It also suggests a misplaced faith that medical school inevitably provides an environment for fruition of emotional maturity and informed sensitivity to ethical issues and human concerns, which are essential to the development of a good physician. An end result of both of these misconceptions is that once they have been selected and provided the requisite cognitive and technical skills, the "twigs" simply grow. Although in fact some may grow without sufficient emotional or ethical maturation, nearly all will enjoy a lifetime mandate for service, responsibility, and the social privilege and power that few other occupations enjoy. It has been reported that "dropout rates have varied from a high figure of about twenty-five percent in the past to a present low of one and one-half percent" (29). Thus today's medical student is almost destined to become and remain a physician. As access to a medical education became increasingly limited and attrition within the medical college dwindled, the need to search for criteria that would select the right "twigs" – and nurture them – became essential to the future of American medicine. It is ironic that the need for new selection criteria is emphasized constantly, but little new is investigated, particularly in areas to which psychiatrists could contribute.

THE UNDERUTILIZATION OF PSYCHIATRY

It is extremely unfortunate that psychiatry is not more involved in attending to the development of students who are selected and in monitoring and assessing that development. We know that some diminution of idealism is a common accompaniment of progress through medical school. We do not know enough about the conditions that foster maturation instead of cynicism, and it may be true that what *is* known is too little applied.

What are the inhibiting factors within psychiatry itself that reinforce its underutilization? In some medical schools, as a result of history, public image, and the structure of medical education – and sometimes their own attitudes – psychiatrists are rarely called in for advice on a specific applicant or student. As long as psychiatrists are viewed only as a court of last resort, their contributions are bound to be minimal.

Psychiatry is a latecomer to medical education, which has been slow to change since the days of the Flexner report. As late as the

1950s, there were few psychiatric beds in teaching hospitals, and psychiatry was in many places part of the outpatient service, which is generally devalued in medical schools.

Among the factors that have tended to place psychiatry in a peripheral position in medical school decision making is the very nature of psychiatry, which permits more independence from medical schools and hospitals than is found in other specialties. The surgeon must have his or her operating theater, and orthopedic surgeons, radiologists, anesthesiologists, etc., must consult and work with one another. In contrast, psychiatrists frequently consult with psychologists or social workers, a pattern that places them in closer alliance with professions outside medical education. Following the patterns of their practice, psychiatrists are not much in evidence in the hospital coffee shops, cafeterias, and doctors' lounges, where many informal but important exchanges lay the groundwork for mutual respect and cooperation. If the medical school does not identify them as central to medical education, psychiatrists themselves all too often do not identify strongly with the medical college. They are seldom well represented in schoolwide events. Although absence from coffee shops and ritual occasions may seem trivial, the consequences of such remoteness from the daily life of medical schools are far from insignificant. One aspect of personal influence in policy decisions in any complex organization is centrality in information exchange. Recommendations are enhanced when the individual who makes them is informed on details of daily problems, alliances, and informal power structures.

There is another factor within psychiatry that interferes with its influence in medical education. The psychiatrist's primary emphasis is concern with people who suffer from emotional problems, and this emphasis may at times adversely affect his or her usefulness on selection and promotion committees. Not infrequently, a psychiatrist may be seen and may function as an apologist or therapist for a student. If the same psychiatrist then serves on promotion committees where the student-patient is discussed, he or she may well become an adversary of fellow faculty members and a champion of the problem student, who may later become a problem physician. The requirements for the role of "gatekeeper to medicine" on behalf of society and those for the role of therapist are very different.

POSSIBLE CONTRIBUTIONS OF PSYCHIATRY

How then can psychiatry contribute more significantly to decision making at crucial junctures throughout the medical education process? Fortunately, psychiatrists are automatically being forced to contribute somewhat more. Centralized services of the Association of American Medical Colleges allow pooling of specific data, and regional screening interviews have been recommended. Public pressure is mounting for attention to the emotional and social qualities of physicians. At the same time, psychiatric knowledge is becoming more essential in the teaching of medical students, which brings psychiatrists into more active participation. Psychiatry departments cannot be effective if they conduct their teaching in an archaically isolated way that is not relevant to the average medical student's immediate interests. Fortunately, the current trend is to teach psychiatry in a way that is relevant to all medical students. Increasing numbers of psychiatrists now serve as active members of medical, surgical, and other departments through psychiatric liaison services. Also, increasing numbers of psychiatrists are becoming active participants in medical school decisions.

Current studies of interviews, interviewers, and the final pooled decisions are beginning to provide data for replication and testing. Interview judgments can be translated into ratings that permit rapid comparisons (33). A study of 79 postresidency students in training found that errors of overestimation of potential growth were more frequent than errors of underestimation (34). Studies of the interviewers also can provide clues to the use of the interview as a selection tool (35). As a study done at the Ohio State Medical School suggested, the selection and training of admissions interviewers is an extremely important task (36). In that study, overreliance on the written file, with its grades and scores, and the use of a barrage of highly directive specific questions were two frequent limitations on the ability of the interview to elicit much more than was already on the record (36). The interview, when developed and recognized as a specific tool, can be a powerful instrument for gaining an estimate of present status and potential for growth in a defined setting. It can also be used throughout the medical college experience.

More active participation of psychiatry in the medical education process will lead to more effective use of psychiatrists' contributions. It does appear that psychiatry has much to offer in terms of the development of self-awareness and perceptiveness in physicians. It also has much to offer as a counterforce to the development of the cynicism that is often reported as a consequence of medical education (37). Psychiatry has an important role in alerting students to ethical issues and reinforcing ethical values.

As psychiatrists demonstrate that they can function effectively with other specialists on medical college committees rather than serving primarily as adversaries or apologists for disturbed students, they will become an essential part of the decision-making process. Both society and medicine will benefit, and so will psychiatry. Psychiatry's place, as Lindsay Beaton said, "is in the mainstream of medicine, not on its banks."

REFERENCES

1. Korman M, Stubblefield RL, Martin LW: Patterns of success in medical school and their correlates. *J Med Educ 43:*405-411, 1968
2. Wingard JR, Williamson JW: Grades as predictors of physicians' career performance: an evaluative literature review. *J Med Educ 48*:311-322, 1973
3. Haley JV: The medical college admission test as a predictor of grade factors. *J Med Educ 48*:98-100, 1973
4. Evans R, Anderson D: The selection of medical students in western Canada. *Can Med Assoc J 96*:473-480, 1967
5. Pasnau RO, Bayley SJ: Personality changes in the first year of psychiatric residency training. *Am J Psychiatry 128*:79-84, 1971
6. Holt R, Luborsky L: Personality Patterns of Psychiatrists. New York, Basic Books, 1958
7. Carter D: *Selection of psychiatry residents at the University of Colorado.* Presented at the 123rd annual meeting of the American Psychiatric Association, San Francisco, Calif, May 11-15, 1970
8. McKee FW: Physicians for the care of the sick. *J Med Educ Supplement,* Nov 1970, pp 122-127
9. Sackett D, Haynes B (eds): *Compliance with Therapeutic Regimen.* Baltimore, Johns Hopkins University Press, 1976
10. Mumford E: The responses of patients to medical advice, in *Understanding Human Behavior in Health and Illness.* Edited by Pardes H, Simons R, Baltimore, Williams & Wilkins, 1977, pp 405-416
11. Davis M: Variations in patients' compliance with doctors' advice: an empirical analysis of patterns of communication. *Am J Public Health 58*:619-625, 1968
12. Korsch B, Nigrete VF: Doctor-patient communication. *Sci Am 227*:66-74, 1972
13. Kasteler J, Kane RL, Olsen DM: Issues underlying prevalence of "doctor-shopping" behavior. *J Health Hum Behav 17*:328-339, 1976
14. Edwards MT, Zimet CN: Problems and concerns among medical students — 1975. *J Med Educ 51*:619-625, 1976
15. Blachly PH, Disher W, Roduner G: Suicide by physicians. *Bull Suicidology 4*:1-18, 1968
16. Vincent MO, Robinson EA, Latt L: Physicians as patients: private psychiatric hospital experience. *Can Med Assoc J 100*:403-412, 1969
17. Glatt MM: Alcoholism and drug dependence in doctors and nurses. *Br Med J 1*:380-381, 1968

18. Leading article: Doctors' disease. *Br Med J 4*:567-568, 1967
19. a'Brook MF, Hailstone JD, McLauchlan IEJ: Psychiatric illness in the medical profession. *Br J Psychiatry 113*:1013-1023, 1967
20. Garb S: Drug addiction in physicians *Anesth Analg 48*:129-133, 1969
21. Coombs, RH: The medical marriage, in *Psychosocial Aspects of Medical Training.* Edited by Coombs RH, Vincent CE, Springfield, Ill, Charles C Thomas, 1971, pp 133-167
22. Raskin M: Psychiatric crises of medical students and the implications for subsequent adjustment. *J Med Educ 47*:210-215, 1972
23. Lewis CE: Illness behavior and academic performance among medical students: implication for preventive medicine. *Arch Environ Health 12*:776-780. 1966
24. Epstein LC, Thomas CB, Shaffer JW, et al: Clinical prediction of physician suicide based on medical student data. *J Nerv Ment Dis 156*: 19-29, 1973
25. Crowley AE: Medical education in the United States 1973-74: introduction. *JAMA Supplement,* 1975, pp 1-2
26. Association of American Medical Colleges: The medical school application process, in Medical School Admissions Requirements 1977-78 – U.S. and Canada. Washington, DC, AAMC, 1977, p 25
27. Gough HG: Nonintellectual factors in the selection and evaluation of medical students. *J Med Educ 42*:642-650, 1967
28. Gough HG, Hall WB: An attempt to predict graduation from medical school. *J Med Educ 50*:940-950, 1975
29. Calkins EV, Richards JM Jr, McCanse A, et al: Impact on admission to a school of medicine of an innovation in selection procedures. *Psychol Rep 35*:1135-1142, 1974
30. Rhoads JM, Gallemore JL Jr, Gianturco DT, et al: Motivation, medical school admissions, and student performance. *J Med Educ 49*:1119-1127, 1974
31. Rosenberg ML: Increasing the efficiency of medical school admissions. *J Med Educ 48*:707-717, 1973
32. Fuchs V: Improving the delivery of health services. *J Bone Joint Surg (Am) 51*:407-412, 1969
33. Zubin J: A brief survey of the interview, in *The Appraisal of Applicants to Medical Schools (pamphlet).* Washington, DC, Association of American Medical Colleges, 1957
34. Klein HR: *Psychoanalysts in Training: Selection and Evaluation.* New York, Columbia University Press, 1965
35. Antonovsky A: Student selection in the School of Medicine, Ben-Gurion University of the Negev. *Br J Med Educ 10*:219-234, 1976
36. Litton Hawes E, MacLean IC, Hines MH: An analysis of the communication process in the medical admissions interview. *J Med Educ 51*:332-334, 1976
37. Becker HS, Geer B: The fate of idealism in medical school. *Am Sociol Rev 23*:50-56, 1958

Hospitalization and Treatment

Chapter 19

PSYCHIATRIC MORBIDITY OF PHYSICIANS

JOHN C. DUFFY AND EDWARD M. LITIN

These are the duties of a physician: First. . . to heal his mind and to give help to himself before giving it to anyone else.

—Epitaph of an Athenian Doctor, 2 AD

PHYSICAL illness in the nation's physicians has been the object of a number of recent investigations.[1-3] For the most part, they have emphasized the need for annual comprehensive medical examinations, particularly with regard to pulmonary function and cardiovascular status. Virtually no studies have been made of psychiatric illness in physicians, the only exception having been in the specific area of drug addiction.

The overall health evaluation of physicians is incomplete without a consideration of psychiatric illness. It is the purpose of this paper to report our experiences with a significant number of physicians whose emotional illness required hospitalization.

With the swell of recent government and public interest in mental illness, it becomes imperative for the medical profession to assess its own mental health. Physicians of all disciplines will be expected to assume a primary role in the overall management of psychiatric patients in the general population. This expectation automatically and justifiably involves the assumption that physicians will be generally an emotionally healthy group. But, is this true?

Our society is becoming increasingly sophisticated in medical matters as a result of medical advances and the widespread dissemination of information about them in the communications media. Because of the demands on the physician's time and knowledge, he constantly feels threatened, not only by his patients but also by his colleagues, to maintain his professional competence. In addition, he is expected to fulfill his obligations as a husband, father, and civic leader. The resulting demand that he be all things to all people is a potentially strong propelling force in the direction of emotional decompensation.

From John D. Duffy and Edward M. Litin, Psychiatric Morbidity of Physicians, *JAMA, 189*: 989-992, September 28, 1964.

Read before the Section on Nervous and Mental Diseases at the 113th Annual Convention of the American Medical Association, San Francisco, June 23, 1964.

DESCRIPTION OF STUDY

Our inpatient psychiatric service is part of a 900-bed general hospital. It is composed of both open-ward and closed-ward units with auxiliary supporting services. There is a total capacity of 30 beds on the closed ward and 20 beds on the open ward. The service is designed to provide diagnostic evaluation and short-term, intensive psychotherapy.

There were 5,925 patients admitted to the psychiatric service during the period from July 1, 1956, through July 1, 1963. During this seven-year period, 93 physicians were admitted to either the open or the closed units of the section of psychiatry. This represents one physician for each 64 admissions, a highly disproportionate ratio when one considers their representation in the population. Unfortunately, we were not able, for comparative purposes, to determine the corresponding ratio for physicians admitted to our medical and surgical services. It must be emphasized that this number (93) represents only those physicians who were sufficiently incapacitated psychiatrically to require hospitalization. Far more were seen in an outpatient diagnostic-therapeutic setting. Each physician's case history was reviewed in detail, with particular emphasis on the longitudinal history of the patient and pertinent factors operating at the time of hospitalization. Each physician-patient was further delineated as to age, type of medical practice, source of the referral for psychiatric study, unit assigned, diagnosis, days hospitalized, treatment, and follow-up information.

FINDINGS

The physician-patients in the study ranged in age from 28 to 86 years. The average patient was in his early 50s. Slightly less than half of the patients were transferred to the psychiatric unit from other services in the hospital. In the referred group, most were seen in consultation, with the recommendation by the psychiatrist that they be transferred to the psychiatric unit (Table 19-I).

The two most frequent reasons for voluntary admission were family pressure directed at the patient and an awareness by the patient of a gross impairment in his clinical ability as a physician. A significant factor in admissions of physicians with drug dependency was the threat of federal action or of revocation by the appropriate state agency of the license to practice medicine.[4]

The high incidence of closed-unit admissions is a fairly accurate reflection of the acute condition of the patient when he was first seen

Table 19-I.—Preliminary Admission Data

Age (years)	
Span	28-86
Mean	54
Source of referral	
Direct	52
Other	41
Prior psychiatric care	
Yes	20
No	73
Unit assigned	
Open	28
Closed	65

in the section of psychiatry. In many instances the precipitating problem which warranted a psychiatric evaluation was one of frankly abnormal behavior by the patient, or serious difficulties in management of the problem by the referring service. Only 20 patients had received some form of psychiatric care before their admission to the service, and they were all direct admissions to the section of psychiatry.

Table 19-II represents a grouping of the physician-patients according to their fields of practice. Although our sampling is small, it is interesting to note that the ratio of general physicians to specialists does not differ markedly from the ratio of their distribution in the medical population[5]; in fact, with few exceptions, our grouping is fairly representative of a cross-section of the practice of medicine today. This is not an unusual finding, and it reflects simply that no person or special group is immune to mental illness. Although this fact is obvious, one still finds evidence of the stereotyped thinking which associates mental illness with one particular group of physicians.

Table 19-II.—Distribution of Patients According to Field of Medical Practice

Practice	Number	Total
General	44	44
Specialty		
Internal medicine	15	
Ophthalmology—Otolaryngology	3	
Neurology	1	
Obstetrics—Gynecology	2	
Pathology	3	
Pediatrics	1	
Psychiatry	4	
Radiology	3	
Surgery	17	49
		93

Psychiatraic diagnosis is, at best, a difficult task, demanding much in the way of objectivity from the psychiatrist. Unfortunately, a psychiatric diagnosis still carries a stigma in many quarters and can be potentially and permanently damaging to a patient's career and future. This is particularly true when the patient is a physician, and as a result we noted a tendency toward assigning a less pathological diagnosis to our colleagues. Unfortunately, this can result in a disservice in the long view, by condoning the self-delusion in the physician-patient that his is not a serious problem.

In general, the most commonly made diagnoses were the affective psychoses, the sociopathic personality disorders, and the psychoneuroses. The organic brain syndromes represented the least frequent diagnoses in the sampling. None of the patients were diagnosed as having a psychophysiological illness. The reason for this is not certain; however, problems of this nature may well be handled directly, without recourse to psychiatry, by other medical specialties and may not be severe enough to warrant hospitalization (Table 19-III).

Table 19-III.—Diagnostic Grouping

Diagnoses		Total	Percent
Brain syndrome			
Acute	5		
Chronic	3	8	9
Psychotic disorders			
Affective	20		
Schizophrenic	7		
Paranoid	4	31	33
Psychoneurotic disorders		19	20
Personality disorders			
Pattern	7		
Sociopathic	28	35	38
		93	100

Figure 19-1 represents the percentage distribution of diagnoses according to the practice categories of surgery, medicine, and general practice. Among the general practitioners, the greatest percentage of illness was in the psychotic and personality disorders. A somewhat more equal distribution of diagnoses is seen in the surgical group, while there were relatively fewer psychotic illnesses in the medical specialties group as compared with the psychoneuroses and personality disorders.

The mean figure for days hospitalized was 12, the shortest duration having been less than one hour, and the longest, 75 days. The treatment in most instances was psychotherapy, medication, and a supportive environment. In 18 cases, electroconvulsive therapy was the treatment of choice. Some form of follow-up information was available in 42 cases, but it tended to be fragmentary and often gave little indication of whether or not the patient had followed through with any recommendations given him at the time of dismissal (Table 19-IV).

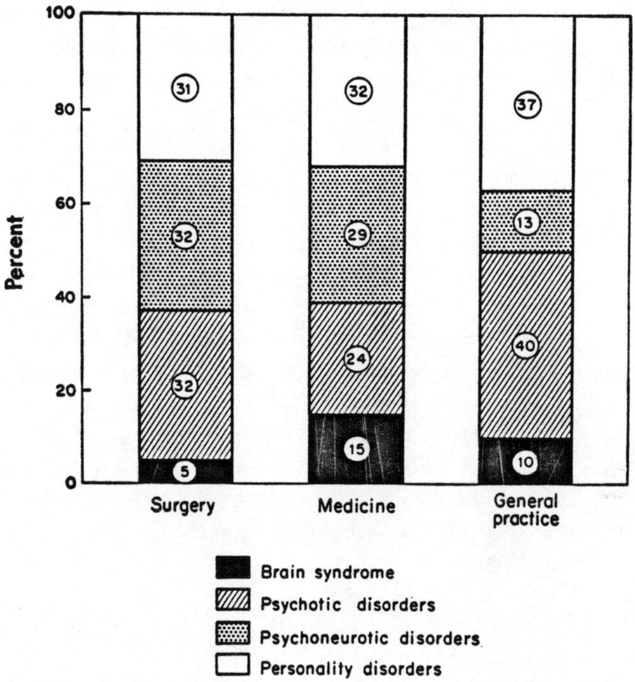

Figure 19-1. Percentage distribution of patients by broad diagnostic groupings and medical practice.

Table 19-IV.—Days Hospitalized. Treatment and Follow-up Information

Days hospitalized	
Span	1-75
Mean	12
Treatment	
Psychotherapy	75
Electroconvulsive therapy	18
Follow-up	
Yes	42
No	51

COMMENT

Our sample is limited and represents preliminary data in which statistically significant findings are not possible. We have no certain way of determining the role of weighting in our sampling, nor is it possible to determine completely the multiple factors which acted on our physician-patients and brought them to us. Many physicians come to our institution because the safe distance from home assures a measure of anonymity and because ours is not identified as primarily a psychiatric center. Within the confines of these limitations there remain clearly defined areas worthy of comment.

It is important to observe that the group involves an inpatient "treated" population and may well represent only a small portion of clinically impaired persons.[6] Pearson and Strecker,[7] in 1960, reviewed their experience over a 15-year period in private practice in the therapy of physicians with psychiatric problems. The total number of physicians studied was 66, and of that number, only 20 required hospitalization at any time during their therapy. In some respects these investigators' findings and formulations were similar to ours, but their group represented a very select sampling and a less "acute" problem in terms of overall psychiatric management.

In our series, 21 patients left against medical advice. This number is high and may be related to the difficulty the physician has in accepting his illness and his status as a patient. The situation is not without strain for the hospital staff, who must cope with their own feelings of insecurity in dealing with the physician as a patient. It is imperative that the staff clearly define their relationship with the patient and emphasize his responsibility in cooperating with them as a patient. Certainly one must avoid special considerations or privileges for the physician, as well as the many other, more subtle, pitfalls in dealing with the "special patient."[8]

Once admitted to the psychiatric service, the physician tended to be quite manipulating of his environment. He generally remained aloof from the other patients and seemed unable to assume the role of a patient in the social structure of the ward. Overt hostility by the patient toward the therapist was common. Once the acute phase of the illness had passed, there was often a demand for immediate dismissal. Denial was a common mechanism in therapy, and any suggestion for follow-up psychotherapy after dismissal was often regarded with ambivalence. Very few physicians returned after dismissal, either for psychiatric or for nonpsychiatric reasons. This may reflect some hostility concerning the circumstances of the admission or an unwillingness to return as a patient after suffering the "stigma" of a psychiatric illness.

In 47 of the cases studied, alcoholism or drug addiction (or both) was an active problem at the time of admission; there were 18 patients with alcoholism, and 37 with some form of drug addiction (21 had both alcoholism and drug dependence as a problem when admitted). There is no simple explanation for this finding, just as there is no single causative factor operating in the alcoholic or the drug addict. However, some consistent patterns were common to the group. The use of alcohol to excess in many cases began early in life, as opposed to drug misuse, whose beginnings were in medical school and the professional years. Often, the use of narcotics was initially justified because of some real or fancied physical complaint. In almost all cases the drinking or the use of drugs represented a defense against intense anxiety feelings. There also was a great deal of difficulty in the control of aggressive drives and little or no gratification of intense dependency needs from the environment.

While it is true that physicians are a heterogeneous group from the standpoint of personality as well as of physical factors, they are all subject to stresses peculiar to the practice of medicine. As mentioned earlier, we noted such factors as the pressing needs of their patients and the maintenance of professional skills as well as family responsibilities, social requirements, and civic commitments playing an important role in our patients' lives. The attempts to fulfill all of these obligations, coupled with their own emotional vulnerabilities, led to serious decompensation.

Physicians need to exercise enlightened compassion with regard to mental illness in their fellow physicians. In the close fraternal ties of the professional, serious emotional illness in a physician soon becomes apparent to all. It would seem that in our group there is a general reticence on the part of other physicians to intervene in the situation, as well as a tendency to be "overprotective" of the involved individual. Equally as destructive for the physician suffering from mental illness is the cold and callous rejection by his medical colleagues as being defective. We condemn such attitudes in the laity, because it postpones definitive care until the situation progresses to an acute decompensation; certainly we should not be guilty of the same naïve thinking within our own professional family.

We regard the study of psychiatric ills of physicians as a preliminary step in the direction of a better understanding of emotional illness as it affects a selected group of individuals and hampers their productivity. There are more questions raised than answered, and many areas are worth exploring in greater detail. The medical profession must be willing to deal directly with the problem of psychiatric illness among physicians, have the courage to diagnose it accurately, and acquire the understanding which must support the physician who returns to the community after "the anguish and folly of madness."

REFERENCES

1. Dowling, H.F.: Physician, Heal Thyself, *GP* 11:69-73 (Jan) 1955.

2. Sharpe, J.C., and Smith, W.W.: Physician, Heal Thyself: Comparison of Findings in Periodic Health Examinations of Physicians and Executives, *JAMA* **182**:234-237 (Oct 20) 1962.
3. Russek, H.I.: Emotional Stress and Coronary Heart Disease in American Physicians, Dentists and Lawyers, *Amer J Med Sci* **243**:716-725 (June) 1962.
4. Quinn, W.F.: Narcotic Addiction: Medical and Legal Problems With Physicians, *Calif Med* **94**:214-217 (April) 1961.
5. Nagan, P.S.: *Medical Almanac,* Philadelphia: W. B. Saunders Co., 1961-1962.
6. Srole, Leo, et al: *Mental Health in Metropolis: Midtown Manhattan Study,* New York: McGraw-Hill Book Co., Inc., 1962.
7. Pearson, M.M., and Strecker, E.A.: Physicians as Psychiatric Patients: Private Practice Experience, *Amer J Psychiat* **116**:915-919 (April) 1960.
8. Pollack, I.W., and Battle, W.C.: Studies of the Special Patient, *Arch Gen Psychiat* **9**:344-350 (Oct) 1963.

Chapter 20

PSYCHIATRIC ILLNESS IN MALE DOCTORS AND CONTROLS: AN ANALYSIS OF SCOTTISH HOSPITALS IN-PATIENT DATA

ROBIN M. MURRAY

INTRODUCTION

THE health of doctors, and the effects of medical practice upon it, have long attracted comment from both within and without the medical profession. Thus, Francis Quarles (1592-1644) optimistically wrote: "Physicians of all men are most happy; what good success soever they have the world proclaimeth, and what faults they commit the earth covereth." Ramazzini (1633-1714) also considered doctors to be healthier than other learned men, and ascribed this "to their cheerful frame of mind when they go home with their pockets full of fees." Bernard Shaw, while doubting the wisdom of allowing doctors to charge fees, was concerned about the effect of their long hours of work and wondered (1911) "why the impatient doctors do not become savage and unmanageable, and the patient ones imbecile? Perhaps they do to some extent."

The General Health of Doctors

There are occasional circumstances in which a doctor's work may hazard his physical health. Ionizing radiation was a considerable danger to the pioneers of radiology (Court-Brown and Doll, 1958), and Reid (1957) noted that pathologists had an increased risk of

---

From Robin M. Murray, Psychiatric Illness in Male Doctors and Controls: an Analysis of Scottish Hospitals In-patient Data, *Brit J. Psychiatry, 131*: 1-10, 1977.

The essential factor in both the planning and execution of this investigation was the unfailing cooperation of the staff of the Scottish Hospitals Research and Intelligence Unit (now known as the Information Services Division of the Common Service Agency). Dr. G. Edwards also provided much needed advice.

tuberculosis. Sixty-one European dialysis units reported outbreaks of hepatitis in 1968-69, and one of 88 affected staff died (Drukker *et al.*, 1969). Women doctors may be at risk of having deformed children as a consequence of exposure to halothane or to rubella infection during pregnancy (Knill-Jones *et al.*, 1972; Harrington, 1975).

These particular hazards should not blind us to the fact that doctors have a life expectancy greater than that of the general population. Figures given in the Registrar General's latest report on Occupational Mortality (1971) show that, overall, doctors have a Standard Mortality Ratio of 89 — i.e. their death rate is 11 percent smaller than that expected from the national death rate. American studies have reached similar conclusions (Emerson and Hughes, 1926; Dickinson and Martin, 1956; Williams *et al.*, 1971; Everson and Fraumeni, 1975).

Williams *et al.* (1971) suggest that much of this improved survival can be attributed to the highly selective process which admits primarily healthy individuals from the middle and upper social classes to medical school. Thereafter, members of the profession have the benefits of high socioeconomic status and easy access to competent and, if necessary, highly specialized medical care. Knowledge of health risks may also contribute; less frequent cigarette smoking amongst English doctors is reflected in their Standard Mortality Ratio from lung cancer being 48 percent of that expected (Registrar General, 1971).

Mental Illness in Doctors

The mental health of doctors has attracted even more attention than their physical health (reviewed by Murray, 1974; 1976a). Research workers have naturally been curious to know whether doctors have a similar advantage in terms of their mental health to that which they enjoy in mortality risk. One method of approaching this question is to study doctors treated for mental illness, and in the 1960s five major studies of series of such doctors were published. These series are not strictly comparable among themselves, since both British studies (a'Brook et al., 1967; Pond, 1969) included in-patients and out-patients, while the three North American series (Duffy and Litin, 1964; Vincent et al., 1969; Small et al., 1969) consisted only of in-patients. Nevertheless, there are interesting similarities, including the mean age of the doctor-patients which ranged only from 42 years to 54 years, and the rates of divorce and separation which varied only from 7 to 13 percent.

In spite of differences in the diagnostic criteria employed, some trends in diagnosis emerge. In four studies,* the percentage of doctor-patients considered psychotic ranged from approximately one quarter to two fifths, and for each doctor diagnosed schizophrenic and each doctor with an organic psychosis there were at least two categorized as suffering from affective psychosis. Drug addiction and alcoholism were disturbingly common; 51 percent of Duffy and Litin's doctor-patients were considered addicted to drugs or alcohol. Doctors with neuroses and personality disorders made up the remaining 18 to 29 percent of patients in the different series.

Deficiencies in the Reported Studies

The results of the reported studies may have been distorted by the special position which doctors occupy in relation to psychiatric treatment. Doctors can not only treat themselves or seek psychiatric advice informally, but if they have a particular complaint they may, because of their professional awareness, seek out a doctor or hospital with special expertise in that condition. The five studies discussed above were carried out at three types of institution — private hospitals, teaching hospitals, and the personal clinics of well known professors; these are likely to have preferentially attracted sick doctors. Consequently these investigations cannot give accurate information about the relative frequency of the different illnesses.

Pond (1969) appreciated this, and indeed demonstrated considerable differences in the age, sex, occupational status and specialty pursued by doctors seen at the three different institutions he studied. He noted that older mentally ill physicians have more often "reached the stage of affluence which enables them to have private treatment." The authors of the other studies give no indication that they understood how potentially unrepresentative their patients might have been. Both a'Brook et al. (1967) and Vincent et al. (1969) attempted to improve the reliability of their conclusions by comparing their doctors with control patients. Unfortunately, they did not sufficiently appreciate that one cannot draw conclusions regarding the frequency of psychiatric illness in doctors and controls from studies of hospital in-patients without knowledge of the size of the populations from which they were drawn.

---

*Small *et al.* (1969) used a category of 'schizophrenic reactions' which is likely to have been much broader than the category of schizophrenia used in the other four studies.

THE PRESENT INVESTIGATION

In order to investigate the occurrence of psychiatric illness amongst doctors in a more meaningful way, it is necessary not only to obtain information regarding a large sample of doctors and controls treated in a variety of different hospitals, but also to know the size of the populations from which they come. Scotland provided the opportunity for such a study.

In 1955 the General Board of Control for Scotland instituted a system of reporting on each patient in mental hospitals and mental deficiency institutions under its control. In 1963 this system was extended to cover psychiatric units in general and teaching hospitals, and came under the aegis of the Scottish Hospitals Research and Intelligence Unit (SHRIU) which from then on collected statistics from all Scottish hospitals other than obstetric ones (Heasman, 1968; Baldwin, 1971; Lockwood, 1971).

Since the SMRMH form on which information regarding each patient is recorded includes a section on occupation, data have been collected regarding all doctors treated in Scottish psychiatric in-patient beds since 1963. Furthermore, the 1961 and 1971 National Censuses for Scotland also included questions on occupation, thus providing an estimate of the population from which these sick doctors were drawn.

METHODS

In-Patient Statistics

DOCTORS. Information was obtained from the SHRIU regarding the first admissions to (for the years 1963, 1965, 1968, 1972) and total discharges from (for the years 1963-72) Scottish mental hospitals and psychiatric units, of male medical practitioners aged 25 years and over. That regarding first admissions consisted of primary diagnosis and age, while that concerning total discharges also included mode of referral to hospital and legal status of admission.

A minimum of 25 years was chosen because of the relatively small numbers of qualified doctors below that age. Female doctors were excluded because of the practice of coding the occupation of a married woman as that of her husband; including them would have led to inaccuracies in the data as a result of the inclusion of some non-medical wives of doctors and the exclusion of some married women doctors.

CONTROLS. There is considerable evidence that social class affects the occurrence and treatment of mental illness (Hollingshead and Redlich, 1958; Brown et al, 1975). As doctors are classified as belonging to social class I (Office of Population Censuses and Surveys, 1970), non-medical social class I males were chosen as controls. There may, of course, be differences between male doctors and non-medical social class I males other than occupation which could influence the occurrence of mental illness. For example, doctors might be more upwardly socially mobile than other social class I males; or, again, doctors developing mental illness might more easily retain their occupational classification. However, non-medical social class I males appear to be closer than any other group to male doctors in social and economic status. Therefore, similar information regarding their admissions to and discharges from Scottish in-patient psychiatric beds was obtained from the SHRIU.

Reliability

The SHRIU regularly check that the number of SMRMH forms received from each hospital are in accordance with the number recorded on the statistical summary form H.S.10; the unexplained discrepancy between the two totals is less than 1 percent. Part of this discrepancy may result from psychiatrists wishing to protect their patients' anonymity and consequently forbidding the dispatch of the SMRMH form. This might occur more frequently with doctors than with other social class I males and so cause an underestimate of the numbers of sick doctors.

The Committee on Hospital Medical Records in Scotland (Scottish Home and Health Department, 1967) recommended that the consultant in administrative charge should be responsible for ensuring the accuracy of hospital in-patient records, including the SMRMH form. It would be unrealistic to assume that all such consultants carry out their duties enthusiastically, or that records clerks do not make errors in transcription and coding. Indeed, in a study of returns to the SHRIU regarding general hospital patients, Lockwood (1971) showed that errors did occur. However, it is likely that the majority of such errors would be equally distributed among the doctors and controls.

General Population Statistics

Information was obtained from the Registrar General for Scotland regarding the age distribution and numbers of all male medical practitioners aged 25 years and over residing in Scotland at the time of the 1961 and 1971 censuses. Similar information was obtained concerning all males of 25 years and over classified as belonging to social class I, and thus the numbers of nonmedical social class I males was calculated. The numbers and age distribution of male doctors and non-medical social class I males were then estimated for each of the years 1963 to 1972, assuming population change to be distributed equally over the years 1961 to 1971, and the same trends were projected to 1972.

Appropriateness of the General Population Statistics

Do the National Censuses for Scotland provide a wholly accurate estimate of the population served by the Scottish in-patient psychiatric beds? Some of the individuals included in the in-patient statistics could have entered Scotland specifically for psychiatric treatment. This may be particularly the case for doctors; some English doctors may have elected to undergo psychiatric treatment in Scotland to prevent their illness becoming public knowledge among their colleagues and patients. On the other hand, some Scottish residents may have had psychiatric treatment at English hospitals for similar reasons of anonymity. There seems no reason to suppose that both doctors and other social class I males moving into Scotland for psychiatric treatment would not be balanced by those moving out of Scotland for the same reason.

Another potential inaccuracy concerns private treatment. Any doctor or other social class I male receiving in-patient psychiatric care outside a National Health Service Hospital would not be included in the SHRIU data. Thus the base populations cited above might be an overestimate of the populations served by the Scottish psychiatrist in-patient beds. However, as there are very few private in-patient psychiatric beds in Scotland, this is unlikely to be a major source of inaccuracy.

RESULTS

First Admissions

A total of 110 male doctors and 379 non-medical social class I males aged 25 years and over were admitted for the first time to Scottish psychiatric in-patient beds during the four years studied.

The primary diagnoses ascribed to the doctors and non-doctors are shown in Table 20-I, and their age distribution in Fig 20-1.

Table 20-1

Primary diagnoses ascribed to doctors and Social Class I controls

Primary diagnosis	Number of first admissions of doctors (% in brackets)	Number of first admissions of social class I controls (% in brackets)
Schizophrenia	6 (6)	27 (7)
Affective psychoses ..	14 (13)	56 (15)
Senile and pre-senile psychosis	5 (5)	41 (11)
Other psychoses ..	4 (4)	15 (4)
Neurotic and functional depression	20 (18)	57 (15)
Neuroses	4 (4)	21 (6)
Personality and behaviour disorders	0 (0)	13 (3)
Alcoholism	42 (38)	121 (32)
Drug dependence ..	5 (5)	7 (2)
Other conditions ..	10 (9)	21 (6)
	110	379

Total rates. The overall mean annual first admission rates were 431 per 100,000 for male doctors and 189 per 100,000 for non-doctors. Rates were higher for doctors than for non-doctors in all age-groups (Fig 20-2), but the disparity was greatest for those aged 65 years and over; the rates were 2.1 times higher for doctors amongst those aged 25-64 years, but 4.4 times higher for doctors amongst those aged 65 years and over.

This greater disparity was not due to any increase in the absolute numbers of elderly doctors admitted (Fig 20-1), but to there being apparently relatively fewer doctors than non-medical social class I males aged 65 years and over in the Scottish population; the ratio of doctors to non-doctors among social class I males dropped from one doctor for every 7.5 non-doctors among those aged 25-64 years to one doctor for every 17.7 non-doctors among those aged 65 years

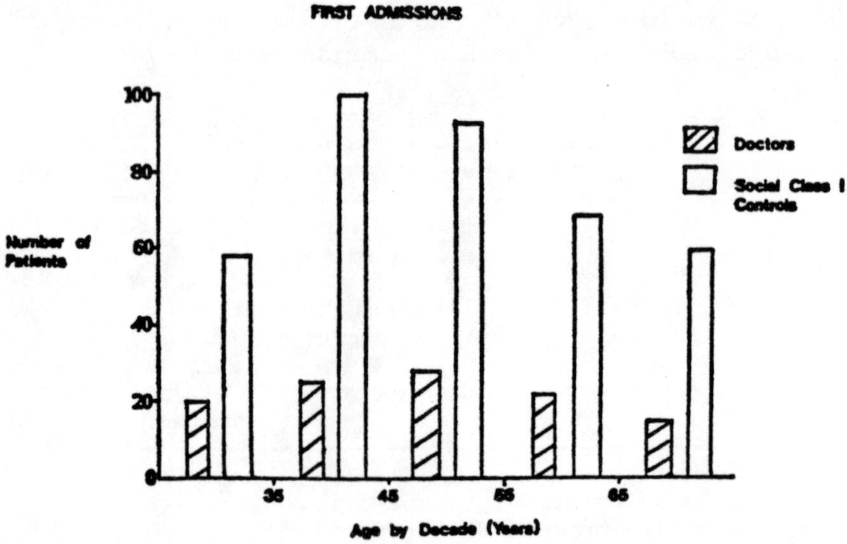

Figure 20-1.

and over. This is unlikely to have been due to increased mortality among doctors, since they have a greater than average life expectancy. Further perusal of the census statistics revealed that the percentage of the population unclassified occupationally rose by a factor of four among those aged 65 years and over. Thus, a substantial number of retired doctors might not have been accredited as such in the national statistics.

RATES FOR THOSE AGED 25-64 YEARS. Because of the likely unreliability of the occupational data for those aged over 64 years, and because the majority of elderly individuals, being retired, would not be subject to the potential stresses of medical practice, the data were reanalysed for those aged 25-64 years. The overall mean annual first admission rate for this age range was 449 per 100,000 for male doctors and 205 per 100,000 for nonmedical social class I males. The rates for all psychotic illnesses were 121 per 100,000 for doctors and 74 per 100,000 for non-doctors, and for all non-psychotic illness 329 per 100,000 and 131 per 100,000 respectively. Thus the first admission rates for all psychotic illness were 1.6 times higher among doctors, while the rates for all non-psychotic illness were 2.5 times higher among doctors.

The rates were higher among doctors for all diagnostic categories with the exception of personaltiy and behaviour disorders, but the differences between doctors and non-doctors were not significant for

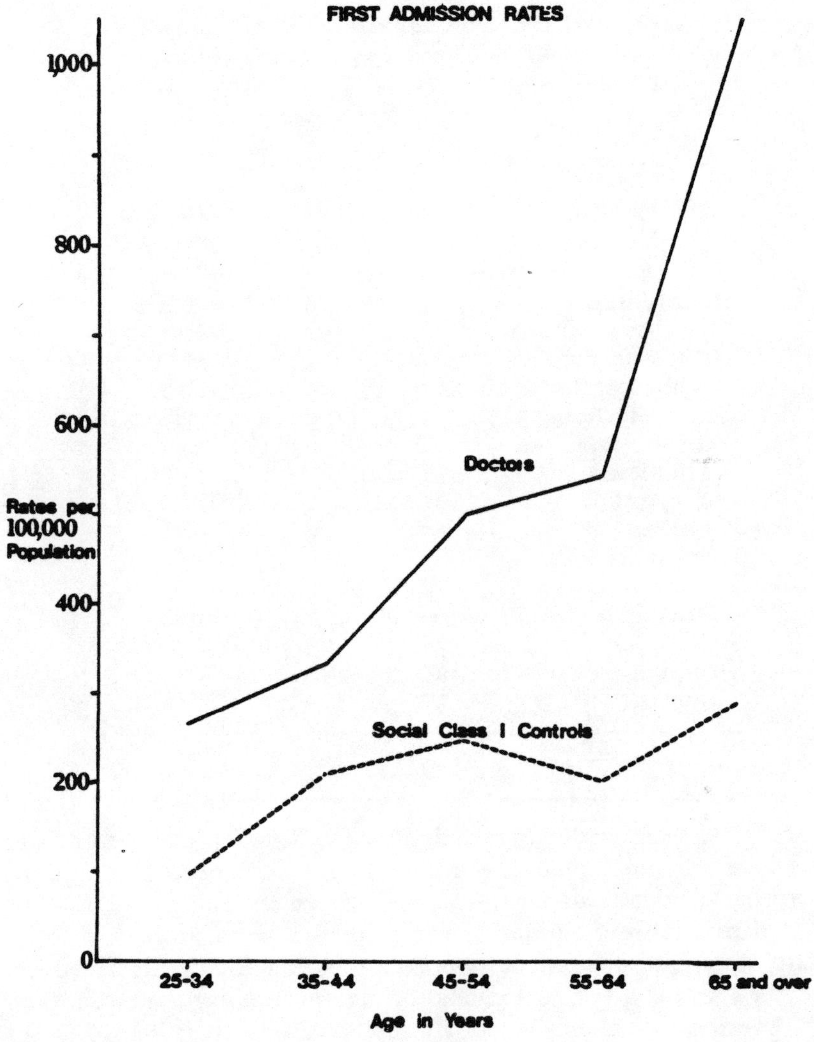

Figure 20-2.

schizophrenia, senile and presenile psychosis, other psychoses and neurosis (Table 20-II). The greatest disparities were in the rates for alcoholism and for drug dependence which were respectively 2.6 and 5.3 times higher among doctors.

Discharges

There were, over the years 1963 to 1972, a total of 686 dis-

Table 20-II

Mean annual first admission rates among those aged 25-64 years for different diagnostic categories

Primary diagnosis	Rates per 100,000		
	Doctors	Social class I controls	Statistical significance
Schizophrenia ..	25	15	NS
Affective psychosis	58	31	$P < 0{\cdot}05$
Senile and pre-senile psychosis	21	19	NS
Other psychosis	17	9	NS
Neurotic and functional depression ..	83	31	$P < 0{\cdot}001$
Neuroses ..	17	12	NS
Personality and behaviour disorders ..	—	7	NS
Alcoholism ..	171	67	$P < 0{\cdot}001$
Drug dependence	21	4	$P < 0{\cdot}01$
Other conditions	37	10	$P < 0{\cdot}001$
	449	205	

charges* of male medical practitioners and 2,008 discharges of other social class I males aged 25 years and over. The primary diagnosis ascribed to doctors and controls are shown in Table 20-III. Age-related trends were similar to those for first admission, with once again the greatest disparities amongst those aged 65 years and over. For the reasons given previously this age-group was then excluded. The overall discharge rates for those aged 25-64 years were 985 per 100,000 for male doctors and 382 per 100,000 for non-medical social class I controls. There were no significant trends in rates over the decade for either group.

Different Diagnostic Categories. The rates for all ten diagnostic categories were higher for doctors than for controls (Table 20-IV). Discharge rates for all psychotic illnesses were 1.8 times higher among doctors and those for all non-psychotic illness 3.1 times higher among doctors. The differences between the two groups did not

*The term discharges is henceforth used to refer to both discharges and deaths.

Table 20-III

Primary diagnoses ascribed to Doctors and social class I controls

Primary diagnosis	Number of discharges of Doctors (% in brackets)	Number of discharges of social class I controls (% in brackets)
Schizophrenia	45 (7)	220 (11)
Affective psychosis ..	81 (12)	351 (18)
Senile and presenile psychoses	21 (3)	136 (7)
Other psychoses ..	33 (5)	53 (3)
Neurotic and functional depression	100 (15)	231 (12)
Neurosis	21 (3)	128 (6)
Personality and behaviour disorders ..	46 (7)	128 (6)
Alcoholism	273 (40)	651 (33)
Drug dependence ..	39 (6)	32 (2)
Other conditions ..	27 (4)	78 (4)
	686	2,008

Table 20-IV

Mean annual discharge rates among those aged 25-64 years for different diagnostic categories

Primary diagnosis	Rates per 100,000		
	Doctors	Controls	Statistical significance
Schizophrenia ..	63	45	NS
Affective psychosis	103	66	$P < 0{\cdot}01$
Senile and presenile psychosis ..	7	4	NS
Other psychosis ..	42	8	$P < 0{\cdot}001$
Neurotic and functional depression ..	122	45	$P < 0{\cdot}001$
Neurosis	32	27	NS
Personality and behaviour disorders ..	76	26	$P < 0{\cdot}001$
Alcoholism ..	439	133	$P < 0{\cdot}001$
Drug dependence	65	6	$P < 0{\cdot}001$
Other conditions ..	17	11	$P < 0{\cdot}001$

reach statistical significance for schizophrenia, senile and presenile psychosis and neurosis, but were highly significant for the remaining diagnostic categories, the greatest differences being in rates for drug dependence, which were 10.8 times higher for doctors (Fig 20-3).

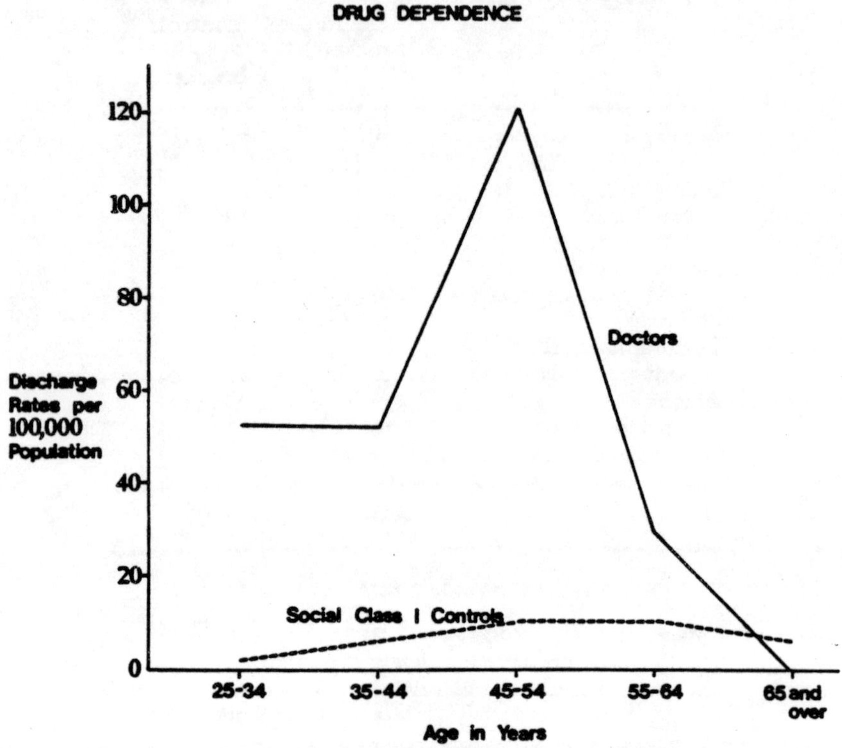

Figure 20-3.

Over the decade a total of 11 male doctors aged between 25 and 64 years died in hospital. Four of these had a primary diagnosis of alcoholism, three a primary diagnosis of drug dependence, and one each of schizophrenia, affective psychosis, senile/presenile psychosis, and "other conditions."

REFERRAL PATTERNS. The pattern of referral to hospital of the male doctors and non-medical social class I males was also examined. The doctor-patients tended to have been more frequently referred by (a) themselves, their relatives and friends and (b) medical sources other than general practitioners, and to have been less frequently referred by (e) general practitioners, (f) local authority agencies and (g) other agencies.

Legal Status on Admission

The percentages of patients admitted under compulsion were almost identical in the two groups, being 7.8 percent for the doctors and 8.0 percent for the controls.

DISCUSSION

The Special Position of Doctors

This study has demonstrated that, in Scotland at least, male doctors are more likely to receive in-patient psychiatric care than other males of similar socioeconomic status. One cannot immediately assume that this is a true reflection of the relative frequency of psychiatric illness in the two groups, because sick doctors may be more likely to come to the attention of psychiatrists for reasons such as their greater familiarity with the referral procedures. On the other hand, some authorities (a'Brook et al., 1967; Simon and Lumry, 1968; Gola, 1972) have suggested that sick doctors are particularly unwilling to accept that they have emotional problems or that they need specialist help. To establish with any degree of certainty the relative prevalence of psychiatric disorder among doctors and their social peers in the community, it would be necessary to undertake a large epidemiological survey of doctors and matched controls without reference to the medical services.

The present more modest investigation has shown that doctors do indeed make use of their greater access to psychiatrists. One cannot be sure, however, that their increased self-referral to hospital contributed to their higher rates of admission. It is possible that the doctors who referred themselves were less ill and therefore, would not have reached psychiatrists but for their ease of access. Alternatively, without such access they might have been referred through more orthodox channels.

Vincent et al. (1969) found doctors very reluctant to accept treatment, and claimed that "all (studies) concur in the extreme reluctance of physicians to admit and to seek help for emotional problems." Of the doctors treated by Vincent and his colleagues 20 percent were admitted under a compulsory procedure compared with only 6 percent of controls. There is no evidence from the present study to suggest that doctors are particularly unwilling to be admitted voluntarily to psychiatric care.

It was of some interest that the ratio of the rates for doctors to non-doctors was not quite as high for first admissions (2.3 : 1) as for all discharges (2.7 : 1). Thus, while the higher rates of all discharges among doctors were not mainly the consequence of their more frequent relapse or readmission, part of the excess might have been so caused. A further possibility is raised (a) by Duffy and Litin's (1964) contention that psychiatrists tend to take an over-optmistic view of the prognosis for their doctor-patients, and (b) by the finding of a'Brook et al. (1967) and Vincent et al. (1969) that sick doctors are particularly likely to discharge themselves precipitately from treatment. These studies suggest that doctors may be less likely to remain in hospital as long-term patients.

To test this possibility, data concerning discharges of first admissions for the years already studied were obtained from the SHRIU. The discharge rates thus calculated were 2.4 times higher for male doctors than for non-medical social class I males. Thus, if preferential discharge operates it is only a minor factor; the bulk of the difference between the doctor : non-doctor ratio for first admissions and that for all discharges appears to be the consequence of more frequent readmission of doctors.

The same ratios were also calculated for each diagnostic category (Table 20-V). The greatest disparities between the doctor : non-doctor ratio for first admission rates and all discharge rates were in respect of drug dependence, alcoholism and senile psychosis.

Three explanations come to mind. (1) The prognosis for these conditions may be worse for male doctors than for non-medical social class I males. (2) Doctors suffering from these conditions may be more likely than non-doctors to be re-referred to psychiatrists. (3) Psychiatrists may more readily readmit doctors than non-doctors suffering from these conditions.

The first explanation is unlikely to apply. The prognosis of senile psychosis is not known to be affected by occupational factors. Small and his colleagues (1969) have suggested that alcoholic doctors fare no worse than other alcoholics, and Putnam and Ellingwood (1966) considered that the prognosis for addict doctors is better than that for other addicts. There is at present no way of ascertaining whether the second explanation applies or not, but the third explanation is worthy of further examination.

The three conditions — senile psychosis, drug dependence and alcoholism — have in common a relatively poor prognosis. Thus, if a substantial proportion of psychiatrists believe, rightly or wrongly, that repeated readmission has little beneficial effect in these conditions they may offer readmission only to a minority of those seeking it. This minority may include a higher relative proportion of doctors because of the psychiatrists' closer identification with them.

Table 20-V

Ratios of rates for doctors as against social class I controls among those aged 24-64 years

	Ratios		
	First admission rates Doctors/non-doctors (A)	All discharge rates Doctors/non-doctors (B)	(B)/(A)
Schizophrenia	1·6 : 1	1·4 : 1	0·9
Affective psychosis ..	1·9 : 1	1·6 : 1	0·8
Senile psychosis	1·1 : 1	1·8 : 1	1·6
Neurotic and functional depression ..	2·7 : 1	2·7 : 1	1·1
Neurosis ..	1·4 : 1	1·2 : 1	0·9
Personality and behaviour disorder* ..			
Alcoholism ..	2·6 : 1	3·3 : 1	1·3
Drug dependence	5·3 : 1	10·8 : 1	2·0
Other psychosis } Other conditions }	2·8 : 1	3·1 : 1	1·1

* No comparison could be made because no doctors had been admitted for the first time with such a diagnosis over the four-year period.

Conditions Possibly More Prevalent Among Doctors

It seems unlikely that the special position of doctors accounts for all of the excess in admission and discharge rates respecting at least the three conditions – drug dependence, alcoholism and depression – for which there were the greatest disparities between doctors and non-doctors. It has, of course, often been said in the past that these are the three conditions which doctors are especially prone to.

Drugs are uniquely available to doctors, and Vaillant and his colleagues (1970; 1972) found that a group of doctors followed up over 20 years took more tranquilizers, stimulants and sedatives than other college graduates. Almost all articles on psychiatric illness in doctors have commented on the frequency of drug dependence, and reviews, e.g. Murray, 1974; Waring, 1974, have concluded that drug dependence is an occupational hazard for those practising medicine. Indeed, although first admission rates for drug dependence in this study were five times higher for male doctors than for other social class I males, the actual percentage of doctor-patients diagnosed as drug-dependent at 5 percent was smaller than that recorded in any other study of mentally ill doctors. This may reflect the relative infrequency of drug abuse in Scotland during the period under study (Scottish Home and Health Department, 1970). There are no published data on comparative attitudes to drug taking among Scottish and other doctors, but Mackay et al. (1973) found that the consumption of cannabis by medical students in Glasgow was much less than that reported for English and North American students.

Alcoholism has been prominent in published series of mentally ill doctors, but a larger percentage of doctors in this study were alcoholic than in all but one (Simon and Lumry, 1968). This is probably related to the particular frequency of alcoholism in Scotland (MacCrae et al. 1972; Sclare, 1975). However, there can be little doubt that numerically alcoholism is a greater problem among doctors than drug dependence, not only in Scotland but elsewhere (Murray, 1976b). It is also less easy to see why doctors should be particularly at risk for alcoholism.

Some researchers have considered that depression, too, was especially prevalent among doctors. Blachly and his colleagues (1968) believed this to be true and suggested that traits such as 'compulsive attention to detail, high aspirations and prolonged deferral of gratification' which are valued in doctors also make them particularly prone to depression. Reports demonstrating that this is indeed true are hard to find, although in their follow-up study Vaillant and his colleagues (1972) noted that at times of crisis doctors were more likely than other college graduates to show "hypochondriasis and turning against self."

Some, e.g. Waring (1974) have assumed that since the suicide rate is higher in doctors than in the general population, this implies that affective disorder is also more prevalent. Such reasoning does not take into account doctors' greater access to drugs and their greater likelihood of knowing the dose of drugs necessary to make a successful rather than an unsuccessful attempt at suicide.

In conclusion, it appears that there is evidence from the literature to suggest that the higher rates of admission to hospital for drug dependence and alcoholism in male doctors which I have described do indeed reflect the greater prevalence of these conditions among doctors. No such supportive evidence has been forthcoming from the literature with regard to depression. Thus, whether the prevalence of, as opposed to admission rates for, depression is greater among doctors remains an open question.

REFERENCES

a'Brook, M. F., Hailstone, J. D. & McLaughlin, E. J. (1967) Psychiatric illness in the medical profession. *British Journal of Psychiatry,* **113,** 1013-23.

Baldwin, J. A. (1971) *The Mental Hospital in the Psychiatric Service: a Case Register Study.* London.

Blachly, P. H., Disher, W. & Roduner, G. (1968) Suicide by physicians. *Bulletin of Suicidology,* 1-18.

Brown, G. W., Bhrolchain, M. & Harris, T. (1975) Social class and psychiatric disturbance in an urban population. *Sociology,* **9,** 225-54.

Court-Brown, W. M. & Doll, R. (1958) Expectation of life and mortality from cancer amongst British radiologists. *British Medical Journal, ii,* 181-7.

Dickinson, F. G. & Martin, L. W. (1956) Physician mortality, 1949-1951. *Journal of the American Medical Association,* **162,** 1462-8.

Drukker, W., Schoutten, W. A. G. & Alberts, Chr. (1968) Report on regular dialysis treatment in Europe, 4. *Proceedings of the European Dialysis and Transplant Association,* **5,** 3.

Duffy, J. C. & Litin, E. M. (1964) Psychiatric morbidity of physicians. *Journal of the American Medical Association,* **189,** 989-92.

Edwards, G. (1973) The alcoholic doctors: a case of neglect. *Lancet, ii,* 1297-8.

Emerson, H. & Hughes, H. E. (1926) Death rates of male white physicians in the United States by age and cause. *American Journal of Public Health,* **16,** 1088-93.

Everson, R. B. & Fraumeni, J. F. (1957) Mortality among medical students and young physicians. *Journal of Medical Education,* **50,** 809-11.

Glatt, M. (1974) Alcoholism among doctors. *Lancet, ii,* 342-3.

——— (1976) The alcoholic doctors. *Lancet, i,* 196.

Gola, N. (1972) The doctor, his illness and the patient. *Australian and New Zealand Journal of Psychiatry,* **6,** 209-13.

Harrington, J. M. (1975) The hazards of being a doctor. *Modern Medicine,* November, pp 26-30.

Heasman, M. A. (1968) Scottish hospitals in-patient statistics: sources and uses. *Health Bulletin,* **26,** 4, 1-9.

Hollingshead, A. B. & Redlich, F. C. (1958) *Social Class and Mental Illness.* New York: Wiley.

Knill-Jones, R. P., Rodrigues, L. V., Moir, D. D. & Spence, A. A. (1972) Anaesthetic practice and pregnancy. *Lancet, i,* 1326-8.

Lockwood, E. (1971) Accuracy of Scottish hospital morbidity data. *British Journal of Preventive and Social Medicine,* **25,** 76-83.

MacCrae, A. K. M., Ratcliffe, R. A. W. & Liddle, S. M. (1972) Alcoholism in Scotland in the 1960s. *Health Bulletin, 30*, 16-22.

McKay, A. J., Hawthorne, V. M. & McCartney, H. N. (1973) Drug taking among medical students at Glasgow University. *British Medical Journal, i,* 540-3.

Murray, R. M. (1974) Psychiatric illness in doctors. *Lancet, i,* 1211-13.

—— (1976a) Psychiatric Illness in Doctors. M.Phil. Thesis, University of London.

—— (1976b) Alcoholism amongst male doctors in Scotland. *Lancet, ii,* 729-31.

Office of Population Censuses and Surveys (1970) *Classification of Occupations.* London: HMSO.

Pond, D. A. (1969) Doctors' mental health. *New Zealand Medical Journal,* **69**, 131-5.

Putnam, P. L., & Ellingwood, E. H. (1966) Narcotic addiction among physicians. *American Journal of Psychiatry,* **122**, 745-8.

Quarles, Frances (1592-1644) *Hieroglyphics, IV. Nicocles.* Reprinted in the Complete Edition included in the Chertsey Worthies Library, 1874.

Ramazzini, B. (1731) *De Morbis Artificium.* Translated by W. C. Wright, Chicago, 1940.

Registrar General (1971) *Decennial Supplement, England and Wales: 1959-1963 on Occupational Mortality.* London: HMSO.

Reid, D. D. (1957) Incidence of tuberculosis amongst workers in medical laboratories. *British Medical Journal, ii,* 1-14.

Sclare, A. B. (1975) Alcoholism in Scotland. *International Journal of Offender Therapy and Comparative Criminology,* **19**, 241-9.

Scottish Home and Health Department (1970) *Drug Misuse in Scotland.* Edinburgh: HMSO.

—— (1967) *Hospital Medical Records in Scotland.* Edinburgh: HMSO.

Shaw, G. B. (1911) *Preface to 'The Doctor's Dilemma'.* Reprinted in Collected Plays with their Prefaces. London: The Bodley Head, 1931.

Simon, W. & Lumry, G. K. (1968) Suicide among physician-patients. *Journal of Nervous and Mental Diseases,* **147**, 105-12.

Small, I. F., Small, J. G., Assue, C. M. & Moore, D. F. (1969) The fate of the mentally ill physician. *American Journal of Psychiatry,* **125**, 1333-42.

Standing Medical Advisory Committee on Alcoholism (1973). London: HMSO.

Vaillant, G. E., Brighton, J. R. & McArthur, C. (1970) Physicians' use of mood-altering drugs. *New England Journal of Medicine,* **282**, 365-70.

—— Sobowale, N. C. & MacArthur, C. (1972) Some psychological vulnerabilities of physicians. *New England Journal of Medicine,* **287**, 372-5.

Vincent, M. O., Robinson, E. A. & Latt, L. (1969) Physicians as patients. *Canadian Medical Association Journal,* **100**, 403-12.

Waring, E. M. (1974) Psychiatric illness in physicians: a review. *Comprehensive Psychiatry,* **15**, 519-29.

Williams, S. V., Munford, R. S., Colton, T., Murphy, D. A. & Poskanzer, D. C. (1971) Mortality among physicians: a cohort study. *Journal of Chronic Disease,* **24**, 393-401.

Chapter 21

MEDICAL PROFESSIONALS WITH EMOTIONAL ILLNESS: A CONTROLLED STUDY OF THE HAZARDS OF BEING A "SPECIAL PATIENT"

E. M. WARING

INTRODUCTION

PREVIOUS studies suggest that psychiatric illness in physicians and nurses is correlated with life adjustment prior to professional training.[12,8,7,5] Despite these empirical findings, an apparently common belief exists that professional medical pressures are sufficient to cause emotional illness. This may reflect a psychological "denial" by health professionals that emotional illness can occur as readily in nurses and physicians as in the general population. Marmor's comment with reference to physicians, "the constant exercise of authority carries with it the occupational hazard of tending to create unrealistic feelings of superiority in the authority figure," seems applicable as an explanation of this common belief.[6] Thus medical and nursing schools have been reluctant to utilize or even consider some form of psychological screening as part of the admission requirements despite considerable evidence that students predisposed to psychiatric illness may be identifiable.

This study was designed to assess a further confirmation of previous empirical research suggesting that positive family histories, development disturbances, and previous psychiatric treatment will occur as frequently in the "medical group" as in the control group.

Previous studies also suggest that depression and drug addiction are the most common psychiatric disorders in the "medical profession."[1,11,3,10] Thus an analysis of the final diagnosis of the physician and nurse group were compared with the control group.

From E. M. Waring, Medical Professionals with Emotional Illness: A Controlled Study of the Hazards of Being a "Special Patient," *The Psychiatric J of the University of Ottawa/Rev. de Psychiatrie del'Univ. d'Ottawa*, Vol. II, No. 4, 1977.

From the Clarke Institute of Psychiatry, University of Toronto, Toronto, Ontario. Research was carried out while the author was a Teaching Fellow at the Institute.

Finally, in a previous paper the author suggests on the basis of his own clinical experience in treating health professionals and a review of the literature that the major "occupational hazard" influencing the form and outcome of emotional illness in physicians is the type and quality of psychiatric care they receive.[13] The author suggested that physicians in general receive poor psychiatric care because: (1) physicians seldom seek professional help early in the course of their disorder, (2) "special patient" status produces negative staff reactions in in-patient units, and (3) transference and counter-transference problems between psychiatrists and medical professionals create difficulties in management.[4,9,1,3,2]

An attempt was made in this study to objectively confirm or reject the above hypothesis. A number of objective but arbitrarily chosen demographic parameters of "quality of care" were selected based on the author's clinical experience, and these parameters were compared with a control group of non-medical psychiatric in-patients. The predictions are listed in Table 21-I.

Table 21-I

RATIONALE FOR PREDICTIONS

1. The length of stay of the doctor-nurse group (D-N) would be shorter than the controls (C).
2. Readmission would be less frequent in the D-N group.
3. The D-N group would receive a greater number of therapeutic drugs than the C group.
4. Discharge against medical advice would be more frequent in the D-N group.
5. Involuntary admission would be common in the C group.
6. Regardless of diagnosis, drug abuse would be more prevalent in the D-N Group.
7. Suicide attempt would be more frequent in the D-N group.
8. More of the D-N group would have out-of-town home addresses.
9. Fewer psychological assessments would be done in the D-N group.
10. Fewer family assessments would be done in the D-N group.

The rationale of the above predictions merits further discussion. As an example it was predicted that the D-N group would have a short hospital stay. Physicians admitted to psychiatric units frequently feel embarrassment and have difficulty accepting a "patient role" and socializing with other patients, creating tension within themselves and on the ward, both with in-patients and staff. The physician or the nurse frequently escapes from this intolerable situation with premature discharge.

It is obvious that the shorter stay predicted (as with the other predictions) could be interpreted as an example of a more rapid improvement in the socially advantaged group. Unfortunately, the objectivity of the parameters chosen, and their ease of recording without observer bias, also makes them open to various interpretations which cannot be validated. It is also questionable whether these parameters reflect only "quality of care." Obviously, positive results in the direction indicated will only confirm that the two groups are different, and it is the author's inference from his own clinical experience that this difference is related to treatment difficulties. However, the author suggests that the predictions are based on clinical experience and have the advantage of being easily reproduced by other investigators. It was felt that (1) greater drug abuse, more suicide attempts would reflect physician reluctance to seek help, (2) a shorter stay in hospital, informal status, fewer family interviews, fewer psychological assessments, more out-of-town admissions, and fewer readmissions in the D-N group would reflect "special status," and (3) greater discharge against advice and higher drug prescribing may reflect transference-countertransference problems.

METHOD

A review was made of all patients admitted to the Clarke Institute of Psychiatry's in-patient unit from 1966 until the total sample had been collected in 1971. All physicians and nurses who were admitted to a total of 30 in each group were selected for study. When an index was identified, the next admission of the same sex, same age (plus or minus five years), and the same initial diagnosis was selected as a control case. The data were collected on precoded data sheet including demographic variables and information regarding the parameters previously mentioned. The doctors' data were compared with their control group using chi-square analysis. This procedure was repeated for the nursing group and their controls and finally the D-N group was similarly compared with the total control group.

RESULTS

The admission rate of one physician admission for 113 nonphysician admissions is somewhat higher than the proportions discussed previously in the paper by a'Brook et al. It is also important to note that the physician admissions declined dramatically from the opening of the Clarke Institute of Psychiatry in 1966 until completion of the study in 1971. This would seem to reflect, in the author's opinion, a generally held perception of the hospital when it was first opened as a special institute for "special patients," and that over a period of time this image of the hospital diminished.

The data regarding family history, of developmental and past history, and previous treatment were not compared statistically between groups. The majority of cases whether "medical" or control had positive family histories of psychiatric illnesses prior to professional study. The author felt that a few case examples might convey more information than a statistical comparison of the doctor-nurse group with their controls showing no difference. In a few cases, the index case or the controls had only two of the three criteria, but this did not differ between the groups. These two histories are presented because they are typical and not unusual, confirming previous research that the major contributing factor to emotional illness in physicians and nurses is the personality that they bring with them into professional training.

CASE #1: This 33-year-old nurse was admitted with a diagnosis of anxiety reaction. Her father had committed suicide when she was eight. Her mother was a diagnosed schizophrenic and one sister was schizophrenic. A brother had died and suicide was suspected. She described her childhood as barren and cold and first sought psychiatric help for anxiety symptoms two years prior to application for nursing school.

CASE #2: A 28-year-old male physician was admitted to hospital following a suicide attempt. There was a family history of schizophrenia in aunts and uncles, but not in first degree relatives. His father went bankrupt, embarrassing the family. One brother committed suicide and a sister was in psychotherapy following a suicide attempt. He was hostile and uncooperative with staff. The diagnosis was depression.

Because the patients are matched with the controls for initial diagnosis, no comparison was possible. However, it is well known that initial diagnosis in psychiatric hospitals are quite unreliable. Thus the final diagnoses in the D-N group were compared with the control group (see Table 21-II). From the table it can be seen that 27 of 60 in the D-N group versus 24 of 60 in the control group had a final diagnosis of depression. Thus, depression was more common in

Table 21-II

COMPARISON OF DOCTOR, NURSE, AND CONTROL TREATMENT VARIABLES

Variables	Nurse N = 30	Nurse Control N = 30	*	Doctor N = 30	Doctor Control N = 30	*	D-N Group N = 60	Control Group N = 60	*
1. Length of Stay	35.3	42.0	N.S.	38.0	38.1	N.S.	40.0	40.0	N.S.
2. Number Readmitted	10	17	N.S.	11	16	N.S.	39	39	N.S.
3. No. of Drugs: Therapeutic (>4)	13	10	N.S.	15	13	N.S.	28	23	N.S.
4. Discharge Against Advice	4	4	N.S.	1	1	N.S.	5	5	N.S.
5. Involuntary Admission	0	5	7.38	3	7	3.89	3	12	8.9
6. Drug Abuse	8	1	7.16	12	2	10.1	20	3	17.0
7. Suicide Attempts	16	11	N.S.	17	6	8.8	33	17	8.9
8. Out-Ot-Town Admission	7	1	5.75	12	4	5.64	19	5	10.7
9. Psychological Testing	9	5	N.S.	7	8	N.S.	16	13	N.S.
10. Family Assessment	7	11	N.S.	10	17	3.33	17	28	4.33
11. Final Diagnosis (Drug Abuse)	2	0	N.S.	4	0	N.S.	6	0	8.63
12. Final Diagnosis (Depression)	15	11	N.S.	12	13	N.S.	27	24	N.S.

* x^2 values for significant difference $p > 0.05$

the D-N group, but not significantly so. Similarly it can be noted that 6 of 60 or 10 percent of the D-N group had a final diagnosis of drug addiction ($p > 0.05$) as compared to no cases in the control group. It should also be noted that the diagnosis of depression and drug addiction made up approximately 57 percent of the diagnoses in the D-N group.

Finally, the results of the hypothesis that the doctor-nurse group is different from the control group was examined (see Table 21-II). In summary, of the ten parameters studied, five were confirmed at statistically significant levels (family interviews, admission status, drug abuse, suicide attempts, out-of-town admissions). In three, the values were in the expected direction but did not quite reach statistical significance (readmissions, length of stay, number of drugs). In two (psychological testing and discharge against advice), no differences were found although only in the cases of nurses' psychological reports, a trend in the opposite direction was noted. Thus, in total, using ten objective parameters of quality of care, some support is lent to the hypothesis that medical patients are considered "special patients." At least, in in-patient psychiatric settings, they may receive different care from other patients.

DISCUSSION

This study supports previous research suggesting that family history of psychiatric illness, childhood deprivation, and previous psychiatric history are the major predisposing variables in emotional illness in medical professionals. In no case was supportive evidence found that being a physician or a nurse was a precipitating factor in admission to hospital. The implications of the above to the selection of applicants to medical and nursing schools have been previously discussed by the author.

Again supporting previous research, drug addiction was shown to be significantly more prevalent in medical professionals than controls. Although depression was more common, this was not a significant finding. Finally the hypothesis that physicians and nurses with psychiatric illness are a "special group" in terms of several arbitrarily chosen objective parameters received some support. These findings suggest that "medical connections" may be a perpetuating factor in the treatment of this group for psychiatric illness in the in-patient setting.

Ironically it would seem that despite convincing the general population that emotional problems are both nothing to be ashamed of and responsive to psychiatric interventions, the findings of decreased physician admission rates over time, the higher prevalence rate of out-of-town admissions and short stays suggests that we have not convinced our medical colleagues. The higher rates of suicide attempts and drug addiction suggests that physicians are reluctant to seek help until desperate. This seems especially frustrating in the light of the finding that 50 percent of the medical group suffered from affective disorders or drug addiction which are currently relatively responsive to psychiatric therapy. Thus the author concludes that previous epidemiological studies showing a higher rate of drug addiction and suicide in physicians, as opposed to other social class I occupational groups, are not a reflection of the higher prevalence of psychopathology, but a reflection of the poor quality of psychiatric care received by medical patients, for reasons discussed previously.

The evidence seems compelling that as a group physicians and nurses do "make the worst patients." This seems to relate to a reluctance on the part of physicians to initiate "help-seeking behaviour." Unfortunately undergraduate psychiatric education, contrary to the hopes and expectations of several authors, does not seem to have had much impact on this attitude. This study suggests "medical connections" may be a perpetuating factor in emotional illness, and that the counter-transference response of the psychiatrist may also be implicated in poor treatment outcome. Hopefully, an increased knowledge concerning the symptoms, causes, and pitfalls of treatment will make this task somewhat easier, and the psychiatrically ill physician will receive more humane treatment than he has in the past.

REFERENCES

1. a'Brook, M. F., Mailstone, J. D., McLaughlin, E. J.: "Psychiatric Illness in the Medical Profession," *Br. J. Psychiat. 113:* 1013-1023, 1967.
2. De Sole, D., Aronson, S., Singer, P.: Suicide and Role Strain Among Physicians, Presented to A.P.A. in Detroit. 1967.
3. Duffy, J. C., Litin, E. M.: "Psychiatric Morbidity of Physicians," *JAMA 189:* 989-992, 1964.
4. Gola, N.: "The Doctor, His Illness and Patient," *Aust. NZ J. Psychiatry, 6:* 209-213, 1972.
5. Hunter, R.C.A., Lohrenz, J. G., Schwartzman, A. E.: "Nosophobis and Hypochondriasis in Medical Students." *J. Nerv. Ment. Dis., 139:* 147-152, 1964.
6. Marmor, J.: "The Feeling of Superiority: An Occupational Hazard in the Practice of Psychotherapy." *Am. J. Psychiat., 110:* 370-376, 1953.
7. Modlin, H. D., Montes, A.: "Narcotic Addiction in Physicians," *Am. J.*

Psychiat., *121:* 358-369, 1964.

8. Pitts, R. N. Jr., Winokur, G., Steward, M. A.: "Psychiatric Syndromes, Anxiety Symptoms, and Response to Stress in Medical Students," *Am. J. Psychiat. 118:* 333-340, 1961.
9. Pollack, I. W., Battle, W. C.: "Studies of the Special Patient," *Arch. Gen. Psychiatry, 9:* 344-355, 1963.
10. Pond: "Doctors' Mental Health Ed. Mental Disturbance in Doctors," *NZ Med. J., 69:* 131-135, 1969.
11. Putnam, P. L., Ellinwood, E. H.: "Narcotic Addiction Among Physicians: A Ten—Year Follow-up," *Am. J. Psychiatry 122:* 745-748, 1966.
12. Vaillant, G. E., Sobowale, N. C., McArthur, C.: "Some Psychological Vulnerabilities of Physicians," *N. Engl. J. Med. 287:* 372-375, 1972.
13. Waring, E. M.: "Psychiatric Illness in Physicians: A Review," *Comprehens. Psychiat. 15:* 519-530, 1974.

Chapter 22

MARITAL THERAPY OF COUPLES IN WHICH THE HUSBAND IS A PHYSICIAN

ROBERT KRELL AND JAMES E. MILES

INTRODUCTION

EMOTIONAL illness in the physician as manifested in such problems as depression, alcoholism, and suicide have received considerable attention in the medical literature. Physician personalities have been scrutinized and described, but relatively little attention has been paid to the physician's marital relationship and his family. The authors of this paper express concern over the relative infrequency with which a physician with a disintegrating marriage comes to psychiatric attention. Few such situations seem to be perceived as worthy of therapeutic intervention, either by the couple in distress or by colleagues who know them, unless an exceptionally critical situation has led to the hospitalization of one or the other partner.

The reasons for not seeking help are many. Certainly, physicians have difficulty channeling themselves to appropriate care. This is particularly unfortunate since physicians do well in marital therapy situations. The physician's personality characteristics as described by Miles et al. (1) of emotional detachment, aloofness, control, rigidity do not speak for an encouraging prognosis in individual psychotherapy.

It has been noted by Vaillant et al. (2) that physicians were more likely than matched controls to have poor marriages, and by Evans (3) that in wives of physicians admitted to a psychiatric hospital, symptoms of depression, somatization, and addiction are prevalent and related dynamically and empirically to the profession of the husband. Miles (1), in a review of hospitalized wives of physicians, noted a high incidence of major marital conflict. A literature review reveals little specifically about individual therapy of physicians and

From Robert Krell and James E. Miles, Marital Therapy of Couples in Which the Husband is a Physician, *Am J Psychother, 30:* No. 2, 267-275, April, 1976.

even less about marital therapy of physician-couples. Pearson and Strecker (4), in a discussion of 66 private patients seen over a 15-year period, conclude that, "emotionally ill doctors do not seek help early enough for themselves, neglecting emotional problems as they do their physical disabilities."

In discussing the high incidence of suicide in doctors, a'Brook et al. (5) state their belief that "ultimate recourse to suicide could be avoided if doctors were less reluctant to seek help from their psychiatrically trained colleagues." They describe the treatment problems of physician colleagues as follows: "The doctor-patient's reluctance to accept his illness and his need for treatment, failure to take medication as prescribed, and a tendency to discontinue treatment prematurely were notable difficulties."

Debates abound in the literature as to whether or not the physician commits suicide more frequently than other professionals. Within the medical profession, colleagues discuss which of their specialty groups are most vulnerable. Some literature states that the physician has easier access to psychotherapy; other articles point out that the physician is reluctant to engage in either his own physical or emotional care.

For purposes of this discussion, information is drawn from 10 physician-couples who were in marital therapy. All physicians were men and all were about to separate or had just separated from their wives. Neither husband nor wife had ever been a patient in a psychiatric hospital. Six of the 10 wives were registered nurses. This is clearly a highly select group, composed largely of physician-husbands and nurse-wives. This may not be a rare situation. Modlin and Montes (6), who discuss 25 physicians addicted to narcotics and admitted to the C. S. Menninger Hospital, note that 24 were married, and of these, nine were married to nurses and one to a physician. Evans (3) hinted at physician-nurse couples in mentioning that "seven wives who at one time had actively participated in the husband's medical practice, stated that they felt excluded and left out after the husband acquired other nursing and office help."

Although the sampling is select, the similarities noted in both the referral and treatment patterns warrant the drawing of some tentative conclusions and the making of recommendations as well. We intend to comment on the peculiarities of the referral process and attendant strategy employed in seeking help, and finally to describe two composite case vignettes.

Referral Sequence

The road to therapy is a rocky one, as evidenced by the circuitous routes into outpatient psychiatric care of the couples under discussion. The maneuvers which dominated the pretreatment period were especially striking and effectively precluded these couples from seeing their problem as a problem of their relationship. Typically, the physician family has two comfortable referral routes, that is, ones less threatening to the physician in that family. One route is through the psychiatric evaluation of a child, where the therapeutic bonus might be "guidance" for the parents. The other is the more serious situation of the admission to the hospital of the physician's wife. The seemingly least comfortable route is one in which the physician himself asks for psychiatric care, although that is certainly more readily requested than marital therapy.

Several factors complicate the physician's attempt to seek therapy for a troubled marriage, and not the least of these is the propensity of some psychiatrists to work exclusively with individuals. This attitude appears to be less prevalent as training programs emphasize marital and family approaches at medical-student and resident levels (7). In addition, few of the physicians in our sample had experienced personal therapy and none was enthusiastic about his own psychiatric learning. They therefore did not seek routinely a psychiatric referral, but approached instead a "colleague-friend" who practiced psychiatry. These friends often provided support and guidance, but felt unable to provide continuing therapy because of their social relationships. These colleague-psychiatrists had encouraged referral for as long as two years before the suggestion was finally accepted.

Characteristic of the medical couple is the attempt to diagnose one or the other as the primary patient. Frequently the physician was successful in convincing his wife that she was emotionally disturbed and needed treatment. Occasionally he sent her to psychiatric colleagues who, upon seeing only her, might confirm such a diagnosis. At other times, the physician-husband, rather than blame his wife, engaged in self-observation of personality and marriage, and pronounced himself in need of treatment. Self-scrutiny was frequently forced by the wife's threat of separation unless the husband went for psychiatric care. In almost all instances, the couples reached agreements where only one partner was to get the blame (emotional illness) and the cure.

Further complications in seeking therapy may arise from the professional role relationship within physician-nurse marriages. Marriage roles are extremely complicated in and of themselves, and many authors have attempted to understand them in order to evolve appropriate treatment techniques (8). In our experience with physicians, the high proportion of nurse-wives drew attention not only to marital roles, but to interwoven, well-understood professional relationships. In such marriages, the nurse-wife invariably maintained partial responsibility for her husband's practice and frequently respected him as a physician no matter how intense her personal loathing of him within the marital relationship. Even in the worst moments she would handle patient calls and fuss over the efficiency of his office.

The degree to which such a physician-nurse team remains functional can complicate the marital disruption. Many such couples, within the throes of marital uncertainty, maintain a professional stance, especially upon conclusion of a diagnostic agreement. Self-diagnosis by such a couple may be followed by self-treatment. Some physicians were on heavy doses of self-prescribed psychoactive medications. Some were giving oral, intramuscular or intravenous medication to their wives. And yet, this medical interplay was often the only mutually agreeable form of communication remaining to these couples. The personal distress was immense and the professional role relationship provided relief from the marital failure.

Case 1

Dr. Smith, a 35-year-old physician, contacted a psychiatrist who had been a long-time friend, to tell him of his "marital problems and sexual inadequacy." He was referred and refused to bring his wife for the initial evaluation, stating the problem was his alone. He described very precisely long-standing sexual problems of impotence and premature ejaculation. He felt restless and unhappy and had separated from his wife with the intent of being cured and then returning to her as a "healthy person." Throughout several sessions, he continued to describe himself with obsessive detail; basically he appeared to be a rigid, defensive person who intellectualized a great deal, but had relatively little understanding. His anxiety had temporarily overcome his usual controls, but he remained competent at work, although he no longer derived pleasure from his work.

The prognosis for individual therapy seemed poor. His desperation increased as his marriage and career were jeopardized. He agreed to an interview of his wife, but did not wish to be present.

Mrs. Smith was an attractive 28-year-old woman who had seen several psychiatrists at her husband's insistence. She had been told she was the cause of the sexual problems. But she did not entirely believe them because the psychiatrists were her husband's "colleagues." She stated the problem was her husband's intense anxiety over possible failure at intercourse. An affectionate touch from her could render him nonresponsive if he thought the touch would lead to having to perform sexually. He soon reinterpreted her affection as "her weapon." She recognized that the problems predated the marriage. They had been married for seven years and had no children because her husband did not want any.

Three weeks after initial contact, Dr. and Mrs. Smith agreed to be seen together. Dr. Smith felt himself to be the inheritor of a long tradition within his family. Men were tough, adventurous, and unemotional in personal relationships. Men were powerful and virile. It bothered Dr. Smith to have so many self-doubts, doubts never expressed to his wife, about his looks, his manners, and his intellect.

Mrs. Smith's home had been warm and casual. Her marital relationship had initially felt comfortable. She attributed the poor sexual adjustment to her husband's work pressures. She, too, worked full-time, and moments together were rare. It was evident that they did enjoy each other and had for most of the marriage.

To begin, they moved back together. Mrs. Smith took a part-time job and her husband reorganized his work days so that they had some time together when both were not physically exhausted. They planned a few holidays and leisure activities.

Both were sexually naive and noncommunicative about such matters. Through discussion and re-education, they worked out a mutually satisfying routine and subsequently had successful intercourse while on holidays. The next focus was on unresolved feelings, incomplete arguments, and poor problem-solving. They were unable to make life decisions and this was largely due to recognition that their marriage might not last. As Dr. Smith revealed his anxieties, his wife confessed her tension was so great that she had to take alcohol and sedatives to keep herself functional.

After 13 conjoint sessions she had dispelled his mythical belief of her need for total, continuous sexual satisfaction. The attendant decrease in anxiety improved sexual funcioning. He, in turn, reassured her that his wish to travel and not have children were simply expressions of his fear about a failing marriage.

Discussion

Dr. Smith's individual seriousness, preoccupations, and concerns reflected personality traits as well as despair. He was a success with his patients, personable with his friends, but a failure within his only intimate relationship. A separation forced him to seek help. Our guess is that a dozen sessions of individual therapy would not have touched him profoundly. His sense of self-esteem and capacity to be a mature sexual being were tied into his marriage, not into himself alone. The early individual sessions were important in setting up a marital treatment situation.

Within this context, his relative lack of affect was nicely balanced by the warmth and emotional capacity of his wife. Rather than deal with his rigid character structure, it became possible to deal with their relationship with its greater flexibility. An educative format decreased the need for insight and dampened the physician's need for intellectualization. The sessions focused on increasing sexual knowledge (generally, and of each other) and on encouraging mutual problem solving. Character traits such as obsessiveness were successfully deployed to better planning of work days and leisure activities.

Case 2

A physician-nurse couple was referred by a psychiatrist-friend because of marital difficulties. Mrs. Jones was a 37-year-old pleasant woman who considered her two teenagers as nearly adult and who wished to renew her academic and professional interests. Dr. Jones was an immaculately groomed 41-year-old physician who complained of a lessening interest in his medical practice and of his wife's lessening interest in him.

For months prior to referral, they had been drinking heavily, had frequent arguments, and finally separated for one month. Throughout this time they fought also over who should go for help and whether the helper should be a social worker, psychologist, or psychiatrist. That dilemma was resolved by the referring psychiatrist, who insisted both be seen together, in this case, by a psychiatrist.

Dr. Jones complained about his wife's "abandonment" of her role as a good mother and obedient wife. And yet, he stated he married her for her "energy, enthusiasm, and unwillingness to be simply a routinized housewife." Mrs. Jones had re-enrolled at the university, was as efficient as ever at home, but expressed dissatisfaction with her marriage. Her husband avoided home, working late at the office to catch up on work he created through poor functioning. His wife tempered her anger with alcohol while she awaited his late-evening arrival. A family interview revealed the distress of their son and daughter as well as the depth of the father's depression and his increasing sense of loneliness.

Throughout the gradually deteriorating marital situation, Mrs. Jones continued to handle emergency calls efficiently, fussed over her husband's practice, and frequently filled in for absent office nurses. While working with him, she knew when he would be home and he was reassured of her company and loyalty. Dr. Jones was threatened with the loss of both his companion-wife and colleague-nurse when she began to develop other interests.

Within marital therapy, Dr. Jones described an impoverished early home life and described his own capacity to feel, enjoy, and relate as impaired. Throughout, he retained a cold, clinical approach to the sessions and a few potentially touching moments made little impact on him. Mrs. Jones maximized these moments and often acted as the interpreter of feelings for both of them. As Dr. Jones became aware of his dependence on his wife as homemaker and nurse, he recognized too his attempts to stifle her maturing into a person capable of pursuing interests beyond her family and his practice. The slight shift in his stance allowed them to work out resonable expectations of each other. Their mood improved when Mrs. Jones felt free of unreasonable demands and he no longer perceived such freedom as a threat to his security.

Discussion

In this situation, the physician-nurse relationship was important. It had provided the husband with the security that his wife would not become too independent of him. He had not considered the possibility that she had other career choices. Mrs. Jones had made a major shift in her percept of how to be a useful, self-respecting individual. While she was enthusiastically engaged with this change, her husband remained static, successful as a physician, but with little opportunity for major life changes. He felt non-productive and non-creative.

Individual therapy for him might have proved difficult. His capacity to express himself as an affective being relied, at least in part, on his wife's contribution to his emotional life. Within the relationship, she possessed affect sufficient for both; but without her he was exceedingly bland. An attempt to nurture that part of his personality, a component missing from most of his life, would have been a near-impossible task. The flexible component which held out hope for a change in both lives was the relationship.

Conclusions and Recommendations

In all physicians of this sample, the pace of life was hectic, the manner of living chaotic. Office hours, appointment schedules, eating and sleeping habits were poorly established or absent. The commitment to work and its attendant responsibilities frequently outweighed the commitment to the family and to personal growth.

Most of these physicians appeared at first, because of their intelligence, verbal ability, and apparent psychologic-mindedness, to be attractive candidates for individual psychotherapy. Too frequently, however, these features were part of a massive intellectual defense system. Almost invariably, the capacity for change was less within the individual than within his relationship with his wife. For many, self-diagnosis led to self-treatment. Psychoactive drugs were frequently used.

Like most of our physician-colleagues who report on treatment approaches, we have described two relatively successful situations. A number of such treatments have not been successful. Into that category fall those cases where hospitalization of one or the other of the marital pair is imminent. No opportunity exists to engage with both partners, for one is at that moment too sick. The illness tends to obscure the marital component, and frequently the patient is treated in isolation.

Treatment problems also arise in those situations where the marital, emotional, and physical split has, in fact, already taken place. The therapist should recognize such a situation and not despair, since useful work can still be accomplished with a couple around such issues as child custody, visitation rights, and the minimizing of further psychologic trauma.

It might be useful to consider a few general recommendations in those instances when a physician or his wife, or both, are referred:

1. Just because the patient is a physician or a physician's wife, do not assume that he or she will recognize the problem, no matter how well it may be described. The long delay between the recognition of problems and actual referral for therapy allows for the development of elaborate intellectual understanding,

but not necessarily for understanding conducive to change.

2. There is a good chance that the physician possesses some personaltiy characteristics related to obsessiveness, a need to control, and a tendency to intellectualize. These characteristics are compatible with being a good physician, but do tend to interfere with psychotherapy. Engaging with prolonged evaluation and therapeutic trials for such persons may result in lost opportunities to meet promptly with the marital pair.
3. Marital distress frequently is reflected in gross disorganization of daily life. Most physicians do have a need for organization and it is helpful to remove the chaos as much as possible. Early structuring of schedules and routines for both the husband and the wife may decrease much irrational activity.
4. Work as an escape must be identified and discouraged. The therapy situation itself offers an opportunity for both partners to discuss life issues away from home and office.
5. Psychiatrists must be prepared to take a firm stand on drug and alcohol abuse. Medication must be handled by the therapist.
6. It helps to see the couple together for the first visit. Aside from the usual alliances which form when one member of a pair sees a therapist, the physician's wife has the additional fear that the M.D.-therapist will side with her M.D.-husband.

It may help to keep in mind that a large proportion of psychiatrically ill physicians and their wives have marital problems. It is also important to note that for the most part we are talking of strong, determined people who seldom stop functioning and, when they do, return quickly to reasonable functioning. The psychiatrist working with a physician-couple must take care not to discontinue therapy too early on the basis of a physician's ability to function. Work is what he does best, often under great stress. Return to work or rapid improvement at work should not be the sole criterion of success with physicians.

There is little question in our minds as to the wisdom of Chessick's (9) suggestions to reintroduce quality into the physician's life. He recommends "keeping up with and contributing to medicine, cultivating the mind through art and music and contemplation of life in terms of first principles, that is — what is true, what is good, what is valuable." No doubt what is true, what is good, what is valuable, include the physician's family.

As for the introduction of quality into the therapist's life, we take to heart Whitaker's and Miller's (10) warning to therapists: "Where the marital tie is weak and divorce threatens, intervention with one of the pair seems routinely to be disruptive. We are impressed that moving unilaterally into a marriage relationship, taking one of the two as a patient and referring or ignoring the mate, is very often a tactical blunder."

We should caution therapists not to despair over the rigid, obsessive individual who responds poorly to individual psychotherapy if that individual has managed to maintain the marital relationship for a number of years. Within this relationship, there is often love and flexibility and there are hopes and dreams which far exceed the individual capacities of the marital partners.

Summary

Physicians do not readily seek either physicial or psychiatric care. The doctor-patient with emotional problems seldom acknowledges the marital component or, if he does, still frequently tends toward individual therapy of himself or his wife. Characteristically, such "medical" couples make a self-diagnosis and may progress to self-treatment. In the 10-couple sampling under discussion, the physicians tended to be obsessive, intellectualized, and emotionally aloof, suggesting a poor prognosis for individual therapy. The prognosis improved dramatically with inclusion of the wife, often the more affective partner.

Therapists must be alert to marital distress when either partner of a physician-wife couple presents for treatment of an emotional illness, and they must move quickly toward inclusion of the spouse.

REFERENCES

1. Miles, J. E., Krell, R., and Lin, T. The doctor's Wife: Mental Illness and Marital Pattern (Abstract). *Sci. Proc.*, 127 Annual Meeting of the APA, 1974, p. 56.
2. Vaillant, G. E., Sobowale, N. C., and McArthur, C. Some Psychologic Vulnerabilities of Physicians. *New England J. Med.*, 287:372, 1972.
3. Evans, J. L. Psychiatric Illness in the Physician's Wife. *Am. J. Psychiat.*, 122: 159, 1965.
4. Pearson, M. M. and Strecker, E. A. Physicians as Psychiatric Patients: Private Practice Experience. *Am. J. Psychiat.*, 116:915, 1960.
5. a'Brook, M. F., Hailstone, J. D., and McLauchlan, I. R. J. Psychiatric Illness in the Medical Profession. *Brit. J. Psychiat.*, 113:1013, 1967.
6. Modlin, H. C. and Montes, A. Narcotics Addiction in Physicians. *Am. J. Psychiat.*, 121:358, 1964.
7. Krell, R., Miles, J. E., and Maurice, W. L. Training in Child Psychiatry: A

Model for Medical Undergraduates. *J. Med. Educ.*, 49:368, 1974.

8. Haley, J. *Strategies of Psychotherapy*, Chapter 6. Grune & Stratton, New York, 1963.
9. Chessick, R. D. On the Quality of the Physician's Life. *Ill. Med. J.*, 136-137:171-174, 1969/70.
10. Whitaker, C. A. and Miller, M. H. A Re-Evaluation of "Psychiatric Help" when Divorce Impends. *Am. J. Psychiat.*, 136:611, 1969.

Prevention and Identification

Chapter 23

REACHING OUT TO THE DEPRESSED PHYSICIAN

Thomas E. Bittker

DEPRESSION, with its secondary manifestations of alcoholism, drug abuse, and suicide, has emerged as a major focus of attention in organized medicine. A priority concern of medical societies since Florida's "sick doctor statute" of 1969 is the effect that illness among physicians has on their ability to practice medicine with reasonable skill and safety to their patients. The term "impaired physician" refers to the physician who is so disturbed that he risks harming patients. The impaired physician is only the end-stage of a problem that affects a much broader spectrum of our profession.

It is difficult to define the magnitude of the problem because of the natural reluctance of physicians to report themselves or their colleagues. Nevertheless, conservative estimates suggest that approximately 17,000, or from 5 percent to 6 percent of the total physician population in this country, is impaired by alcoholism, drug abuse, or mental illness.[1] At least 100, and perhaps up to 300 physicians kill themselves each year.[2] Ross[3] has emphasized that in the United States, suicide accounts for more physician deaths than automobile accidents, plane crashes, drownings, and homicides combined. Among medical students, suicide is the second most common cause of death. This trend continues, at least through middle age. White male physicians under the age of 40 years commit suicide at a rate four times that of their counterparts over the age of 25 years. Studies of physician family relations are equally alarming. Vaillant's controlled studies conclude that 47 percent of physicians have unsatisfactory marriages.[4] Among the wives of physicians, depression accounts for the largest percentage of those emotionally disturbed.[5]

From Thomas E. Bittker, Reaching out to the Depressed Physician, *JAMA 236:* 1713-1716, 1976.

From the Dept. of Neuropsychiatry, Arizona Health Plan, Phoenix. Christine Bittker, Mary Lynn Matilsky, and Phebe Thompson assisted in preparation of this article.

ORIGINS OF PROBLEM

Many of the character traits that contribute to physician success become risk factors for depression when amplified. The qualities of self-sacrifice, perseverance, competitiveness, and even, to some degree, denial of feelings are essential for the passage of the physician through the stages of student to mature professional. The superhuman expectations of the physician were most eloquently voiced by Osler:

> You cannot hope, of course, to escape from the cares and anxieties incident to professional life. Stand up bravely, even against the worst. Your very hopes may have passed on out of sight, as did all that was near and dear to the Patriarch at the Jabbok ford, and like him, you may be left to struggle in the night alone. Well for you, if you wrestle on, for in persistency lies victory, and with the morning may come the wished for blessing. But not always; there is a struggle with defeat which some of you will have to bear, and it will be well for you in that day to have cultivated a cheerful equanimity. Remember too that sometimes "from our desolation only does the better life begin." Even with disaster ahead and ruin imminent, it is better to face them with a smile, and with the head erect, than to crouch at their approach.[6]

A balanced personality must be endowed with the capacity to play, to indulge the child in oneself, to attend to feelings of rage and dependency, to express these feelings, and to comfortably seek nurturance from others. The drive toward achievement may subvert these latter needs in many physicians. That there is a relationship between these achievement needs and physician problems is in part supported by the studies of Bissel and Jones,[7] indicating that more than half of 98 alcoholic physicians interviewed graduated in the upper third of their medical school class. More than 23 percent were in the upper tenth, and only 5 percent of the doctors reported being in the lower third of their class.

Obligatory achievement is one manifestation of the obsessive character more likely to occur in those reared by autocratic and restrictive parents. Overachievement emerges when the child feels that he can maintain self-esteem only by satisfying the demands of others. Inherent in the socialization of physicians are factors that reinforce this overachievement; in some cases, these factors help produce doctors who can maintain self-esteem only through compulsive self-denial. These physicians have particular difficulty satisfying their demands for nurturance and typically will experience guilt whenever they receive help from others. Some solace can be achieved by satisfying the demands of patients; identification with the dependent patient may vicariously satisfy nurturance needs of these physicians.

Unaccustomed to appreciating personal needs, the physician can saturate his life with professional obligations while at the same time leaving little opportunity for the cultivation of recreational skills or relationships with friends or with family. Ultimately, frank depression emerges. The depression may be heralded by the loss of a significant friend or family member, physical illness, awareness of aging, or simply by the perceived failure to satisfy highly valued expectations. So plagued, the physician may attempt to bolster his failing self-esteem by a frenzied pursuit of stimulus. He may work even longer hours, seek material satisfaction, or attempt to restore his mood through the use of drugs or alcohol.

Given the guilt associated with receiving nurturance from others and the shame provoked by feelings of being weak and needing help, the physician will only reluctantly turn to colleagues for professional assistance. When seeking help, his behavior is thoroughly permeated with ambivalence. Often the initial request for help is veiled by out-of-context remarks regarding "sick friends." At other times, the initial request may occur incidental to professional business, in the hospital hallway or while mingling with friends at a cocktail party. As with other depressed patients, the depressed physician becomes overwhelmed by feelings of despair, fear, and uncertainty. Aware that his usual coping methods have failed, he becomes burdened by thoughts of guilt and overwhelming anxiety. His judgment and reality testing become poor, and his attempts to meet his responsibilities yield decreasing efficiency and success. Thoughts of suicide may be entertained as a respite from suffering rather than as a clear decision to die.[8]

TREATMENT OF PHYSICIANS

Notoriously reluctant to seek help, the emotionally disturbed physician presents an enormous challenge to family, colleagues, and therapists. Since many of his defenses have been mobilized to deny awareness of his dependency needs, the physician may seek treatment only when his capacity to practice is imperiled. Reluctance is further magnified by realistic fears of stigma associated with the role of the psychiatric patient. However the depressed physician comes to treatment, several key issues need to be confronted.

First, he must be approached in such a way that guilt about past behavior or indiscretions is minimized. Initial rapport can be facilitated by listening to the patient in a nonjudgmental way, achieving as complete an understanding of the problem as possible, and enlarging the avenue of trust between the physician-patient and the helping physician. Even if a referral to another physician is being considered, it is imperative that the helping physician achieve a clear, mutually-understood treatment contract with his depressed colleague. An effective treatment contract includes (1) a shared understanding of the problem, (2) an agreement as to who will be involved in the evaluation and treatment of the problem, (3) limit-setting on self-destructive behavior, (4) a plan as to what to do next.

Second, having defined that the therapist and not the sick physician is to be principally responsible for the management of the case, the therapist should then perform a more detailed assessment of the dimensions of the physician's problem, of his coping, and of his interpersonal resources. The following factors must be considered in evaluating suicide potential: (1) What is the degree of the depression? (Depression will manifest itself in the affective, somatic, cognitive, and adaptive spheres. Affective manifestations include hopelessness, worthlessness, sadness, and guilt. Somatic concerns relate to fatigue, decreased libido, anorexia, insomnia, and vague somatic complaints. Cognitive manifestations include inability to plan for the future and inability to cope.) (2) Does the patient harbor conscious suicidal preoccupations or intent? (3) Does the patient have a suicidal plan? (4) Are his depressive symptoms worsening? (5) Does the patient have a history of impulsivity? (6) To what degree has the patient already exhausted his intra- and interpersonal resources? (The patient without money, job, friends, or future prospects has less to live for than the financially and socially successful patient.) (7) Is there evidence of alcoholism and drug dependence? (8) Is death identification operating here? (Individuals who identify either with someone significant who has committed suicide or who have been exposed to death in childhood of a parent or close family member are at considerable risk.) (9) What method of suicide has been considered? (In general, the more violent and painful the method considered or chosen, the greater the ultimate risk of suicide.)

EMERGENCY PSYCHOLOGICAL SUPPORT

During the crisis phase of working with the disturbed professional, the therapist should: (1) Reflect to the patient an awareness that he appreciates both the intensity and depth of the patient's problems. This is done most effectively by focusing on the patient's feelings as he talks about his experiences. (2) Convey an appreciation of the seriousness of the patient's problem. (3) Remind the patient of his identity. In the midst of crisis, most depressed people lose their anchors in time. That is, they are neither aware of themselves as they have functioned in the past nor can they conceive of the possibility of functioning better in the future. Patients can recapture this sense of self in the process of offering a detailed history of their past life as well as a careful examination of their plans. (4) Stimulate the patient toward constructive action. Prescribe behavioral assignments that the patient can accomplish prior to the next encounter with the therapist. Such activities should be relatively simple and achievable given the patient's resources. (5) Involve the patient's family whenever possible. Although the question of involving the family for long-term treatment remains negotiable, it is critical to involve at least the spouse in the crisis management of the depressed physician. (6) Develop an anti-self-destructive contract. This is essential to the emergency psychological support of all patients, and through this the therapist sets limits on the patient's self-destructive behavior. The critical elements of the contract include an agreement by the patient that no matter what happens he will not involve himself in self-destructive behavior whether that be by suicide, drinking, or drug taking, and a time limit on the contract. Whereas most patients in difficulty will be unable to sustain a contract indefinitely, they can successfully refrain from self-destructive behavior for an agreed on period of time, whether that be three hours, one day, one week, or one month. Note that contracts will only be valid for those patients who enter them in a non-psychotic state and in clear consciousness.[9]

LONGER-TERM THERAPY

When the physician-patient leaves the hospital or emerges from the crisis that initially caused him to seek treatment, a reevaluation should be made with a view toward involving the patient in a treatment program that will remedy the underlying problem: his obligatory overachievement. The therapist should have secured from the patient an understanding that the overall thrust of treatment would be to assist the patient in cessation of the self-destructive behavior pattern and to substitute for this more adaptive patterns. Again, family involvement may prove critical. Simply by involving the spouse, the therapist will enhance his leverage on the patient's behavior and diminish the patient's sense of responsibility for his illness. In addition, it will enhance the chances for securing a more reasonable style of living by dealing with a couple or family system rather than by dealing with the patient alone. Whether or not the patient is ultimately dealt with individually, in a group, or in couple or family therapy, the following issues should be considered: (1) What is it that needs to be changed? (2) What is the patient, couple, or family willing to risk in order to change? (3) How will one know when change has been achieved, and what behavioral indices can be used to assess change? (4) What part is psychotherapy going to play in the change process?

SPECIAL PROBLEMS

LOCATION OF TREATMENT. During the evaluation process, initial consideration should be given as to whether or not the physician-patient should be treated locally or away from his practice. Obviously, this decision becomes more critical when hospitalization is being considered.

DENIAL OF PATIENTHOOD. The sick physician will tend to deny his patienthood. Often when the crisis passes, such a compulsive individual will no longer acknowledge the need for help and will resume those behaviors that initially precipitated the symptoms. While the patient still feels considerable distress, the therapist should openly anticipate this "flight into health" and obtain an agreement preempting the flight. The therapist should evaluate the working and family environment of the patient. Unless the therapist can secure an agreement that ultimately he is in control of treatment, the treatment is bound to fail. As a part of this agreement, the physician-patient should cease prescribing drugs for himself or his family.

FLIGHT FROM TREATMENT. There is a great deal of pressure on the part of the physician-patient to flee the treatment situation, avoid the implication of his crisis, and resume prior obligations. Such flight may initially seem rewarding both to patients and therapists, since the patient may achieve a brief remission of depressive symptoms. In the long run, it will be better to confront the depression and to set limits on the unceasing obligations that a patient presents for himself. Although self-esteem should be supported by encouraging the patient to resume working, careful consideration should be given to altering the work setting as necessary and to the examination of each future obligation as it arises.

SCHEDULING OF RECREATIONAL ACTIVITIES. At the insistance of the therapist and with an awareness that pleasure may not be immediately forthcoming, the physician-patient should regularly schedule recreational activities. Athletic endeavors are a key part of this recreational regimen. When indicated, athletic activities might require the close supervision of the therapist or of a cardiology consultant.

PREVENTION

I doubt that medical schools will be successful in selecting physicians less vulnerable to the problems of depression. However, medical schools can take steps to prevent the growth of this problem. First, the faculty should be alerted to the need to model a more balanced life-style. No longer should the 70-hour week be reinforced as exemplary conduct among faculty members. Clearly, there are some who may be able to satisfy personal needs and professional and family obligations while working such extraordinary schedules. Although we may marvel at their capacity, the young physician should be cautioned that modeling such behavior may present significant risks for him. Second, self-awareness groups focused on the problem of adaptation to the physician's role should begin in medical school "with opportunities, following graduation, to participate in such groups provided by local medical societies."[10] These groups should provide not only cognitive awareness of the physician's problems but should permit participants to increase their capacity to tolerate feelings within themselves, to listen to others effectively, and to reexamine their position vis-à-vis their life goals. Organizers of national medical meetings should consider including similar experiential learning groups. Third, medical societies are excellently positioned to identify consultants who could educate their colleagues in the prevention and recognition of depression among physicians. If needed, these consultants could serve as a first line of assistance to emotionally disturbed physicians. Fourth, although we are accumulating a large body of knowledge on how to cope with stress, rarely is this shared with or practiced by physicians. Beginning in medical school and continuing on through their professional life, physicians could benefit by cognitive and experiential instruction in such coping skills as (1) accurate appraisal of the stressful situation, (2) effective information-seeking and utilization, (3) contingency planning, (4) rehearsing of behavioral alternatives, (5) sustaining pleasurable activities under stress, and (6) maintaining contacts with reference groups.[11]

Comment

Depression is an outgrowth of characterological qualities that have proved adaptive for most physicians. When amplified, however, these qualities (self-sacrifice, altruism, achievement orientation, and denial of feelings) expose the physician to high risk of clinical depression and its manifestations (alchoholism, substance abuse, and suicide). The depressed physician is burdened by an obsessive behavioral style that serves to ward off dependency feelings, and he represents a considerable challenge to the psychotherapist. Some key concepts in the treatment of depression in the physician are (1) definition of the physician-patient relationship, (2) assessment of suicidal risk, (3) provision of emergency psychological support, and (4) negotiation for long-term treatment. As for prevention, physicians must foster efforts to improve self-awareness, tolerance of feelings, and coping skills for dealing with stress in themselves and their spouses.

REFERENCES

1. The Impaired Physician: An Interpretive Summary, Department of Mental Health. AMA Conference on Impaired Physician, San Francisco, April 11, 1975.
2. Blachly PH, Disher W, Roduner G: Suicide by physicians. *Bull Suicidology* December 1968, 1-18.
3. Ross M: Suicide among physicians: Psychologic study. *Dis Nerv Syst* 34:145-150, 1973.
4. Vaillant GE, Sobowale NC, McArthur C: Some psychological vulnerability of physicians. *N Engl J Med* 287:372-375, 1972.
5. Evans JL: Psychiatric illness in the physician's wife. *Am J Psychiatry* 122:159-163, 1963.
6. Osler W: *Aequanimitas*. Philadelphia, Blakiston Co, 1947, pp 7-8.
7. Bissell L, Jones R: Disabled doctors: Ignored by peers. Read before the AMA Conference on the Impaired Physician, San Francisco, April 11, 1975.
8. Kiev A: Psychotherapeutic strategies in the management of depressed and suicidal patients. *Am J Psychother* 19:345-354, 1975.
9. Drye RC, Goulding RL, Goulding ME: No-suicide decisions: Patient-monitoring of suicidal risk. *Am J Psychiatry* 130:171-174, 1973.
10. Scheiber SC: A comprehensive state-wide approach to the sick doctor. *Ariz Med* 32:933-935, 1975.
11. Hamburg DA, Coelho GV, Adams JE: Coping and adaptation: Steps towards a synthesis of biological and social perspectives, in Coelho GV, Hamburg DA, Adams JE (eds): *Coping and Adaptation*. New York, Basic Books Inc Publishers, 1974.

Chapter 24

CLINICAL PREDICTION OF PHYSICIAN SUICIDE BASED ON MEDICAL STUDENT DATA

LYNN CHAIKIN EPSTEIN, CAROLINE BEDELL THOMAS, JOHN W. SHAFFER AND SEYMOUR PERLIN

THE purpose of this investigation was to determine whether there are recognizable psychological characteristics of predictive value in identifying future physician suicides. A retrospective-prospective design was used. The 33 subjects were a subset of the 1198 medical students who were both participants in the long-term Study of the Precursors of Hypertension and Coronary Disease and graduates from the medical school. The group consisted of nine suicides, two matched controls for each suicide, and six distractors. Using a wide range of materials collected for other purposes, a psychiatrist, blind to the number of the suicides and controls, as well as to the criteria for selection of controls, was able to identify the nine suicides correctly.

On a rank ordering of the 33 subjects for suicide potential, the suicides occupied the first nine places. There was also a highly significant correlation between the reviewer's rating for suicide potential and the dichotomy, suicide-nonsuicide. The reviewer's ratings on eight categories from the Lorr Outpatient Mood Scale and on five selected dimensions adapted from the Katz Adjustment Scales significantly separated the suicides from the controls. Psychopathology scores were higher for the suicides from the controls, and the Minnesota-Hartford Personality Assay revealed

---

From Lynn Chaikin Epstein et al., Clinical Prediction of Physician Suicide Based on Medical Student Data, *J Nerv Ment Dis* Vol. 156, No. 1, 1973.

This research was supported in part by the National Institute of Mental Health Grant MH18819 and the Clayton Fund of the Johns Hopkins University.

The authors would like to express their appreciation to Ms. Karen R. Duszynski and Mrs. Peter Brown for their valuable assistance.

that the suicides were related significantly higher than the controls on many personality factors, particularly self-destructive tendency, depression, and guilty self-concept. These findings are briefly discussed and possible explanations for the success in identifying the nine suicides are suggested. The results are provocative and strongly imply that the suicide group differs in many identifiable ways from the control group of medical students.

Objective analysis of physician suicide has been hampered by the reluctance of both the lay and professional community to acknowledge its occurrence openly. In the past, articles on physician suicide offered theories of presumed causality, with little data to go on, and it is only recently that more substantive studies have been conducted. For example, in 1903, an editorial in the *Journal of the American Medical Association* bemoaned the death of physicians by suicide and ascribed the etiology to over-abundance of and competition among physicians, their familiarity with death, and their easy access to lethal methods (12). The solution proposed entailed augmented self-interest plus professional organization and regulation.

Many formulations have been expressed regarding physicians suicides (3,13,19,34). A recurrent theme is the notion of stress combined with opportunity and toxicological knowledge as causative factors (4). Knopf (16) emphasized the importance of certain personality traits of the physician, including illusions of wealth and fame, variable degrees of anhedonia, self-neglect, and masochism. DeSole et al. (6) underscored the significance of the professional role and the "gap between expectations and performance" (p. 299). Such hypotheses create the need for further studies.

Controlled investigation of physician suicide has met with the same obstacles as other areas of suicide research. Gathering statistics on the occurrence of physician suicide is an arduous task, which requires ingenuity and persistence. There is some disagreement in the literature over the frequency of suicide in physicians relative to comparable age-, sex-, and race-matched members of the general population, as well as for specifically delineated socioeconomic groups (1,2,5,7,24,28,33). In a recent review of the literature, Ross (25) presents demographic data on these facets of physician suicide. Accurate reporting notwithstanding, valid reconstruction of the premorbid personality after the suicide is problematical. An important advance in this regard is the application of the *Katz Adjustment Scales — R Forms* to suicides and driver fatalities (27).

Advance identification of suicides using psychological and

predictive scales has proved a formidable and often impractical task (17). Current practice in this area, as, for example, in the work of Pokorny (22, 23), is to use data from the history and psychiatric evaluation. Thus, clinical reseach in physician suicide has focused on those doctors who have been under psychiatric care (8,29). The implications of such studies are limited by their retrospective design and the fact that in most cases the identity of the suicides is known to the investigators. Furthermore, it is risky to generalize from observations made on physicians treated for psychiatric illness to the greater numbers of doctors who have never received such care. A promising alternative which circumvents many of these obstacles is offered by combining the retrospective design with the "uninformed" or "blind" reviewer. This approach was employed to predict suicide in schizophrenic patients with some success (21).

The present study attempts to approximate the situation of prospective identification of physicians who later commit suicide by reviewing data on former Johns Hopkins medical students, with one of the investigators (L.C.E., hereafter called the reviewer) uninformed ("blind") as to the number and identity of the suicides in the study sample as well as in the population from which they were drawn. The purpose of this investigation is twofold:

1. to determine whether a psychiatrist can distinguish medical students who later committed suicide from nonsuicide medical student controls, using a wide range of material collected for other purposes; and
2. if so, to define which features or concepts make the task possible.

METHOD

Subjects

All subjects were participants in the Study of the Precursors of Hypertension and Coronary Disease, a longitudinal investigation of Johns Hopkins medical students in classes graduating between 1948 and 1964. Of a total of 1337 students registered in these classes at some time, 1198 were active participants in the Precursors Study while in medical school and graduated. The high incidence of suicide in the total population has been previously noted (31).

A subset of 33 graduates from among the Precursors Study participants was selected by two of the authors (C.B.T., J.W.S.) for the purposes of this study. These consisted of nine subjects who were known to have committed suicide at some time after graduating from medical school, two matched controls for each suicide, and six "distractors." The controls were living graduates matched for age, sex, race, class in medical school, marital status in medical school, and psychologist administering the psychological tests. The distractors consisted of two subjects who had died prematurely of ambiguous causes where the possibility of suicide was present,[2] and four additional subjects to make the matching by sex and class less obvious. The reviewer was informed only that there were 33 records for study and that these included at least one completed suicide and suitable controls.

All suicides were Caucasian; seven were men, two were women. Their ages at death ranged from 27 to 48 years. The mean age at death was 34.7 years, the median age was 31 years. Death from suicide occurred 1 to 18 years after graduation from medical school. The mean interval between graduation and death was 7.8 years, the median interval was 6 years.

Source Material

A variety of Precursors Study data obtained during medical school was available for each subject, which included general background, photograph, family history, medical history, physical examination, laboratory tests, work history, habits of sleep, diet, smoking, drinking, drug usage, and nervous tension, as well as family attitudes, reports of interviews with Dr. Thomas, and Rorschach and Figure Drawing tests. This material was quite complete for all but the earliest classes in which interviews and figure drawings were not obtained. In addition, the Dean's Office record on each student provided access to admissions information, medical school grades, rank in class, comments by faculty, and loan and scholarship information. From both of these sources, only material up until the time of graduation was made available to the reviewer for study.

Review Procedure

The order in which subjects' records were reviewed was determined by using a table of random numbers. The reviewer first read all of the available material on a given subject (with the exception of

[2]One was later determined to have committed suicide in the course of a disabling illness.

the projective test interpretations) and made systematic notations. She next assigned ratings for the selected scales. Only then were the interpretations of the projective tests considered; the reviewer recorded brief comments as to whether she agreed or disagreed with them and gave an additional score in red to any previously scored item if it seemed warranted. Finally, the reviewer evaluated each subject for suicide potential.[3] Upon completion of each subect's evaluation, all material pertaining to that subject was locked in a cabinet by a research assistant. Thus none of the investigators had access to it until completion of the study. After all the subjects had been characterized, the reviewer ranked the 33 subjects for suicide potential from most suicidal to least suicidal.

Methods of Characterization

The technique used to describe and classify each subject included the following:

(1) *The Social Readjustment Rating Scale* (11): Each item on the Social Readjustment Rating Scale was scored as being either present or absent as determined from available records, and the standard values developed by Holmes were subsequently assigned. Any item for which there was no information was considered to be absent. As employed here, this scale was adapted to give a general measure of known stress in a subject's life up to the time of graduation from medical school.

(2) *The Lorr Outpatient Mood Scale (LOMS)* (18): After examining a number of instruments designed to describe general mood, this scale was selected by the reviewer as the most appropriate for the purposes of this study. The mood scale consists of 60 adjectives which have been intercorrelated and factored. The 60 adjectives, or individual items, within each of the eight factors are scored on a four-point scale: 0 = not at all, 1 = a little, 2 = quite a bit, 3 = extremely. Numerical scores for the items within each factor were summed and the resulting score was used for data analysis. The eight factors and their constituent items are listed in Appendix 1.

(3) *A Modification of Five Dimensions Suggested by The Katz Adjustment Scales (KAS)* (14): Five sets of rating scale items were adapted for this study on the basis of their suspected effectiveness in separating suicides from normal subjects (Appendix II). These dimensions represented aspects of personality which were not included in the

[3]The Minnesota-Hartford Personality Assay forms were checked by the reviewer after evaluating each subject for suicide potential.

LOMS. Again, a four-point scale was used. The items were individually scored and the scores for each set were then summed.

(4) *Clinical Characterization:* The reviewer had compiled three lists of characteristics to describe the subjects with respect to (a) general psychopathology, (b) ways of expressing anger, and (c) ways of handling anxiety or stress (Appendix C). These items were scored on the four-point scale mentioned above, but they have not been included in the statistical analyses. Rather, they served to provide the reviewer with a rough guide for recording her own thinking as she went through the sometimes voluminous data.

(5) *Individual Potential for Suicide as Judged by the Reviewer:* Suicide potential was again rated on a four-point scale, based on all the foregoing methods of appraisal. In so doing, the reviewer summarized her evaluation of the probability of future suicide for each subject.

(6) *The Minnesota-Hartford Personality Assay (MHPA)* (10): This was added to the battery of tests after each subject had been evaluated for suicide potential by means of the steps outlined above. Using the appropriate form (male or female) of the Doctor's Subset, the reviewer rated each of the items on a seven-point scale, low to high, after which the forms were mailed to the Institute of Living Research Laboratories in Hartford, Connecticut, for computer scoring on 20 personality dimensions. The MHPA overlaps information contained in the other scales but was included to provide a carefully standardized profile of each subject.

(7) *Rank Ordering for Suicide Potential:* Rank ordering was achieved by first sorting the 33 subjects into four groups on the basis of their suicide potential as judged by the reviewer, and then ranking the subjects within each group.

Results

When the 33 subjects were placed in rank order for overall suicide potential, the nine suicides occupied the first nine places and were thus correctly classified (Table 24-I). All suicides were rated either 3, extremely suicidal, or 2, quite a bit suicidal (Table 24-II). The matched control who ranked tenth was the only nonsuicide with a rating of 2, and thus might be considered a false positive. All other matched controls and distractors were rated 1, a little suicidal, or 0, not at all suicidal. The two distractors who died under ambiguous circumstances were ranked 13th and 14th and rated 1. There was a fivefold difference in mean ratings for suicides and matched controls, and a threefold difference between mean ratings for suicides and distractors, a mixed group.

Table 24-I

REVIEWER'S RANK ORDERING FOR SUICIDE POTENTIAL

Group	N	Rank as to Suicide Potential*
Suicides	9	1 through 9
Matched controls	18	10-12, 16, 17, 19, 21-23, 25-33
Distractors	6	13-15, 18, 20, 24

*Ranked from most suicidal (rank 1) to least suicidal (rank 33).

Table 24-II

REVIEWER'S RATING FOR OVERALL SUICIDE POTENTIAL ON FOUR-POINT SCALE

Rating*	Number in Group Receiving Rating		
	Suicides ($N = 9$)	Matched controls ($N = 18$)	Distractors ($N = 6$)
3	5	0	0
2	4	1	0
1	0	7	5
0	0	10	1
Mean	2.56	0.50	0.83
SD	0.53	0.62	0.41

*3 = extremely suicidal; 2 = quite a bit suicidal; 1 = a little suicidal; 0 = not at all suicidal.

Means for the scales on which these overall ratings were based and their standard deviations are given in Table 24-III. The *F* ratios were calculated for suicides and matched controls using the randomized block design for unequal but proportional replication[4] (15). On the modified Social Readjustment Rating Scale, the mean for the suicide group did not differ significantly from that of the control group, although the difference was in the expected direction.

[4]The p values determined using the randomized block design were similar to those obtained using uncorrelated t tests.

Table 24-III

COMPARISON OF SUICIDES AND MATCHED CONTROLS BASED ON SELECTED DIMENSIONS FROM THREE PSYCHOLOGICAL RATING SCALES

Scale	Suicides ($N = 9$)		Matched Controls ($N = 18$)		p Value*
	Mean	SD	Mean	SD	
Social Readjustment Rating Scale (modified)	329.00	141.84	253.06	121.79	N.S.
Lorr Mood Scale factors					
Cheerful	9.78	6.44	11.50	4.95	N.S.
Energetic	11.33	2.87	10.50	4.08	N.S.
Inert-fatigue	2.78	3.49	2.17	2.62	N.S.
Thoughtful	14.22	2.28	9.28	3.14	<.001
Relaxed-composed	5.67	3.39	6.00	3.09	N.S.
Anger-hostility	9.89	3.18	4.28	3.59	<.025
Tense-anxious	9.11	3.55	6.22	3.06	N.S.
Depressed	16.33	3.61	4.78	4.25	<.001
Dimensions modified from the Katz Adjustment Scales					
Negativism	8.78	2.28	4.06	2.82	<.005
Suspiciousness	5.33	2.34	2.06	1.11	<.005
Verbal expansiveness	6.78	2.99	3.44	2.79	<.005
Dependency	10.78	3.23	4.94	3.21	<.001
Impulsivity	3.89	1.45	1.39	1.68	<.005

*For bidirectional test, where p was calculated using a randomized block design for unequal but proportional replications. N.S., not significant.

Three categories from the LOMS separated the suicide group from the control group. The suicides were rated significantly higher in the areas of *thoughtfulness* ($p < .001$), *anger-hostility* ($p < .025$), and *depressed* ($p < .001$). For the categories *cheerful, energetic, inert-fatigue, relaxed-composed,* and *tense-anxious,* there were no significant differences between the suicide and control groups. All five of the categories suggested by the KAS significantly differentiated the suicides from the controls. Suicides received higher scores in the areas of *negativism* ($p < .005$), *suspiciousness* ($p < .005$), *verbal expansiveness* ($p < .005$), *dependency* ($p < .001$), and *impulsivity* ($p < .005$).

The raw scores for the items on the lists drawn up by the reviewer (Appendix C) are summarized in Table 24-IV. In each instance, the means for the suicides were higher than those for the nonsuicides, particularly with respect to general psychopathology.

The mean MHPA scores for the suicide and control groups are shown in Table 24-V, where they are listed in order of their differentiating power. The suicides had significantly higher scores than the controls for many of the factors; of these, *self-destructive tendency, depression,* and *guilty self-concept* were the most significant.

DISCUSSION

The results are striking and clearly show that the reviewer was able to differentiate medical students who later committed suicide from a control group of medical students when approaching descriptive material blind to the identity of the suicides. In view of the correlation between previous suicide attempts with later suicide, it should be mentioned that only one of the 33 subjects had made a suicide attempt known to the reviewer (21). That subject was one of the suicides and stood second in rank order for suicide potential.

The task of predicting suicide in the context of this study appears more straightforward than the more usual clinical task of determining which psychiatric patients will ultimately commit suicide (9,30). The most likely explanation for our success relates to the high base rate of suicide within the study sample. To separate out nine suicides from a population of 33 represents an artificial situation established for the purpose of studying the feasibility of this approach. Identifying nine suicides within the population of 1198 graduate participants would be a far more difficult task and would undoubtedly result in a larger number of "false positives." These considerations are more elaborately described in the paper on prediction of suicide in schizophrenics (21).

Table 24–IV

SUMMARY OF REVIEWER'S OWN CHARACTERIZATION

Characteristics	Suicides ($N = 9$)		Distractors ($N = 6$)		Matched Controls ($N = 18$)	
	Mean	Range	Mean	Range	Mean	Range
General psychopathy (56 items)	55.1	37-79	27.7	11-49	16.0	1-46
Ways of expressing anger (32 items)	36.7	31-40	28.7	24-35	26.2	19-37
Ways of handling anxiety or stress (23 items)	29.7	26-34	21.7	18-30	20.2	16-30

Table 24-V

COMPARISON OF SUICIDES AND MATCHED CONTROLS ON 20 MINNESOTA-HARTFORD PERSONALITY ASSAY FACTORS

MHPA Factors	Suicides ($N = 9$)		Matched Controls ($N = 18$)		t*	p Value
	Mean	SD	Mean	SD		
Self-destructive tendency	73.00	3.00	48.33	5.87	11.53	<.001
Depression	81.11	4.91	49.00	8.87	10.05	<.001
Guilty self-concept	77.22	10.10	50.67	8.32	7.28	<.001
Dissociative concern	65.33	5.72	47.06	6.44	7.20	<.001
Thinking disorder	47.78	1.72	44.78	0.88	6.07	<.001
Lack of insight	35.67	8.05	22.17	6.55	4.68	<.001
Paranoid thinking	53.11	5.28	45.28	5.11	3.72	<.005
Hostile aggressive behavior	62.89	6.23	49.89	10.03	3.54	<.005
Overt anxiety symptoms	68.11	9.36	54.94	10.76	3.12	<.005
Dependency	62.33	8.68	52.83	7.08	3.05	<.005
Homosexual concern	47.67	13.45	39.00	0.03	2.79	<.025
Disturbance of affect	66.33	9.21	58.17	7.31	2.51	<.025
Dissociative tendency	47.67	3.71	44.56	2.73	2.48	<.025
Social isolation	84.56	6.60	75.22	11.78	2.20	<.05
Lack of social communication	60.89	8.74	54.22	8.09	1.97	N.S.
Lack of social conformity	71.56	7.16	64.56	11.70	1.64	N.S.
Anhedonia	67.33	8.20	62.22	9.84	1.34	N.S.
Somatic concern	44.00	5.22	41.67	4.56	1.19	N.S.
Compulsivity	64.78	8.42	61.83	9.66	0.78	N.S.
Disorientation	51.56	10.25	52.00	14.20	0.08	N.S.

*The uncorrelated t test was used here.

In a separate study of suicides within the Precursors Study population, it was found that a list of 25 habits of nervous tension checked by the medical students themselves differentiated the suicides from matched controls with a high degree of accuracy[5] (32). By using multiple discriminant function analysis, 83.3 percent of the suicides and 87.5 percent of the controls in that study were correctly classified. When the suicides were compared with 1107 living subjects who completed the checklist, 66.7 percent and 78.8 percent, respectively, were correctly classified. Thus, comparison with the larger, unmatched population was, as expected, less precise, but was nevertheless significant. Hence, systematic analysis of the Habits of Nervous Tension Questionnaire which formed but a small portion of the material available to the reviewer resulted in a similar but less complete differentiation. It should be noted that, in a much larger study of characteristics of former college students which were predictive of suicide in later life, Paffenbarger and Asnes (20) found that brief personal interviews had been less conclusive than self-assessed appraisal. In the present study, of course, both self-administered questionnaires and interviews were available to the reviewer.

The practical implications of this study are to suggest that, given appropriate information, a clinician probably can identify a subset of medical students at high risk for suicide. It is entirely possible, however, that one would really be differentiating a group at high risk for emotional difficulties of various forms of which possible suicide is just one. It is noteworthy in this regard that the suicides received substantially higher scores than the controls in the area of general psychopathology as shown in Tables 24-IV and 24-V. Akin to this is the recent study comparing the drivers of single car and multiple car accident fatalities (26). There appear to be many parallel characteristics between the drivers of single car accident fatalities and completed suicides, although the suicides appear to be the more deviant groups (27).

The results are provocative in suggesting areas which differentiate the suicides from the control group. The suicide group received significantly higher scores on the LOMS in the categories *thoughtful*, *anger-hostililty*, and *depressed* and on the KAS for *negativism*, *suspiciousness*, *verbal expansiveness*, *dependency*, and *impulsivity*. These findings are generally confirmed by the significant factors from the MHPA. This agreement among the instruments of characterization

[5]These analyses were not available to the reviewer of the present study until after the blind code was broken.

is to be expected, since the same reviewer filled out all of them.

The relatively poor showing of the Social Readjustment Rating Scale is not surprising when it is remembered that the life events scored by the reviewer did not occur within a fixed time interval of the event of suicide, although this was how the scale was intended to be used. In addition, many of the 43 items proved to be relatively useless in this study, either because the item was checked for all 33 subjects (9 items), was not checked for any subject (10 items), or was checked for only one subject (10 items checked, 5 for suicides and 5 for nonsuicides). Of the remaining 14 items, only a few, such as "outstanding achievement," could be both accurately defined and showed substantial differences between the suicide and matched control groups. Thus, one should not draw any inferences concerning the utility of the Social Readjustment Rating Scale from these data.

The question remains as to how the reviewer arrived at these distinctive profiles on the basis of a wide variety of sources. The cues were contained in the rough notes she had made as she went through the often voluminous source material. That her deductions from these rough notes were largely correct was demonstrated to one of the authors (C.B.T.) and another observer (K.R.D.) many months after the notes were made and after the blind code had been broken, when the reviewer's notes and deductions were compared with detailed information received by the Precursors Study concerning two of the suicides after their deaths. Thus, she was able to piece together these fragmentary, irregular bits of information, often no more than hints, into profiles of each subject.

APPENDICES

Appendix A

Factors and Items from Lorr Outpatient Mood Scale

Cheerful (10 items)
- elated
- on top of the world
- excited
- lighthearted
- carefree
- gay
- cheerful
- happy-go-lucky
- pretty good
- optimistic

Energetic (7 items)
- active
- energetic
- full of pep
- alert
- vigorous
- lively
- enthusiastic

Inert-Fatigue (7 items)
- weary
- tired
- sluggish
- lethargic
- lazy
- listless
- languid

Thoughtful (7 items)
- introspective
- thoughtful
- contemplative
- pensive
- earnest
- serious
- preoccupied

Relaxed-Composed (6 items)
- calm
- at ease
- composed
- relaxed
- serene
- nonchalant

Anger-Hostility (8 items)
- furious
- annoyed
- angry
- spiteful
- resentful
- ready to fight
- bad-tempered
- grouchy

Tense-Anxious (7 items)
- nervous
- anxious
- shaky
- worried
- jittery
- tense
- on edge

Depressed (8 items)
- hopeless
- helpless
- worthless
- unhappy
- lonely
- blue
- frightened
- apathetic

For each item: 0 - not at all, 1 - a little, 2 - quite a bit, 3 - extremely.

Appendix B

Dimensions Suggested by the Katz Adjustment Scale

Negativism (8 items)
- critical of others
- critical of self
- disagrees with everything
- selfish
- sarcastic
- lies
- stubborn
- has trouble with law

Suspicousness (6 items)
- distrustful
- cautious
- fears close relationships
- think people are talking about him
- acts as if he's suspicious of people
- feels people try to get him to do things against his will

Verbal Expansiveness (6 items)
- puts on front
- loud, boisterous
- talks too much
- brags
- interrupts
- competitive

Dependency (6 items)
- feels inadequate
- passive, submissive
- dependent on others
- needs to be accepted
- can't take criticism
- fragile

Impulsivity (3 items)
- must have immediate gratification
- often says things and regrets them later
- often does things he later regrets

For each item: 0 = not at all, 1 = a little, 2 = quite a bit, 3 = extremely.

Appendix C

Items Used by Reviewer for Characterization of Subjects

General Psychopathology

- inadequate
- self-critical
- self-conscious
- anxious
- manipulative
- conversion symptoms
- obsessive-compulsive
- submissive
- dependent
- tries to please
- sad, pensive
- pities self
- depressed
- suicidal
- hypochondriasis
- psychosomatic illness
- fragile
- threatened by women
- impotent
- fears close relationships
- suspicous
- hostile
- cautious
- impulsive
- irresponsible
- superficial
- arrogant
- pretentious
- overbearing
- conceited
- acts out
- sarcastic
- drug abuse
- sexual excess
- sexual perversion
- derogatory attitude
- feelings of ugliness
- withdrawn
- idealistic
- ambivalent
- autistic
- inappropriate affect
- loose associations
- wide mood swings
- delusions
- hallucinations
- confusion
- bizarre
- disoriented
- psychiatric outpatient care
- psychiatric inpatient care
- authoritative
- trouble with authority
- trouble with the law
- lies
- steals

Way of Expressing Anger

- denial
- repression
- projection
- sublimation
- rationalization
- intellectualization
- depression
- hyperactivity
- somatization
- anxiety
- confusion
- depersonalization
- withdrawal
- obsessive-compulsive
- direct expression to person
  - verbally appropriate
  - verbally abusive
  - physically abusive
- indirect expression to person
  - sarcasm
  - act out
- expression to substitute person or object
  - verbally appropriate exchange
- verbally abusive
  - physically abusive
- self-punishment
  - self-deprivation—pleasures
    - food
    - sleep
  - verbal self-depreciation
  - physical self-abuse—drugs
    - alcohol
    - other/accident
- suicidal thoughts
- suicidal attempts

Way of Handling Anxiety or Stress

- denial
- repression
- projection
- sublimation
- rationalization
- intellectualization
- depression
- confusion
- withdrawal
- depersonalization
- obsessive-compulsive
- hyperactivity
- somatization
- verbal abuse of others
- physical abuse of others
- anger
- act out
- realistic modification of situation
- self-punishment
  - self-deprivation
  - verbal self-depreciation
  - suicidal thoughts
  - suicidal attempts
- accident

For each item: 0 = not at all, 1 = a little, 2 = quite a bit, 3 = extremely.

REFERENCES

1. Blachly, P. H., Disher, W. and Roduner, G. Suicide by physicians. *Bull. Suicidol.*, 1-18, December, 1968.
2. Blachly, P.H., Osterud, H. T. and Josslin, R. Suicide in professional groups. *New Eng. J. Med.*, *268*: 1278-1282, 1963.
3. *British Medical Journal.* Mental disturbance in doctors, *2*: 448, 1969.
4. *British Medical Journal.* Suicide among doctors, *1:* 789-790, 1964.
5. Craig, A. G. and Pitts, F. N., Jr. Suicide by physicians. *Dis. Nerv. Syst.*, *29*: 763-772, 1968.
6. DeSole, D. E., Singer, P. and Aronson, S. Suicide and role strain among physicians. *Int. J. Soc. Psychiat.*, *15*: 294-301, 1969.
7. Dublin, L. I. and Spiegelman, M. D. The longevity and mortality of American physicians 1938-1942. A preliminary report. *J.A.M.A.*, *134*: 1211-1215, 1947.
8. Duffy, J. C. and Litin, E. M. Psychiatric morbidity of physicians. *J.A.M.A.*, *189*: 989-992, 1964.
9. Flood, R. A. and Senger, C. P. A retrospective examination of psychiatric case records of patients who subsequently committed suicide. *Brit. J. Psychiat.*, *114*: 443-450, 1968.
10. Glueck, B. C., Jr., Mechl, P. E., Schofield, W. and Clyde, D. W. *Minnesota-Hartford Personality Assay.* The Institute of Living, Hartford, Connecticut.
11. Holmes, T. H. and Rahe, R. H. The social readjustment rating scale. *J. Psychosom. Res.*, *11*: 213-218, 1967.
12. *Journal of the American Medical Association.* Suicide of physicians and the reasons. *41*: 263-264, 1903.
13. *Journal of Medical Education.* Suicide by physicians in training, *43*: 1196, 1968.
14. Katz, M. M. and Lyerly, S. B. Methods for measuring adjustment and social behavior in the community: I. Rationale, description, discriminative validity, and scale development. *Psychol. Rep. Monogr.*, *13*: 503-535, 1963.
15. Kempthorne, O. *The Design and Analysis of Experiments.* Wiley, New York, 1952.
16. Knopf, S. A. Suicide among American physicians—Its causes and suggestions for prevention. *New York Med, J.*, *117*: 84-87, 1923.
17. Lester, D. Attempts to predict suicidal risk using psychological tests. *Psychol. Bull.*, *74*: 1-17, 1970.
18. Lorr, M., Daston, P. and Smith, I. R. An analysis of mood states. *Educ. Psychol. Meas.*, *27*: 89-96, 1967.
19. Margolis, P. M. M.D. suicides. Why? *Mich. Med.*, *67:* 589, 1968.
20. Paffenbarger, R. S., Jr. and Asnes, D. P. Chronic disease in former college students. III. Precursors of suicide in early and middle life. *Amer. J. Public Health*, *56:* 1026-1036, 1966.
21. Perlin, S., Shaffer, J. W., Schmidt, C. W., Jr. and Stephens, J. W. *The prediction of suicide in schizophrenia.* Presented at the 125th Annual Meeting of the American Psychiatric Association, Dallas, Texas, May, 1972.
22. Pokorny, A. D. Characteristics of 44 patients who subsequently committed suicide. *A.M.A. Arch. Gen. Psychiat. (Chicago)*, *2:* 314-323, 1960.

23. Porkorny, A. D. Suicide rates in various psychiatric disorders. *J. Nerv. Ment. Dis., 139:* 499-506, 1964.
24. Powell, E. H. Occupation, status and suicide: Toward a redefinition of anomie. *Amer. Sociol. Rev., 23:* 131-139, 1958.
25. Ross, M. Suicide among physicians. *Psychiat. Med., 2:* 189-198, 1971.
26. Schmidt, C. W., Jr., Perlin, S., Towns, W., Fisher, R. S. and Shaffer, J. W. Personality characteristics of single car driver fatalities: A comparative study. *Arch Gen. Psychiat.* (Chicago), in press.
27. Shaffer, J. W., Perlin, S., Schmidt, C. W., Jr. and Himmelfarb, M. Assessment in absentis: New directions in the psychological autopsy. *Johns Hopkins Med. J., 130:* 308-316, 1972.
28. Simon, J. L. The effect of income on the suicide rate: A paradox resolved. *Amer. J. Sociol. 74:* 302-303, 1968.
29. Simon, W. and Lumry, G. K. Suicide among physician-patients. *J. Nerv. Ment. dis., 147:* 105-112, 1968.
30. Temoche, A., Pugh, T. F. and MacMahon, B. Suicide rates among current and former mental institution patients. *J. Nerv. Ment. Dis., 138:* 124-130, 1963.
31. Thomas, C. B. Suicide among us: Can we learn to prevent it? *Johns Hopkins Med. J., 125:* 276-285, 1969.
32. Thomas, C. B. Suicide among us: II. Habits of nervous tension as potential predictors. *Johns Hopkins Med. J., 129:* 190-201, 1971.
33. Tuchman, J., Youngman, W. F. and Kreizman, G. Occupation and suicide. *Industr. Med. Surg. 33:* 818-820, 1964.
34. Van Dellen, T. R.: Suicide among physicians. *Illinois Med. J., 133:* 622, 1968.

Chapter 25

SUPPORT GROUPS FOR WOMEN IN MEDICAL SCHOOL: A FIRST-YEAR PROGRAM

ELAINE HILBERMAN, JUDY KONANC, MARIA PEREZ-REYES, ROSEMARY HUNTER, JOAN SCAGNELLI, AND SHIRLEY SANDERS

AS women, faculty members, clinicians, and parents, the authors have had long-standing concerns about the conflicts which plague women as they enter medical careers and the lack of opportunity within the traditional structure of medical education for women to recognize and deal with these issues. This report describes a support system for first-year women medical students at the University of North Carolina School of Medicine as they negotiate the process of entry into medical school and establish the beginnings of a professional identity.

While some of this process is universal, there is increasing evidence to support the notion that women, by virtue of sex-role socialization patterns, as well as a minority status in medicine, have a more formidable burden of conflict resolution than do their male peers. A major barrier to a woman's achievement of excellence and commitment is the expectation that her career pattern will be identical to that of men when, in fact, the usual pattern for women includes multiple roles, dual commitments, and occasional interruptions (1). The woman who would aspire to a career and retain her femaleness is often excluded, not because of an active program to keep her out of medical school but because the inflexibility of the traditional medical curriculum is incompatible with the maintenance of dual roles (2-4).

It can be assumed that the women currently entering medical school are products of traditional sex-role socialization (5) in which femininity is equated with passivity and child bearing/rearing ac-

---

From Elaine Hilberman et al., Support Groups for Women in Medical School: A First-Year Program, *Journal of Medical Education, 50:* 867-876, Sept., 1975.

The project evaluation was supported in part by the University of North Carolina School of Medicine Faculty research grant AF 448.

tivities, and in which a woman's gratification of intellectual strivings is achieved only indirectly by identification with the successes of her husband and children. Notman and Nadelson (6) describe the spectrum of conflicts stemming from traditional socialization values. Entry into medical school usually occurs before issues of identity and sex role are fully resolved. The young woman student who has identified with a male professional may encounter difficulties in resolving her own female identity; in addition, failure to identify with a traditional woman may be perceived as a betrayal of her mother' values. Invariably, medicine is presented as a field which is incompatible with family life. Further, successful student behavior (assertiveness, competitiveness) is at odds with the usual definitions of feminity, and so men are bright, young "go-getters" while women are "pushy." The absence of nontraditional female role models is a major deterrent to resolution of these identity issues and also perpetuates and reinforces maladaptive coping mechanisms.

Several authors (6,7) have addressed the issue of coping mechanisms in women medical students. The woman student can deny that there is any difference between herself and her male colleagues; she identifies with men and becomes "one of the boys" and, therefore, different from (and better than) most women. Alternatively, she can dispel some of her anxieties about her femaleness by adopting almost a caricature of the traditional female role, with a seductive, helpless, and dependent stance. Both of these patterns are often reinforced by male colleagues, who have had little exposure to women professionals and who allay their own anxieties by relating to women students as either "neuters" or sex objects. Another variation on these themes is for the woman student to become a "superwoman" with the goal of compulsive excellence in both career and family roles and a continual need to prove her competence in all areas.

As an alternate route the woman student may recognize the unfairness of her milieu, which puts her in an equally difficult position. Anger and frustration are prominent and may lead to significant isolation from her peers. Constructive support or the establishment of liaisons with other women students as well as empathetic male students may help in bridging the isolation and, hopefully, lead to corrective action by bringing these issues to the attention of the institution. A number of authors (5-9) suggest the importance of a support system for women students in order to provide role models and opportunities for mutual sharing and solving of problems, but the availability of such support is quite rare. In this paper the authors review the process of formation of such a support system and present an evaluation of the program by means of faculty assessment of the group process and a year-end student critique.*

GROUP FORMATION

A letter was sent to all entering women medical students in the summer of 1973 as part of their orientation packet, and an informal meeting was held with all interested women during their orientation. The following issues were identified and discussed as being potentially conflictual: scarcity of female role models in medicine, stereotypic views of women physicians and their impact on self and career definition, direct or covert communication of sex role bias by male peers or faculty, family-career conflict and the acquisition of dual roles, intensification of role conflicts by the inflexible medical school curriculum, and definition of medicine as a "masculine" field. The women students were then given the option of meeting weekly in small informal discussion groups. The 18 first-year women participants (of a total of 23 women in the first-year class) and one second-year woman student were assigned randomly to one of three groups, with two faculty women in each group. Groups met during the day for one to two hours, not only to avoid conflict with nightly family responsibilities but also because supportive services for minority students were felt to be an essential, legitimate part of medical education. The six authors (the participating faculty) met separately at weekly intervals to detail group process via written process notes and recall. All faculty were from the Department of Psychiatry, the only department in the medical school with a sizable female membership.

FACULTY ASSESSMENT

From the beginning each group assumed its own distinct personality and tempo. Group A was the most reticent, with the majority of members experiencing significant personal and interpersonal conflict. Group B was a verbally expressive, lively, and highly competitive group in which the minority of more reserved members tended to be ignored. Group C evolved more slowly from a small

*A more formal program evaluation by means of preparticipation and postparticipation testing of both group members and a control group at a neighboring medical school failed to find significant differences. Future efforts might be directed toward a study of changes in the woman medical student's image of female physicians and of herself as a physician, as well as the value of women role models. Further information is available from the authors.

irregularly attended group to a larger regular meeting of equally involved members. There were many similarities and some differences in the evolution of group relationships and content among the three groups, and what follows is the shared process of these groups.

Early meetings were characterized by high levels of anxiety, as each group went through a "getting acquainted" phase. Members asked about family backgrounds, motives for choosing a medical career, and reactions to the availability of a support group. There was a wide variation in self-assessment; some felt "special" and bright, while others more nervously labeled themselves as different, weird, and neuter, in comparison with nonprofessional women as well as their male colleagues. Group structure and goals at that time were undefined.

For each group, a sense of cohesiveness evolved in response to a different "challenge." Two members in Group B with previous experiences in psychotherapy promoted an intimate, insight-oriented group model which was accepted and led to an early sense of cohesiveness and purpose. Group A united in anger towards both an unsupportive and competitive group member and a lecturer with a gross sex bias. The members took action by way of verbally protesting the lecturer's behavior, sensing their common reaction to the other member and gradually moving to focus on group goals. At an open meeting of all groups, initiated and persuasively led by Group B six weeks into the year, Group C was confronted with the possibility of dissolving itself. In reaction to the threat of dissolution, Group C coalesced as a group.

By the end of the second month all groups began exploring a number of identity issues. They openly wondered why they chose medical careers. Few felt that they did so through identification with their mothers. In one group a majority of the participants felt that their career decisions reflected a reaction to the perceived emptiness of their mothers' roles. While families were often supportive of their choices, the mothers seemed to indicate that their daughters must choose between career and marriage: "Don't marry. Do something with your life." "Don't waste your life. You are too talented to give up a career for marriage." A recurring and collective fantasy emerged of what it would be like to be a medical student or physician. There would be an end to bright clothing, laughing, dancing, romantic pursuits, and emotional expressiveness, all of which would be replaced by "serious thinking" and a total devotion to medicine. One student described herself as a "dropout from femininity." In short, many members believed they were supposed to emulate the stereotypic cold, rational male, with a medical career and femaleness fearfully viewed as mutually exclusive.

A prominent and allied identity issue concerned the image of the omniscient, super physicians the women students were to become versus the frequently overwhelmed, fallible individuals they felt themselves to be. Again, the women described themselves as being different from their male peers, but now the difference was given an openly negative connotation. During this early period, the leaders collected data for an evaluation of the program, and it was apparent that some of the students felt quite threatened; that is, they feared the test results would show that they had no business being in medical school. It was clear that they had an idealized image of what physicians are like from previous life experiences. Two aspects of that image, to be male and to be omniscient, would never be possible; and over the year this image was adaptively revised.

Acknowledgement that professional identities were shaky led to increased anxiety levels and a strengthening of group cohesiveness. Focus shifted to male-female relationships, with feelings and conflicts concerning marriage being perhaps the most problematic. There was ample evidence that the students defined themselves as deviant females because of professional aspirations, and they adopted various modes of compensation in their relationships with men. Many students assumed that if they behaved naturally, they would be perceived as threatening and unfeminine. Thus, they became perfect wives who maintained all domestic responsibilities and kept medical studies secondary and remote from their relationships. This obligation to play the traditional passive role in relationships with men resulted in a large reservoir of chronic anger, guilt, and conflict, both within themselves and in their relationships with their men. Single women experienced similar feelings and, in addition, had special problems with respect to how to meet men. They had a minimum of free time to meet and date men outside of school and were in reality quite isolated. All of the women were often resentful that their male peers regarded them only as buddies or laboratory partners rather than as women and equal professionals.

Feeling of isolation were conspicuous in all groups for all women, particularly in the early months; and these seemed to be a partial reflection of the loss of emotional support by family and friends as a result of the move to the medical school community. Opportunities to make new friends were limited. Except for the groups, the women had little chance to talk with other women medical students, and male classmates were ambivalently regarded. A more troublesome source of isolation stemmed from their minority status in the medical school. Isolation was intensified by sporadic incidents in which male faculty members made derogatory remarks and jokes demeaning both women physicians and women patients. Students used the groups to ventilate their anger about such incidents, and eventually one group directly confronted a professor about his behavior. Male peers did not offer much support to the women at these times, a fact which painfully increased their sense of isolation and difference.

Special problems with identity issues were evidenced by the black women in each group, who were contending with the double pressures of being both black and female. There was a tendency for some black members to be less active and absent more as the year progressed, although other black students moved from listening to active participation.

All groups shifted in focus following the semester break, each assuming a different direction. Group B seemed to feel more interpersonal distance, with discussions centering on impersonal, global concerns such as death and dying and government-financed health care. Group C, in contrast, was now a very cohesive unit which began to handle more personal problems in its meetings. That group initiated a social gathering at the home of a staff member; this both reflected and fostered the growing intimacy between students and staff members. Group A focused on themes of competitiveness, especially among women.

Each group dealt with feelings about being female, with increased recognition of the ways in which women have devalued themselves and other women by virtue of judging females by male standards and the male company they keep. Group members explored a variety of possible roles for women and in doing so reflected again on their own backgrounds, the roles of their mothers, and the marriages of their parents. There were widely differing views of marriage and parenting, with considerable discussion about the relationship between an unhappy role and inadequate parenting. The faculty women, who represented a wide spectrum of life-styles and interests, functioned prominently as role models during this time of exploring ways to combine personal and professional goals.

The students' new experience with patients (taped interviews in the second semester) prompted reworking of their professional identities. They expressed concerns about their acceptance by patients, particularly male patients, with a focus on anticipated reactions of male patients to them as women physicians, for example, embarrassment about physical examinations, avoidance of sexual concerns, or seductive behavior. In defining their probable roles in relation to patients, the students were also trying to derive their own roles as individuals separate from that of being physicians. There was a strong wish to maintain a personal identity with significant relationships and interests outside of medicine. They hoped to care for others and for themsleves without either an impersonal, selfishly materialistic emphasis or total self-denial.

Toward the end of the academic year, the women seemed to feel more comfortable about being both female and competent. In contrast to earlier discussions which focused on internal and personal conflcts impeding identity development, attention was now turned to institutional barriers. As an example, the rigid third-year schedule was seen as preventing adequate parenting. Usually, student requests for schedule modifications were handled on an individual basis with each clinical service, thus leaving each student feeling guilty about her special favor and resented by her colleagues. Many of the first-year women, and this time some men, formally suggested to the administration that a restructured more flexible curriculum would be beneficial to both sexes.

As final examinations approached, anxiety levels rose within the groups, and attendance for the first time began to wane. Groups with more competitive members perceived discussion of these pressures as escalating rather than decreasing their anxiety. Despite this, the *esprit de corps* remained. Members wished the groups might continue the following year and expressed sadness about ending. A myriad of personal questions directed to the leaders seemed to reflect the intense need for role models and the desire for greater, continuing closeness. The women organized a postexaminiation social gathering for the final termination of two of the groups. The affectionate congratulations of one another for having passed the examinations verified the development of close personal friendships and the women's increased comfort in their roles as medical students. The groups had provided an experience in closeness and female support which now continued outside the groups. The faculty leaders, too, felt increased closeness as well as considerable appreciation and respect for these young women who chose, despite sizable obstacles, to become physicians.

Role definition of the faculty leaders was a complex and problematic issue. There was lengthy discussion about how the leaders might relate to the groups with the options including the roles of therapist, faculty member, role model, and peer. In retrospect, it appeared that the leaders were called on to be all of these at different times, depending on each group's need. In contrast to the authors' usual role as therapist, it seemed most important to be themselves in the groups so that the students would have an opportunity to share the leaders' histories, identities, and modes of adjustment. At times, however, the leaders did function more as therapists in dealing with intragroup and intrapsychic dynamics. Faculty roles became more prominent in confronting situations which required administrative action. The essential and unique feature of the groups, however, seemed to be the opportunity to share personal feelings and conflicts of every sort in an empathetic gathering of students and faculty. Attention had been focused on one's person and not one's performance.

Certain unavoidable problems in the project design were regretted. For example, although the need for black role models was obvious, there were none in the medical school. It is relevant that in the subsequent academic year the black women themselves requested and obtained funds to bring in black women physicians as speakers. Similarly, the participation of women physicians from other specialties would have been welcomed and would have provided a richer matrix of role models.

STUDENT ASSESSMENT

All group members anonymously completed a specially designed evaluation form at the end of the academic year. Table 25-I lists in rank order the concrete needs/expectations students had as they entered the groups and the extent to which they felt their expectations had been met. The two most important initial reasons given for joining the groups involved exploration of the problems and identities of professional women. In retrospect, the students rated the groups as only moderately helpful in meeting these original expectations and rated getting to know and becoming close friends with women classmates as the two most helpful functions of the group. This composite perception by the women reflected an apparent shift in goals that evolved with the development of group needs and experiences. This shift is reflected in the following statements by two students:

> It seemed appropriate to become more personal in our conversations after getting to know each other better and getting to be a stable group.
>
> I made two shifts. In the beginning I was mainly interested in having some outlet for personal feelings and problems. Later I realized that the most important thing for me in the group was developing closer relationships with other women. I've developed some strong friendships partly because of group. Without the group I might not have taken the time.

Table 25-I

PERCENTAGES OF STUDENTS RANKING IMPORTANCE OF EXPECTATIONS BEFORE TAKING PART IN SUPPORT GROUPS AND HELPFULNESS OF GROUPS IN FULFILLING THESE EXPECTATIONS*

Needs	Importance				Helpfulness of Groups			
	Very	Moderate	Mild	Not	Very	Moderate	Mild	Not
† Better understanding of problems of professional women	50	25	25	0	16.7	66.7	16.7	0
Better idea of what being professional woman is like	50	16.7	25	8.3	16.7	50	25	0‡
† Becoming closer friends with women classmates	41.7	16.7	33.3	8.3	41.7	33.3	16.7	8.3
Help with personal difficulties/frustrations	33.3	41.7	16.7	8.3	33.3	25	33.3	8.3
† Getting to know self better	25	41.7	25	8.3	16.7	66.7	8.3	8.3
† Getting to know women classmates socially	25	25	50	0	50	33.3	16.7	0
Better understanding of interpersonal relationships	16.7	66.7	8.3	8.3	16.7	58.3	16.7	8.3
Help with school difficulties/frustrations	16.7	50	25	8.3	25	33.3	25	16.7
Getting to know women faculty better	16.7	41.7	33.3	8.3	8.3	66.7	25	0
Help with family and career problems	8.3	41.7	16.7	33.3	8.3	33.3	33.3	25
Help with anxieties about starting school	8.3	33.3	25	33.3	16.7	33.3	0	0‡
Social activist involvement in school	8.3	8.3	58.3	25.0	0	33.3	41.7	16.7‡

* Both the importance of expectations and the helpfulness of the group in fulfilling them were ranked subsequent to participation in the groups.

† Needs most fulfilled by the groups.

‡ Figures do not add to 100 percent because not all respondents replied to question.

Despite the apparent modification of group goals, however, the original goals appeared to remain important, and the group was considered to be moderately helpful to the majority of group members in their understanding of personal identities and the problems and identities of women professionals. It is also probable that the student reports of finding the group highly important as a means for developing closeness with other women classmates represents another more indirect continuing process which enables women to help each other establish a professional identity.

All the women had well-defined reasons for participating in the group. No one joined simply to "follow the crowd." In addition, social activism was neither highly sought after nor strongly promoted within the groups. A majority of the women indicated that they were satisfied with the frequency and length of the meetings and the attendance and participation of classmates and faculty. They recommended mixing the groups by sex, minority representation, advanced and incoming students, and nonpsychiatric faculty. They further indicated that more structure might have helped in group discussions. On the whole, however, the students expressed satisfaction with the supportive nature of the groups and a wish that such a program be provided for new first-year students as well as continued for themselves.

CONCLUSIONS

The students who participated in the first-year program of support groups explored an impressive array of issues related to being women and physicians. These included relationships with parents, colleagues, patients, and significant men and women in their lives. There was increasing awareness of internal (self-concept) and external (institutional) obstacles to the development of a satisfactory professional identity and resolution of role conflict. Their feelings of isolation in medical school, anxiety about course demands, and anger over sex discrimination were aired, shared, and in part resolved, at times by establishing new friendships, discussing mutual fears, or actively protesting biased behavior. Professional identity was developed and enhanced. The students expressed overall satisfaction with the groups and special appreciation for the support and closeness provided. They were enthusiastic about getting to know and befriend other women classmates and sharing in the development of personal and professional identity. It is likely that their established friendships with each other will continue to be mutually gratifying and helpful.

Women who enter medical school appear to be bright, capable individuals who experience considerable professional and personal pressures as they adjust to the process of medical school education. They must deal with issues of universal concern to medical students, for example, the doctor-patient relationship, and death and dying, and those of special concern to women, for example, heterosexual roles, and achievement. Support groups seem to provide a needed, constructive setting within which exploration of personal and professional concerns can occur. Women at other medical schools might profit by involvement in comparable groups.

It should, however, be firmly stated that role conflicts are not peculiar to women professionals. Male classmates of the women group participants frequently expressed their own need for a similar program. The apparent absence of family-career conflict in men is attributed to social norms, in which the traditional male resolves or denies such conflict by choosing one role, that of the professional, thereby burdening his wife with the major responsibility for maintaining a home, family, children, and marriage. Statistics relevant to the personal lives of all physicians, for example, suicide rate, alcoholism, drug abuse, and divorce, suggest that support groups for both men and women physicians in training might be an important preventive health measure. As more women aspire to and attain an equal status with men and enter into occupations and professions outside the home, male physicians are likely to experience many of the difficulties presently encountered by women including increased pressure on men to assume more responsibility for home and child-rearing activities. Hopefully, more medical schools in the future will provide support groups for all students, men and women alike.

REFERENCES

1. White, M. S. Psychological and Social Barriers to Women in Science. *Science*, **170**:413 416, 1970.
2. Williams, P. A. Women in Medicine: Some Themes and Variations. *J. Med. Educ.*, **46**:584 591, 1971.
3. Bunker, J. P., and Pool, J. G. The Case for More Women in Medicine: The Stanford Program. *N. Engl. J. Med.*, **285**:53, 1971.
4. Kaplan, H. I. Women Physicians: The More Effective Recruitment and Utilization of their Talents and the Resistance to It — The Final Conclusions of a Seven Year Study. *Wom. Physician*, **25**:561-570, 1970.
5. Lopate, C. *Women in Medicine*. Baltimore, Maryland: Johns Hopkins Press, 1968.
6. Notman, T., and Nadelson, C. C. Medicine: A Career Conflict for Women. *Am. J. Psychiatry*, **130**:1123-1126, 1973.
7. Campbell, M. A. *Why Would a Girl go into Medicine? Medical Education in the U. S.: A Guide for Women*. Old Westbury, New York: the Feminist Press, 1974.
8. Goldstein, M. Z. Preventive Health Efforts for Women Medical Students. *J. Med. Educ.*, **50**:289-291, 1975.
9. *Women in Medicine: Action Planning for the 1970's*. Philadelphia: Center for women in Medicine, The Medical College of Pennsylvania, 1974.

Chapter 26

SPECIAL REPORT

Medical Society of the State of New York: Physicians' Committee

PHYSICIANS have for centuries, by oath and by tradition, accepted responsibility for the care of their colleagues who became ill. They have also agreed to the difficult and often painful duty of policing their own ranks. Usually accepted gladly is the opportunity to treat physical disease, but those illnesses that carry moralistic overtones or might result in a colleague's loss of freedom to practice medicine have been approached with uncertainty and discomfort.

In 1973, the council on Mental Health of the American Medical Association[1] published a report on the problem of the mentally ill, alcoholic, and drug-addicted physician in which local medical societies were urged to develop methods for helping these sick physicians. Model legislation toward this end was also suggested.[2]

On September 12, 1974, at the Council meeting of the Medical Society of the State of New York, a plan was presented and approved for dealing with the problem of the sick physician in New York State. This plan was devised after much study and many meetings by a joint ad hoc committee of the committees on Alcoholism, Drug Abuse, and Mental Health. Jackson W. Riddle, M.D., executive secretary of the State Board for Medicine, and Mr. Peter Milana, acting director of the DPC (Division of Professional Conduct) of the State of New York Department of Education, had met with this group, were aware of the proposals contained in the plan, and fully approved them.

PROBLEMS

This plan attempts to solve some of the problems that have beset similar efforts in the past. Among these difficulties have been the following.

1. Confusion as to whether the sick physician should be regard-

---

From Special Articles, the *New York State Journal of Medicine*, pp 420-423, February, 1975.

ed as "ill" or as "bad," so that plans often combined two opposing philosophies in such a way that neither approach could be taken effectively or consistently.

2. Divided responsibility in New York State where the public assumes that physicians determine the right to practice of other physicians but where, in fact, the power to grant or revoke a license is held by the Department of Education, which must also monitor many other licensed professions. It attempts to do so with a very small staff and inadequate budget.

3. Reluctance on the part of physicians to report a colleague for fear that their attempt to help might result in punishment instead.

4. Concern that intervention in a colleague's personal affairs might lead to unpleasant social, legal, and professional consequences for the would-be helper.

5. Dissatisfaction with the speed and efficiency of presently available methods for intervention so that these methods are not regarded as reliable, rapidly responsive, and worth invoking except in extreme and clear-cut cases.

6. Ignorance of actual methods of reporting and precedures available.

7. Lack of consensus among groups of physicians as to what course of action should be followed so that ambivalence waits hopefully for unanimity and is rewarded instead with indecision and delay.

EXTENT OF PROBLEM

Unfortunately accurate statistics are not available for the incidence of mental illness, alcoholism, and drug addiction among physicians in the United States. Even if such figures were available, they might not apply to New York State. If incidence were known, it would still be difficult to predict how many of the total population of sick physicians would be recognized as in need of help during any given year. What is clear is that physicians have no special immunity against these illnesses. Whether the incidence is higher among physicians than the general public is probably not as important as the fact that such physicians do exist and that organized medicine is the first professional group to address itself frankly and openly to these problems within its own ranks and to attempt to devise solutions. Hopefully, if physicians are able to develop workable methods for reaching and assisting each other, other professions may follow suit.

PROPOSED PLANS

Two completely separate approaches to the sick physician are to be available. One, the noncoercive approach, is already operational in the form to be described later. The other approach which is frankly coercive is described as it is recommended, not as it presently exists.

It is important, if the reader is to understand the proposed plan and use it effectively, to make a clear distinction between these two approaches which are quite separate and whose functions do not overlap. The noncoercive approach provides a means by which the sick physician can be offered help by a colleague, but, by this method, if that help is refused, there is no further action. The coercive method provides for a series of increasingly stern measures to get the sick physician who is felt to be dangerous to his patients into treatment whether he wishes it or not.

Noncoercive Approach

A committee has been formed by the MSSNY known as the Physicians' Committee. Its members are physicians with skill in dealing with alcoholic, drug-addicted, or mentally ill patients. Committee members may or may not be members of other MSSNY committees. They serve without pay and remain, as far as possible, anonymous, so as to avoid their being approached or questioned outside of the agreed-on channels of communication. There is no public recognition of their service nor opportunity for financial gain. This committee is in operation and has already begun its work.

To illustrate how the committee operates, a hypothetical case might be useful. Assume that Dr. X is alcoholic and that Dr. A and Dr. B who work with him are seriously concerned. They are reluctant to discuss him with the chief of his service who sometimes overreacts or with hospital administration since it is a matter of medical competence. They are hesitant to speak to Dr. X himself, because if he responds with anger and denial future work relations may be even more strained, and he has other friends on the staff who might also be upset by what could be perceived as an attack on Dr. X rather than as an expression of concern.

Dr. A and Dr. B then decide to contact the Physicians' Committee. Dr. A calls the MSSNY, asks to speak to a secretary regarding a sick physician. He gives his own name, address, and phone number but does *not* give the name of Dr. X. Dr. A states whether the problem appears to be with alcohol, drugs, or mental illness. He is then told that an appropriate physician will call him for further details.

Dr. C, having been called by the secretary, contacts Dr. A. If Dr. A is willing for his name to be used as a source of information when Dr. X is seen, his call alone activates the committee. If he prefers that his name not be used, he will be asked to have a second complainant, Dr. B, contact Dr. C and thereby minimize the risk that someone merely wishes to harass Dr. X. With the second call, Dr. C designates two committee members to approach Dr. X. Dr. C will not do this himself nor will he identify the original caller to them. Dr. C will have no report on what transpires between Dr. X and the other committee members. He will know for certain only that an attempt to make contact has occurred. Dr. C will urge Dr. A and Dr. B to call him again in some six weeks' time to report whether or not there has been an observable change in Dr. X's behavior. Thus the committee may be able to judge its own effectiveness. Dr. C will also explain that while Dr. X will be offered help, he will remain entirely free to refuse it. If he does refuse it and denies that there is in fact any problem, the committee will take no further action. If Dr. A and Dr. B wish to attempt to coerce Dr. X into treatment, they are free to do so at any time, before, during, or after the Physicians' Committee attempts to make contact.

The Physicians' Committee keeps no records and makes no reports to anyone. Its members relate to the sick physician as physicians to patients. Under no circumstances can they then take steps to do him harm. In fact, their membership on this committee binds them not to accept appointment to any disciplinary committees before a significant period of time has elapsed so that they will not carry with them into other settings information gained as Physicians' Committee members.

When Dr. C has satisfied himself that Dr. A and Dr. B are acting in good faith, he contacts Dr. D and Dr. E of the alcoholism group. If either Dr. D or Dr. E knows Dr. X they will not as a rule contact him. Assuming they do not know him and can therefore approach without the anxiety and discomfort they might feel were Dr. X a personal friend, they proceed to make personal contact with him. They explain that two of his colleagues are sufficiently upset at what they perceive to be a serious drinking problem that they have seen fit to activate the committee. Dr. D and Dr. E are not there to sit in judgment of Dr. X nor to ask him for a confession. There only desire is to be of help if he needs and wants it. If he does want help, they know exactly where and how it can be obtained since they are proficient in the area of his illness. They cannot themselves take Dr. X into treatment.

If Dr. X agrees, he is helped into treatment. If he refuses, he will know that Dr. D and Dr. E are available for help at a later date, should he change his mind. Whether or not Dr. D and Dr. E call on Dr. X more than once is a matter left to their judgment. If Dr. X does not wish treatment his desires are respected.

Clearly the noncoercive route can only help. It can fail, but it cannot do harm. Concern is often expressed that every man "accused" of illness has a right to face his accuser and that the sick physician has a right to know who called about him. That would certainly be true if this committee were to collect records, make reports, or in any way interfere with Dr. X's privacy or his freedom. Another concern expressed is dismay that if Dr. X refuses to accept treatment he will be free to continue as before. The answer to that is that Dr. A and Dr. B have always been free to invoke coercive methods and remain free to do so whether the Physicians' Committee is successful in its approach or not. The committee on the other hand will be used by people who will not invoke coercive means but who first wish to try a gentler approach. Its strength is in fact derived from its weakness.

Coercive Approach

The coercive approach (not as yet implemented) will utilize no more than modifications of the existing structure by which the DPC of the State of New York Department of Education now operates. The major changes will be the introduction of the concept of "monitored treatment" and will make use of the speed and efficiency with which changes may be acted on. The sick physician is to be given the opportunity to enter monitored treatment at each and every step of his licensure difficulties. Acceptance of such therapy would stop the progress of his legal problems at the level then attained.

Monitored Treatment

The committee agreed that an obvious problem in previous approaches to the physician coerced into treatment has been that of combining a treatment and monitoring role in the same person. Clearly a sick physician who continues to act out with drugs or alcohol or in other ways will not feel free to admit these behaviors to the same person who may have to report him. Also, it is difficult to trust a therapist to whom one has been assigned, yet free choice of a reporting physician may well lead the sick physician to choose a friend whom he knows will be lenient. A solution to this problem would be to assign the job of monitor to a physician who would agree to fill this role but who would not attempt to do treatment. The monitor should be as competent as the treater. His methods are his own but with the DPC staff available to him for help if needed. He should not be able to demand that the treating physician breach the confidence of his physician patient. His responsibility is simply to determine whether or not the sick physician's behavior permits his continuing in the practice of medicine without endangering the welfare of his patients, and his reports should be to the DPC on at least a quarterly basis. While the monitor would be assigned, the sick physician would have free choice of the person to whom he entrusted himself for treatment. While both treating and reporting physicians might be psychiatrists, in the case of alcoholism and drug addiction problems, they might be of other medical disciplines. The duration of monitored treatment would remain at the discretion of the Board for Medicine, or the Court, in the case of a restraining order.

Steps in Implementing Suggested Coercive Approach

1. A complainant both calls, for speed, and writes, for documentation, directly to the Division of Professional Conduct of the State of New York Department of Education.
2. Within thirty days the DPC will investigate. If the complaint appears valid, charges are filed through the attorney general with the sick physician himself.
3. The sick physician has twenty days in which to reply. He has two options: (1) he can elect to go into monitored treatment without this constituting an admission of guilt or acceptance of a diagnosis, in which case the physician monitor assumes responsibility for notifying the DPC if their help is needed beyond this stage; or (2) he can fail to reply or deny charges, in which case the DPC will reinvestigate within thirty days.
4. If on second investigation the physician is still in trouble and appears imminently dangerous, the DPC requests the attorney general to seek an immediate restraining order, within a maximum of ten days. If at this point the sick physician accepts monitored treatment, charges again can be dropped. At all times the physician

is fully protected by the right of due process including the right of appeal. On the other hand, a restraining order can be sought whenever circumstances appear to warrant.

5. If no urgency exists for interrupting the physician's professional activities, charges are presented before a hearing panel consisting at the present time of five or more members of the committee on professional conduct of the New York State Board for Medicine. The present sequence of appearance before the committee on discipline of the Board of Regents, review by the full Board of Regents, and, if desired, by the appellate division of the Court may still be followed in such a circumstance. Following such a procedure, a punitive verdict entailing curtailment of licensure privilege may be arrived at, and monitored treatment would then achieve the official status of probation (finite period).

Conclusion

The two methods here outlined provide a means for reaching out to New York State's sick physician. The noncoercive approach brings a skilled and tactful confrontation and the offer of help without the need for disciplinary measures. This mechanism was accepted and funded by the Council of MSSNY in September, 1974. It became operational in November, 1974.

The coercive method as described represents a more rapidly responsive and streamlined version of the present system; it could be implemented without the need for passage of new legislation. It would, however, require appropriate and more adequate budget than that presently offered to the Division of Professional Conduct. The MSSNY has strongly urged the State to avoid any failure to fulfill the responsibilities which the legislature assigned to the Department of Education. The physicians of this State, in their willingness to assist the sick physician and serve to protect the best interests of their patients, can do no more than urge the public and the legislature to give their full cooperation and assistance.

REFERENCES

1. The sick physician. Impairment by psychiatric disorders, including alcoholism and drug dependence, *J.A.M.A. 223*: 684 (Feb. 5) 1973.
2. Disabled Physician Act, a Bill for an act concerning the practice of medicine, model law proposed by Legislative Department, American Medical Association, 1973.

Suggestions for Further Reading

GENERAL

Annas, G.J.: Who to call when the doctor is sick. *Hastings Cent Rep, 8*:18, 1978.

Dorsey, R.E.: Mental disorders among physicians. *Ohio State Med J, 73*:744, 1977.

Duffy, J.C., Litin, E.M.: Psychiatric morbidity of physicians. *JAMA, 189*:989, 1964.

Duffy, J.C.: The emotional health of physicians. *Arch Intern Med, 69*:1319, 1968.

Duffy, J.C., Litin, E.M.: *The Emotional Health of Physicians.* Springfield: Charles C Thomas, Publisher, 1967.

Ellard, J.: The disease of being a doctor. *Med J Aust, 2*:318, 1974.

Gold, N.: The doctor, his illness and the patient. *Aust NZ J Psychiatry, 6*:209, 1972.

Green, R.C., Carroll, G.J., Buxton, W.D.: *The Care and Management of the Sick and Incompetent Physician.* Springfield: Charles C Thomas, Publisher, 1978.

King, H.: Health in the medical and other learned professions. *J Chronic Dis, 23*:257, 1970.

Murray, R.M.: Psychiatric illness in doctors. *Lancet, 1*:1211, 1974.

Murray, R.M.: The health of doctors: A review. *J R Coll Physicians Lond, 12*:403, 1978.

Niven, R.G.: Physicians' perceptions and attitudes toward disabled colleagues, in *The Impaired Physician, Proceedings of the Third A.M.A. Conference on the Impaired Physician.* Minneapolis, MN., 1978, pp. 21-25.

Report of the AMA Council on Mental Health: The sick physician: Impairment by psychiatric disorders, including alcoholism and drug dependence. *JAMA, 223*:684, 1972.

Steindler, A.M.: *The Impaired Physician: An Interpretive Summary of the AMA Conference on the Disabled Doctor. Challenge to the Profession.* Dept. of Mental Health, American Medical Association, April 11-12, 1975.

Waring, E.M.: Psychiatric illness in physicians: a review. *Compr Psychiatry, 15*:519, 1974.

Wilkins, J.T., Marvin, N.G.: The physician as a person. *J Fam Pract, 7*:379, 1978.

ALCOHOLISM AND DRUG ABUSE

Ayers, P.R.: The physician alcoholic. *Ohio State Med J, 73*:737, 1977.

Borsay, M.A., Leff, A.M.: Physician drug addiction: A challenge to medical educators. *Ohio State Med J, 73*:740, 1977.

Burrows, T.: Helping the impaired physician. *Can Doctor, 46*:76, 1980.

Connelly, J.C.: The alcoholic physician. *J Kansas Med Soc, 79*:601, 1978.

Edwards, G.: The alcoholic doctor. A case of neglect. *Lancet, 2*:1297, 1975.

Gilbert, J.A.L.: Alcoholic and drug addicted physicians: the scope of the problem.

Can Fam Physician, 26:851, 1980.

Glatt, M.M.: Alcoholism among doctors (C). *Lancet, 2*:342, 1974.

Goby, M.J., Bradley, N.J., Bespalec, D.A.: Physicians treated for alcoholism: A follow-up study. *Alcoholism: Clinical and Experimental Research, 3*:121, 1979.

Hall, R.C., Stickney, S.K., Popkin, M.K.: Physician drug abuse. *J Nerv Ment Dis, 166*:787, 1978.

Harrison, J.: Alcohol and the impaired physician. *Alcohol Health Research World, 3*:2, 1978.

Henry, S.: Alcohol and drugs: the doctor's own prescription. *Can Med Assoc J, 120*:989, 1979.

Murray, R.M.: Characteristics and prognosis of alcoholic doctors. *Br Med J, 2*:1537, 1976.

Putnam, P.L., Ellinwood, E.H. Jr.: Narcotic addiction among physicians: a ten-year follow-up. *Am J Psychiatry, 122*:745, 1966.

Sclare, A.B.: Alcoholism in doctors. *British Journal of Alcohol and Alcoholism, 14*:181, 1979.

Thomas, C.B., Santora, P.B., Shaffer, J.W.: Health of physicians in midlife in relation to use of alcohol: a prospective study of a cohort of former medical students. *Johns Hopkins Med J, 146*:1, 1980.

MARITAL AND FAMILY DISCORD

Barrand, J.: Masochism, masturbation and matriarchy: the doctor's family. *Aust Fam Physician, 39*:71, 1979.

Eagle, J.R., Smith, B.M.: Stresses of the medical student wife. *J Med Educ, 43*:840, 1968.

Gravey, M., Tuason, V.B.: Physician marriages. *J Clin Psychiatry, 40*:129, 1979.

Maddison, D.: Stress on the doctor and his family. *Med J Aust, 2*:315, 1974.

Nelson, S.B.: Some dynamics of medical marriages. *J R Coll Gen Pract, 28*:585, 1978.

Peer, M.: Social and cultural influences on the doctor's family. *Am J Psychoanal, 39*:71, 1979.

Savoy, J.N.: Group discussions with doctors' wives. *J R Coll Gen Pract, 29*:173, 1979.

SUICIDE

Blachly, P.H., Disher, W., Roduner, G.: Suicide by Physicians. *Bull Suicidol,* Dec., 1968.

Blachly, P.H., Osterud, H.T., Josslin, R.: Suicide in professional groups. *N Engl J Med, 268*:1278, 1963.

Craig, A.G., Pitts, F.N.: Suicide by physicians. *Dis Nerv Syst, 29*:763, 1968.

Everson, R.B., Fraumeni, J.F.: Mortality among medical students and young physicians. *J Med Educ, 50*:809, 1975.

Pasnau, R.O., Russell, A.T.: Psychiatric resident suicide. An analysis of five cases.

Am J Psychiatry, 132:402, 1975.

Powell, E.H.: Occupation, status, and suicide: towards a redefinition of anomie. *Am Social Rev, 23*:131, 1958.

Rich, C.L., Pitts, F.N.: Suicide by male physicians during a five-year period. *Am J Psychiatry, 136*:1089, 1979.

Rockwell, D.A., O'Brien, W.: Physicians' knowledge and attitudes about suicide. *JAMA, 225*:1347, 1973.

Ross, M.: Suicide among physicians: a psychological study. *Dis Ner Syst, 34*:146, 1973.

Sakinofsky, I.: Suicide in doctors and wives of doctors. *Can Fam Physician, 26*:837, 1980.

Thomas, C.B.: Suicide among us: can we learn to prevent it? *Johns Hopkins Med J, 125*:276, 1969.

Thomas, C.B.: Suicide among us: II. Habits of nervous tension as potential predictors. *Johns Hopkins Med J, 129*:190, 1971.

Von Brauchitsch, H.: The physician's suicide revisited. *J Nerv Ment Dis, 162*:40, 1976.

STRESS

Boyle, B.P., Coombs, R.H.: Personality profiles related to emotional stress in the initial year of medical training. *J Med Educ, 46*:882, 1971.

Burrows, J.D.: Stress and distress in middle age — the mental health of doctors. *Aust Fam Physician, 5*:1203, 1976.

DeSole, D.E., Singer, P., Aronson, S.: Suicide and role strain among physicians. *Int J Soc Psychiatry, 15*:294, 1969.

Evans, C.E.: Physician survival: should the doctor come first? *Can Fam Physician, 26*:856, 1980.

Mawardi, B.H.: A career study of physicians. *J Med Educ, 40*:658, 1965.

Pitt, F.N., Winokur, G., Steward, M.A.: Psychiatric syndromes, anxiety symptoms and responses to stress in medical students. *Am J Psychiatry, 118*:333, 1961.

Raskin, M.: Psychiatric crises of medical students and the implications for subsequent adjustment. *J Med Educ, 47*:210, 1972.

Wilkins, J.T., Marvin, N.G.: The physician as a person. *J Fam Pract, 7*:379, 1978.

PERSONALITY

Baird, L.L.: The characteristics of medical students and their views of the first year. *J Med Educ, 50*:1092, 1975.

Betz, B.J., Thomas, C.B.: Individual temperament as a predictor of health or premature disease. *Johns Hopkins Med J, 144*:81, 1979.

Hackman, J.D., Low-Beer, J.R., Wugmeister, S., Wilhelm, R.C., Rosenbaum, J.E.: The premed stereotype. *J Med Educ, 54*:308, 1979.

Myckatyn, M.M., Miles, J.E.: A profile of today's medical student. *Can Med Assoc J, 109*:1118, 1973.

Schlageter, C.W., Rosenthal, V.: What are "normal" medical students like? *J Med Educ, 37*:19, 1962.

Thomas, C.B., Duszynski, K.R., Shaffer, J.W.: Family attitudes reported in youth as potential predictors of cancer. *Psychosom Med, 41*:287, 1979.

Thomas, C.B.: Precursors of premature disease and death, the predictive potential of habits and family attitudes. *Ann Intern Med, 85*:653, 1976.

MEDICAL EDUCATION

Berg, J.K., Garrard, J.: Psychosocial support of residents in family practice programs. *J Fam Pract, 11*:915, 1980.

Cliff, M.M., Cliff, T.M.: Attitudes of medical students towards medical school and their future careers. *J Med Educ, 47*:534, 1972.

Coombs, R.H., Vincent, C.E.: *Psychosocial Aspects of Medical Training*. Springfield: Charles C Thomas, Publisher, 1971.

Cramond, J.L.: Psychosis in young doctors. *Br Med J, 1*:560, 1978.

Hawkins, D.R., Hawkins, E.W.: The role of psychiatry in Western European medical education. *J Med Educ, 54*:408, 1979.

Hunter, R.C.A., Prince, R.H., Schwartzman, A.E.: Comments on emotional disturbances in a medical undergraduate population. *Can Med Assoc J, 85*:989, 1961.

Kausch, D.F.: Medical students' attitudes towards the mental health field: a longitudinal study. *J Med Educ, 44*:1051, 1969.

Kelly, W.A.: Suicide and psychiatric education. *Am J Psychiatry, 130*:463, 1973.

Kligfield, M., Hoffman, K.I.: Medical student attitude towards seeking professional psychological help. *J Med Educ, 54*:617, 1979.

Light, D., Jr.: The impact of medical school on future psychiatrists. *Am J Psychiatry, 132*:607, 1975.

Neilson, A.C.: The magnitude of declining psychiatric career choice. *J Med Educ, 54*:632, 1979.

Rezler, A.G.: Attitude changes during medical school: a review of the literature. *J Med Educ, 49*:1023, 1974.

Russell, A.T., Pasnau, R.D., Taintor, Z.C.: Emotional problems of residents in psychiatry. *Am J Psychiatry, 132*:263, 1975.

Valko, R.J., Clayton, P.J.: Depression in the internship. *Dis Nerv Syst, 36*:26, 1975.

TREATMENT

a'Brook, M.F., Hailstone, J.D., McLauchlan, I.E.J.: Psychiatric illness in the medical profession. *Br J Psychiatry, 113*:1013, 1967.

Franklin, R.A.: One hundred doctors at the Retreat: a contribution to the subject of mental disorder in the medical profession. *Br J Psychiatry, 131*:11, 1977.

Jones, R.E.: A study of 100 physician psychiatric inpatients. *Am J Psychiatry, 134*:1119, 1977.

Linn, L.S., Lewis, C.E.: Attitudes towards self-care among practising physicians.

Med Care, 17:183, 1979.

Meissner, W.W.: Treatment problems of the hospitalized physician. *Int J Psychoanal Psychother, 7*:437, 1978-79.

Osmond, H., Siegler, M.: Doctors as Patients. *Practitioner, 218*:834, 1977.

Pearson, M.M., Strecker, E.A.: Physicians as psychiatric patients: private practice experience. *Am J Psychiatry, 116*:915, 1960.

Small, I.F., Small, J.G., Assue, C.M., et al.: The fate of the mentally ill physician. *Am J Psychiatry, 125*:1333, 1969.

Vincent, M.O., Robinson, E.A., Latt, L.: Physicians as patients: Private psychiatric hospital experience. *Can Med Assoc J, 100*:403, 1969.

IDENTIFICATION AND PREVENTION

British Medical Association Special Committee on the Registration of Doctors Suffering from Mental Disorder: Interim Report, February, 1972. *Br Med J, 2*:169, 1973.

Cohen, S.: The conspiracy of silence. *Cam Fam Physician, 26*:847, 1980.

Goldstein, M.Z.: Preventive mental health efforts for women medical students. *J Med Educ, 50*:289, 1975.

Help for the Alcoholic Physician: A Seminar, *Alcoholism: Clinical and Experimental Research, 1*:129, 1977.

Kansas Medical Society. K.M.S. impaired physician program: statement of purpose. *J Kansas Med Soc, 80*:27, 1979.

Nicholson, J.F.: The impaired physician: some coping mechanisms. *Can Fam Physician, 26*:833, 1980.

Sargent, D.A., Jensen, V.W., Petty, T.A., et al.: Preventing physician suicide. The role of family, colleagues, and organized medicine. *JAMA, 237*:143, 1977.

Talbott, G.D., Holdenfield, H., Shoemaker, K.E., et al.: The disabled doctors plan for Georgia. *Alcoholism: Clinical and Experimental Research, 1*:143, 1977.

Talbott, G.D., Richardson, C., Atkins, E.: The MAG disabled doctors' program: A two-year review. *J Med Assoc Ga, 66*:77, 1977.

Vincent, M.O.: The impaired physician and you. *Can Fam Physician, 26*:861, 1980.